PENGUIN
ARKANA

Chiron and the Healing Journey

The ancient science of astrology, founded on the correlation between celestial movements and terrestrial events, recognizes the universe as an indivisible whole in which all parts are inter-connected. Mirroring this perception of the unity of life, modern physics has revealed the web of relationship underlying everything in existence. Despite the inevitable backlash as old paradigms expire, we are now entering an age where scientific explanations and models of the cosmos are in accord with basic astrological principles and beliefs. In such a climate, astrology is poised to emerge again as a serious study offering a greater understanding of our true nature. Arkana's Contemporary Astrology Series offers, in readable books written by experts, the insight and practical wisdom the world is now ready to receive from the newest vanguard of astrological thought.

Melanie Reinhart was born in Zimbabwe, whose night skies inspired her vocation of astrology. She holds a BA in Music and Drama. An award-winning Diploma-Holder of the Faculty of Astrological Studies, she has been a professional astrologer since 1975 and has a rich background of training and participation in various psychological and spiritual disciplines. Her individual practice is based in London, where she teaches for both the faculty of Astrological Studies and the Centre for Psychological Astrology. She has travelled extensively in South Africa, Europe, Australia and New Zealand, giving lectures, workshops and readings. Her special interest in Chiron was prompted by a visionary experience, and this book is the result of five years' intensive research, which has recently extended to further groundbreaking material on the Centaurs. Her other published work includes numerous journal articles, contributions to *Modern South Africa in Search of a Soul* (1990), *Wilderness and the Human Spirit* (1997) and the books *To the Edge and Beyond* (1996) and *Incarnation* (1997).

CONTEMPORARY ASTROLOGY
Series Editor: Erin Sullivan

CHIRON *and the* HEALING JOURNEY

An Astrological and Psychological Perspective

MELANIE REINHART

ARKANA
PENGUIN BOOKS

PENGUIN BOOKS

Published by the Penguin Group
Penguin Books Ltd, 27 Wrights Lane, London W8 5TZ, England
Penguin Putnam Inc., 375 Hudson Street, New York, New York 10014, USA
Penguin Books Australia Ltd, Ringwood, Victoria, Australia
Penguin Books Canada Ltd, 10 Alcorn Avenue, Toronto, Ontario, Canada M4V 3B2
Penguin Books (NZ) Ltd, Private Bag 102902, NSMC, Auckland, New Zealand

Penguin Books Ltd, Registered Offices: Harmondsworth, Middlesex, England

First published 1989
Reprinted with revisions 1998

4

Copyright © Melanie Reinhart, 1989, 1998
All rights reserved

The permissions on page 422 constitute an extension of this copyright page

Printed in England by Clays Ltd, St Ives plc
Filmset in Linotron Bembo

For my late parents, Val and Rosemary,
all my ancestors, and the Spirit of Zimbabwe

Contents

Acknowledgements

Many people have contributed in their own ways to the process of writing this book, and I offer here my grateful thanks to them all. Howard Sasportas brought the opportunity and encouraged me along the way. Although I felt deep sorrow at his death in May 1992, his absence from my life has also poignantly highlighted his generosity of spirit. I am so grateful for all he gave to me, as a friend, colleague and teacher. Christine Murdock's perceptive editorial help, supportive clarity and sense of humour were much appreciated. Ronald Cohen kindly loaned me the computer on which I had begun storing research material several years previously, and made available his extensive library. Enjoyable and stimulating discussions with colleagues, especially Darby Costello and Steven Sinclair, helped me to formulate my ideas; Mike Harding patiently answered many a technical question. Changes Bookshop never failed to obtain obscure publications needed for research, and David Fisher supplied information from the Astrological Association's data bank.

This book is the outcome of a personal journey during which I have been influenced by numerous people to whom I am indebted: some I have known personally, while others inspired me with their ideas. Freda Kroeger and Lama first set me on the inner path, and the late Fazal Inayat-Khan was an exemplar of 'crazy wisdom' for me. Elizabeth Burke awakened my love of words, and Godfrey Chidyausiku reconnected me with my roots. I have learned much from Diana Whitmore, and also from the work of C. G. Jung, and Stanislav Grof. Dane Rudhyar first inspired my commitment to astrology, which was later nourished by Alan Oken, Liz Greene, Howard Sasportas, Steven Arroyo, Geoffrey Cornelius and many others. I also wish to acknowledge all those who have dedicated time and energy to studying Chiron and made available their ideas, whether known or unknown to me.

Special acknowledgement and gratitude is due to the many clients, colleagues and friends, who over the years have told me of their suffering and also of their healing journeys. Through their openness I learned much of what is in this book, and many have generously given permission for me to include anecdotal material from their horoscopes and their lives.

Much of your pain is self-chosen.
It is the bitter potion by which the
    physician within you heals your sick
    self.
Therefore trust the physician, and drink
    his remedy in silence and tranquillity:
For his hand, though heavy and hard, is
    guided by the tender hand of the
    Unseen.

Kahlil Gibran, *The Prophet*

Introduction

The discovery of a new outer planet is a momentous event, suggesting that an archetypal pattern, another facet of the divine, is being activated within the collective psyche, stirring below in the unconscious depths and seeking recognition. Jung believed that the human consciousness was indispensable for the fulfilment of Creation, and in this sense we are all co-creators of the process of being and becoming, just as we are created by the process. When a new planet is discovered, many synchronous events occur which express its archetypal theme; a distinct cluster of images and mythic figures can be seen at work within historical and political events and general trends within the collective, the meaning of which may also have enormous impact upon the individual psyche.

Chiron, named after the Centaur in Greek mythology, was discovered in 1977, at about 10.00 am on 1 November, by Charles T. Kowal of the Hale Observatories at Pasadena, California. Although a photographic record going back to the 1890s was assembled from observatories in various countries, the planet had never before been noticed, perhaps because we were not ready to respond to the archetypal pattern which Chiron represents, that of the Wounded Healer. However, several astrologers had made predictions heralding something about to be discovered. Dane Rudhyar postulated a 'Higher Moon', between Saturn and Uranus; Charles Jayne predicted that a new planet would be found in 1975, near its own Node, with an orbit of about fifty years. Chiron was found within 4° of its South Node, only two years later than the predicted discovery time, and its orbital period is indeed fifty years.

Chiron's position, size and behaviour are unusual: it is large for an asteroid, small for a planet and found where one was not expected according to previous mathematical models, notably Bode's Law.[1] Perplexed as to how Chiron should be classified, astronomers coined the term 'planetoid', meaning 'planet-like'. For simplicity, however, I will use the word 'planet', which is derived from the Greek for 'wanderer'.

Astronomically, Chiron wanders with a periodicity of about fifty years, through a most elliptical orbit steeply inclined to the ecliptic; astrologically the theme of the wanderer, outsider, loner or maverick is relevant to Chiron. Some astronomers believe that Chiron may one day be ejected from our solar system, having strayed in from elsewhere like a comet and been trapped.[2] However, it is certainly here to stay for our lifetime, and proving to be of increasing interest to astrologers the more its meaning unfolds.

The student of astrology will be familiar with popular astrological beliefs of earlier times, where the planets were linked with the animal, vegetable and mineral kingdoms in a comprehensive system of correspondences, and believed literally to cause events, illnesses and life conditions. Man was largely seen as being at the mercy of the fate described by his horoscope, although he could perhaps counteract an evil fate through charms, talismans and the like. Since the advent of 'Humanistic Astrology', pioneered by the work of Dane Rudhyar, the view of the horoscope as a process and a map of potentials waiting to be developed has become popular. We might consider the former view as Saturnian, where individual freedom of choice is negligible and issues are considered very concretely; in terms of scientific paradigms it is dominated by the Newtonian–Cartesian view of the universe, preoccupied with the mechanisms of cause and effect. In contrast, the latter is rather more Uranian, recoiling warily from the idea of immutable fate and orienting instead towards 'self-actualization'; here the discoveries of Einstein and the recent explorations of the New Physics provide the scientific paradigm.

Against the classical concepts of permanence and identity the realization that all living is a dynamic process of transformation from which no entity escapes now stands backed up by the whole edifice of scientific research. On the ruins of the world of thought dogmatically extolled by nineteenth century minds we witness the reappearance of ancient concepts which were for millennia the foundations of human knowledge.[3]

Chiron was discovered between Saturn and Uranus, and the astrological perspective it represents, in my opinion, is one that includes both these views, and embraces the resultant paradox. In other words, while moments of inspiration confirm the truth of the above vision of life as a ceaseless process of transformation, we also live in the world of separate forms, structure, limitation and suffering. On the one hand, the psyche is fixed in time and place by fate, in the guise of parental and ancestral influences, social and educational conditioning, and perhaps also by the spiritual inheritance and karma we bring with us to this life; yet on the other, the psyche is also limitless, fluid and always in process. In physics, matter can be seen as comprising either particles or waves, depending on how it is viewed; this is perhaps a useful analogy for our purposes. The individual horoscope represents that portion of the universe which we are given to work with, so to speak; although its pattern is fixed at the moment of birth, it is also continually in a process whose unfolding is indicated by the cycles of transits and progressions. Thus our relationship to what is symbolized in our natal horoscopes, and the way in which we integrate and express this in our lives, is both unique to each one of us and also evolves and changes over time.

Synchronous with the discovery of Chiron, there has developed within astrology an approach that includes the perspectives of depth psychology. Dane Rudhyar pioneered this approach, which has recently been expanded by the work of astrologers such as Liz Greene, Steven Arroyo and others; however, its roots lie in historical precedents going back almost a thousand years – for example, in the *Centiloquy*, ascribed to Ptolemy.[4] Astrological patterns are recognized in terms of the *meaning* that we bring to inner and outer experiences, although we are perhaps in turn predisposed to the quality of our experiences by the patterns themselves. However, rather than trying to pre-empt fate, to ward it off or pretend it does not exist, we may perhaps work with it as consciously as we are able: thus we participate in the alchemical *opus*, the hero's journey, the search for the philosopher's stone, or the finding of the long-lost kingdom.

. . . Necessity governs the soul's movements as well as the motions of the stars. As souls pass beneath her seat, so on her lap turns the spindle ruling the planetary motions. What happens to soul and to stars is on the same web. So one tries to puzzle out the compelling necessities of the soul by consulting the motions of the planets . . . But astrologers have taken this correspondence literally, rather than imaginally. For it is neither the stars nor the astrological planets that are the rulers of personality. Astrology is a *metaphorical* way of recognizing that the rulers of person-ality are archetypal powers who are beyond our personal reach and yet are involved necessarily in all our vicissitudes.[5]

In the ten or so years since Chiron's discovery, there has been an unprecedented response in the astrological world: excitement flared up immediately, and volumes of research, speculation, information, books and articles about Chiron have appeared. Now, an increasing number of astrologers are beginning to integrate Chiron into their work, finding it particularly useful in the areas of counselling and psychologically oriented work. Given the nature of the archetypal pattern behind the planet Chiron, this is not surprising, for at its very core lies the issue of the meaning which our personal suffering may eventually yield up to us, and which roots us firmly in the soil of our own lives, sufficiently perhaps to be able to fulfil our individuality by being of service to others. It is often our 'Chiron issues', especially as they become set off by transits, that first prompt us to seek help; many a successful cycle of healing has been started under auspicious transits of Chiron.

In this book, I have emphasized to some degree the question of our woundedness as represented by the position of Chiron, for reasons which I trust will become obvious through the chapters which comprise an exploration of Chiron's archetypal meaning. If we go helter-skelter towards self-actualization, struggling to manifest our potential without also embracing our woundedness, we may fall prey to the tragic one-sidedness that we can see in the lives of those people who were famous but unhappy, notorious and powerful but deeply unfulfilled, or, less glamorously, were simply deceiving themselves. As long as our suffering is projected out on to others, or indeed the world at large, personal healing may be impossible, and ideals of service to humanity may degenerate into misery and self-sacrifice. Admitting one's own suffering into consciousness for the first time may itself initiate a cycle of healing; it is in this spirit that the observations on Chiron by house, sign and aspect are offered.

This book is in the nature of a mosaic; the long process of researching and writing it has been rather like the experience of trying to piece together a jigsaw for which initially there was no picture, and eventually several different pictures! The reader will find many irreconcilables sitting here side by side, sometimes with no attempt to resolve them. The archetypal nature of Chiron himself is also thus: the opposites of horse and human being are yoked uncomfortably into one form, awaiting the more inclusive synthesis that only a journey into the depths of his own inner nature can bring. Latching on to ready-made philosophies does not necessarily work where Chiron is involved, for this archetypal pattern suggests the need, and brings the opportunity, for each of us to make our own personal and unique quest for the meaning of our lives. During this process, we inevitably come up against many imponderables, paradoxes and unanswerable questions.

In Part I of this book the archetypal background to the planet Chiron at work in the horoscope is described as fully as possible given the limitations of space. It is my intention here to create a resource bank of images, associations and themes pertaining to the somatic, psychological and spiritual aspects of the journey represented by the planet Chiron. In addition, immersing ourself in the mythological and archetypal background of a planet often has the effect of bringing it alive in our life, and thus stimulating a spontaneous process of learning from observation and experience. Richard Tarnas expresses this eloquently:

The sustained study of astrology grants human consciousness the experience of clear and overwhelming indications of divine intelligence of infinite complexity, power, and beauty . . . By having one's limited rational framework repeatedly demolished by powerful synchronicities, one's vision of the universe opens to an intimate knowledge of the numinous.[6]

The larger archetypal background provides a context within which all the different meanings attributed to the planet Chiron can be seen to have coherence. Its underlying structure is like the warp and woof threads on a loom; in each individual life the design woven upon this will be unique. With some sense of this, when we approach Chiron within the horoscope, we may be more able to appreciate how these threads of meaning are being woven, to see the pattern that is forming, and perhaps even to begin to enjoy the weaving of it.

Although I have detailed some of the many manifestations of Chiron which I have observed in the lives of individuals, ultimately the process of understanding Chiron in enough depth to make it truly part of our astrological vocabulary requires each of us to make our own journey of exploration. I believe this to be what the planet itself represents: a spirit of philosophical independence, compassion in the face of our suffering, and an ongoing process of learning to trust the Inner Teacher or Guide. The Chironian way of learning is to prepare oneself to listen to the Inner Teacher, whose classroom is no less than our own life experience and whose skills develop over time by allowing meaning to emerge organically. Thus I hope this book will stimulate this process of personal discovery symbolized by Chiron, thereby being of practical use both for those astrologers who work with clients in a counselling capacity, and also for those who use their horoscope as a guide to understanding their own inner journey as it unfolds.

PART ONE

THE MYTHIC IMAGE

I · Shamanism: The Roots

Somewhere beyond the walls of our awareness . . . the
wilderness side, the hunter side, the seeking side of
ourselves is waiting to return.

Laurens van der Post[1]

Before exploring the central story of Chiron, let us look at its
root-system – a network of material from various pre-Hellenic
sources. A major theme symbolized by the planet Chiron is the
reconciliation and healing of the fundamental split between the
spiritual and the instinctual in ourselves; this in turn serves as a
prototype for the many other pairs of opposites which live within
the psyche. By the time most of the Hellenic myths were formulated by Hesiod and Homer, around 750 BC, this split was already
becoming institutionalized, as patriarchal social and religious
forms replaced their earlier matriarchal counterparts. Before this
time, in the areas now comprising Europe and the Near East, the
Great Mother was worshipped in a multitude of different forms.
Being synonymous with fertility and the instinctual life, the
suppression of her worship meant the feminine in general became
devalued; with the advent of Christianity, the world of the senses
was relegated to the realm of the Devil, the enemy of God. We
remain thus divided against ourselves, but if we are to heal this
split, if we are to invite the mythic image of Chiron to speak
afresh to us, we must delve deeper and look further back to
palaeolithic times and to the dawning of human consciousness,
for here lie the origins of his story.

The Horse in Myth and Ancient Folklore

Chiron had a horse's body and legs, with human torso and arms.
The symbology of horses is rich, suggesting raw vitality and

instinctual energy, a wild but potentially tameable libido. Their plunging unbridled movement suggests free and ecstatic sexual expression, but also the dangers of frenzy and madness; bridled, they represent cultivated instincts, power channelled by discipline and consciousness, and harmony between man and his animal self.

Horse-worship was a feature of many pre-Hellenic cultures. In Mycenae, for example, mare-headed Demeter is said to be the mother of the Centaurs; her priests were castrated and wore female dress. In North Africa and around the Black Sea, the Amazons worshipped the goddess in her mare form, and were said to have been the first to tame horses;[2] men who entered their territory uninvited were sacrificed to the mare-goddess. As we shall see later, the figure of the Amazon is one which also accompanies the mythology of Chiron.

Since prehistoric times, in Britain the horse has been a sacred animal, associated with ancient fertility rites and rebirth. In Ireland, as late as the twelfth century, pagan horse-worship co-existed with Christianity,[3] and before assuming kingship Irish kings were symbolically reborn from the white mare Epona, whom Robert Graves equates with mare-headed Demeter.[4] Devotees of this cult carved her gigantic image into a chalky hillside at Uffington in Berkshire, where it can still be seen today. Horses featured in British folk customs, some of which still survive: the hobby-horse of the morris dancers is a wooden horse-head on a stick, sometimes called the cock horse, revealing its ancient associations with fertility rites. In Wales, between Christmas and New Year, a pantomime horse accompanies revellers who go from farm to farm bringing good tidings. Lady Godiva, who rode naked on horseback through the streets of Coventry, although a real woman, was later mythologized and linked with the goddess of earlier pagan rituals who was held to ensure fertility during the following season.[5]

In Scandinavia, horses were considered essential to the funeral rites of great warriors, and a hero's horse would often be sacrificed and buried with his master in the belief that it was needed to carry its master to heaven. In the Happy Hunting Grounds, the after-death realm of the North American Indians, warriors enjoy flight mounted on magical horses; similarly, in the Chinese heaven the moon-coloured horses of foreknowledge enable warriors to visit past, present or future. In Islam, the prophet Muhammad is said to have ridden a mythical mare named Buraq.

The horse is frequently associated with the World Tree, the Tree of Life, which connects the human realm with the upper and lower regions of spirit and the Underworld, the realms of Death. The Centaurs are often represented in Greek art together with a cut pine-tree, suggesting again the linking of the life and death. In his quest for wisdom, the Norse god Odin hung and bled for nine days and nights on the World Ash Tree called *Yggdrasil*; in Old Norse, *drasil* means both 'gallows tree' and 'horse', and *Yggr* was Odin's name as Lord of Death, when he rode an eight-legged horse, a mythic creature that also features in other shamanic cultures. The Valkyries, who were the semi-divine daughters and emissaries of Odin, would appear on horseback, announcing to doomed warriors their imminent death.

However, the roots of this European horse mythology may lie in Vedic India. Ghandarvas were the Indian equivalent of the Centaurs, and arose from the blood wedding of the Earth Mother and the Horse's Penis.[6] This involved the ritual sacrifice and dismemberment of a horse, whose penis would be cut off and ceremonially buried at a hallowed place, to ensure a rich harvest. The Ghandarvas were reputed to be powerful wizards and expert healers; they were skilled in music and dance, and were not above abducting young virgins from their husbands. They represent the chthonic and phallic counterpart of the orthodox priesthood, and were very similar in character to the Greek Centaurs. In addition to their renown for fertility, Ghandarvas were also thought to represent the part of the soul which continued through different reincarnations,[7] a detail which we shall explore later on.

This brings us to the central 'tap root' into which all these diverse sources feed, one which penetrates deep into the realm of archetypes, and converges in Greek times to form the story of Chiron, where we again meet the figure of the shaman, the archetypal pattern of the Wounded Healer. Synchronous with the discovery of Chiron, there has been increasing interest in other cultures, their religious beliefs and cosmologies; many fascinating accounts of personal journeys of shamanic initiations have recently been published by Westerners.[8] Although the details of shamanic practices vary from one culture to another, there is an underlying consistency in terms of meaning which I feel is relevant to an understanding of Chiron.

Shamanism: A Historical and Cultural Perspective

Historically, shamanism flourished in palaeolithic hunter-gatherer societies; today there are few primarily shamanic cultures still surviving, exceptions being found amongst indigenous tribes in Africa and the Americas. In his book *Up From Eden*, Ken Wilbur describes as 'typhonic' any figure represented as half animal and half human; he also uses this word to describe the mode of consciousness which prevailed around 200,000 to 50,000 years ago. The mythic image of Chiron is obviously derived from this ancient mode of consciousness. It provides a clue to its astrological meaning in the horoscope, a meaning which is supported by observation of what happens during its major transits: it suggests the re-emergence of an ancient world-view, one that lies dormant in the substrata of our own individual psyches, and one that we are perhaps being called upon to re-embrace.

The typhonic mind or sensibility, and the shamanic initiation, are both characterized by a direct experience of the force-field lying beneath the myriad forms perceived by our senses. Rational consciousness specializes in discriminating, analysing and separating things; by contrast, this consciousness is holistic and able to intuit directly the significance of personal events, as well as the numinosity and interconnectedness of the whole of life, including the realms beyond physical death. So-called 'primitive' consciousness embraces paradoxes that would totally confound a linear and rational Western consciousness steeped in the Newtonian–Cartesian world-view:

Since the mind is not yet developed, it does not have the capacity to differentiate itself from the body, and thus the self likewise is embedded in and undifferentiated from the body . . . man did not learn to clearly distinguish self from body until quite late in his evolutionary career – in fact he would develop a severe lesion between self and body, ego and flesh, reason and instinct. But prior to that time, self and body were more or less fused and confused – they were totally undifferentiated. The angel and the animal, the man and the serpent, were one.[9]

Historically, then, the shamanic period is characterized by tribal living, man's individuality being embedded in a totality comprising his family, his ancestors, the world of nature, and indeed the whole of life, often seen as a reflection of various cosmological deities. Hence, a person's individuality does not exist in isolation, but has its validity *in relation to the community and his or her place in it*. It is precisely this lack that is our wound, the illness of our industrialized Western society. Jung expresses this poignantly:

As scientific understanding has grown, so our world has become dehumanized. Man feels himself isolated in the cosmos, because he is no longer involved in nature and has lost his emotional 'unconscious identity' with natural phenomena. These have slowly lost their symbolic implications. Thunder is no longer the voice of an angry god, nor is lightning his avenging missile. No river contains a spirit, no tree is the embodiment of wisdom, no mountain cave the home of a great demon. No voices now speak to man from stones, plants and animals, nor does he speak to them believing they can hear. His contact with nature has gone, and with it has gone the profound emotional energy that this symbolic connection supplied.[10]

The shaman is one initially set apart from his or her tribe by the force and immediacy of personal religious experience and vision: 'hierophantic realization' is achieved, 'the realization of something far more deeply interfused, inhabiting both the world outside and also one's own interior experience, which gives everything a sacred character'.[11] Once having accepted his vocation, however, the shaman is highly regarded within his group, exercising considerable influence by virtue of his vocation as healer, intermediary, diviner and visionary. Shamans have often brought warning visions to their people, and have functioned as a source from which the spiritual life of the collective can be renewed and replenished. Amongst the Zulu, the chief of a *kraal* (settlement) is also a priest and, in consultation with a diviner, safeguards the well-being of his clan group; the 'heaven-herd' is responsible for bringing rain. In Zimbabwe, every traditional Shona family includes a spirit medium to help maintain a harmonious network of relationships between the living and the dead, which they consider to be essential for the health of both the land and those who live on it.

Thus the shaman is the custodian of a heritage of direct access to realms of the sacred inaccessible to most people, and the guardian of the soul-history of a people. Specific knowledge may be passed from one shaman to another, and the record of his or her personal inner journey may be communicated through various art forms, such as painting, music, dance and story-telling. However, the substance of the shaman's experience and its transformative impact are unique to the individual and not transmissible.

Shamanic Vocation: Crisis and Call

The spontaneous signs of vocation can appear at any age, and are usually accompanied by the onset of physical or mental illness, or both. As a child, the candidate may have been nervous, withdrawn and dreamy; he or she may have a physical deformity or disability. In some cultures, notably Eskimo and African, epilepsy is regarded as a sign of shamanic vocation. Amongst the Shona, if an illness does not respond to conventional forms of treatment (usually herbal), a *nganga* (shaman) will be called in. If he determines the illness to be a sign of vocation, he will intercede on behalf of the spirit who is trying to possess the person; if he or she agrees to act as its medium, recovery will follow acceptance of the vocation.[12] Refusal is considered by most shamanic societies to be a serious mistake almost certain to end in death.

As the process of initiation deepens, rupture of normal life and withdrawal from the everyday world may follow; this can occur several times, over a prolonged period. For example, it takes about seven years of full-time preoccupation with the process to qualify as a *sangoma* (diviner and healer) in Southern Africa. In every shamanic tradition, the candidate must undergo a period of intense psychological, physical and spiritual trial, a 'night sea journey' into the unconscious, to use a Western term. He has died to his former self; he communes with the spirits and the world of nature as a prelude to his future role as intermediary between the realms of nature, human life and the spirits, for 'the shaman is the channel for interspecies communication'.[13] He must be able to traverse the land of the dead and return to acquire and consolidate the skills necessary for his future work.

Shamanic Cartography

In order to describe some of the archetypal features of the journey undertaken by the shaman, let us first consult the map of the cosmological territory through which he will travel. Ancient shamanic practices often involved an elaborate cartography of the Underworld.[14] In Western cultures our understanding of this has until recently been somewhat rudimentary by comparison. Many extra-ordinary states of consciousness which were recognized by shamans to be of potentially healing value if handled correctly are pathologized by us, labelled, suppressed with drugs or negative attitudes, and perhaps even somatized into fatal disease.

Collectively, we have been sorely lacking a flexible spiritual and psychological topography which can creatively address the potentially transformative experiences which many people go through. The Christian heaven and hell are domains to which one is sent for all eternity after death. The finality and literalness of these images may impoverish rather than enrich our human life; it becomes a terrifying necessity to ensure our place in heaven (by obeying the Church); there are no second chances, so every action brings either doom or glory in its wake. By contrast, the corresponding realms in shamanic traditions (and in Eastern religions such as Hinduism and Buddhism) are recognized as *timeless*, non-physical dimensions of consciousness, which ordinarily are traversed by the soul after death, but which are also encountered during the process of shamanic initiation or expansion of consciousness; they naturally accompany the evolutionary journey of the soul, rather than threatening it with damnation for all time.[15]

In the typical shamanic view, consistent across many widely different cultures, the world is divided into three realms. The Middle Realm is where we live our earthly life, and is the only terrain bound by the laws of linear time and three-dimensional space; 'above' is the Celestial Realm, and 'below' the Infernal Realm. Relating this to our astrological model, we can say that the planets up to and including Saturn are primarily concerned with the Middle Realm, while the Celestial and Infernal Realms belong to the outer planets. We will expand this analogy in the chapters on aspects and transits.

The Journey of Suffering, Death, Rebirth and Return

The mythological realms traversed on the inner journey are outside time and space, and may be experienced in dreams, visions, and altered states of consciousness. In many cultures, hallucinogenic or narcotic plants are ceremonially used to induce ecstasy; the plant itself is considered to be sacred, synonymous with the god with whom the shaman communes, and from whom he learns inwardly. Externally, many sacred sites and places of pilgrimage act as powerful evocations of this inner terrain, and are considered as the dwelling-places of spirits, demons or gods. Likewise, trials of initiation may include ordeals of physical and psychological endurance intended to evoke inner experience. During the famous Sun Dance of the Sioux Indians of North America the candidate is strung up by eagle's claws attached to his pectoral muscles, as portrayed in the film *A Man Called Horse*.

Departure on the journey may be accompanied by images of thresholds, crossroads, womb-like doors, holes or openings such as caves, grottoes and underground places. Periods of psychological rebirth frequently evoke biological and spiritual memories and resonances of our actual birth.[16] A period of incubation, enwombment or gestation follows, during which the future shaman may be physically and/or mentally ill, when he descends into the terrain of 'death'. He may be called upon to battle demons, endure various psychic trials, or encounter spirits which have possessed him and thus initiated the journey. The imagery of death may symbolize a former world-view, self-concept or phase of life which must die if rebirth is to occur. For example, the shaman may be eaten down to the bone by demons or hungry spirits; his intestines may be removed and replaced by quartz crystals; he may be tortured, burnt alive or dismembered. If all goes well, however, he will be resurrected and these tormenting spirits, whether animal, ancestral or archetypal, may later become his allies and assist him in his work through 'a covenant forged in death *and* in spirit between the eater and the eaten'.[17] In communion with the forces of nature, the shaman represents the bridge which links one level of reality with another.

Time for return to the world may be signalled by dreams of birds or flying creatures; revitalization and rebirth occur as the spirit returns to the body. The peaks of sacred mountains, the heart of the sun and various images of centring, reconnection, re-memberment and the meeting and reconciliation of opposites all feature during the period of restitution. The World Tree or *axis mundi* at the centre of the universe symbolizes the harmonious interchange, between the Underworld, the everyday world and the celestial realms, which has been opened up during the inner journey.

After disengaging from society during this period of illness and initiation, the shaman eventually must return to take up his or her vocation and serve within it. Too long a sojourn in the world of the spirits may make creative return impossible. Although elaborate ceremonies may mark his graduation, it is only endorsement by the community which eventually qualifies a person to be recognized as a shaman. 'The shaman . . . has a social rather than a personal reason for opening the psyche as he or she is concerned with the community and its well-being.'[18] '. . . shamans are trained in the art of equilibrium, in moving with poise and surety on the threshold of the opposites, in creating cosmos out of chaos. The Middle Realm then is still a dream that can be shaped by the dreamer.'[19]

The Horse in Shamanism

To return to our image of the horse, we find it frequently occurring in shamanic cosmology and ritual practices, for in many cultures the horse is literally and/or symbolically present in the shamanic seance. It depicts the ecstatic 'flight' of the shaman in trance, and facilitates what Eliade terms a 'breakthough in plane', the passage from this world to other worlds. The horse represents a bridge between the world of form and the world of the unseen. It also carries the deceased to the afterlife and enables the shaman to search for the lost souls of those whose are ill: it is a funerary animal and *psychopomp*, a guide or one who shows the way. In Central Asia, when a shaman is recalling an errant soul, a horse will be tethered nearby; its shivering signals the return of the soul. White horse hairs may be burnt during rituals, thus evoking the magical animal; the shaman may sit on a mare-skin; he may induce ecstasy by beating a drum with a horse-headed stick or by dancing astride the stick, the symbolic means of his magical flight during which he performs divinations and healing.

Let us now follow this image into the central story of Chiron, exploring how the ancient figure of the Wounded Healer was represented by the Greeks. As mentioned at the beginning of this chapter, the split between the spiritual and the instinctual was already occurring within the Hellenic culture of this time. The development of the heroic ego was well under way, as man struggled to separate himself from uroboric unity with the Great Mother and all organic life by fighting against it.

2 · Chiron in Greek Mythology

The Centaurs

Chiron's relationship with the Centaurs, the mythical beasts who were half human and half horse, is described in a variety of ways by different sources. He is sometimes their ancestor, sometimes their priest and ruler, and sometimes he is merely seeking their companionship in revelry and merry-making. Although the origin of the Centaurs themselves is also variously described, two common accounts say that the Centaurs were either descended from Centaurus, son of Apollo and Stilbe, or from Ixion and Nephele (a cloud made by Zeus to resemble Hera).[1] Mount Pelion in Thessaly was their home and the stories about them feature their wars with their neighbours, the Lapiths, also descended from Ixion.

These wars underline a theme central to the mythology surrounding Chiron: that of the conflict between the 'civilized' and the 'uncivilized'. The Centaurs were notoriously unruly and lecherous, and were traditionally part of the retinue of Dionysus, while the Lapiths were quite the opposite in temperament and were even said to have invented the bridling of horses;[2] together they provide a most appropriate image for the juxtaposition of wild 'unbridled' instinctual responses with behaviour that is more controlled.

Chiron and His Origins

In the most common version of Chiron's birth, he is the son of Cronus (Saturn) and the nymph Philyra, daughter of Oceanus and Tethys. Cronus first found Philyra in Thessaly while searching for his baby son Zeus, whom his wife Rhea had concealed from him, weary of his repeated devouring of their offspring. Philyra changed herself into a mare (cf. mare-headed Demeter) to try and escape from Cronus, who began ardently pursuing her. However, Cronus in turn deceived her, by changing himself into a horse; and thus he succeeded in mating with her. Eventually, a child of this union was born to Philyra: he was Chiron the Centaur, who had the body and legs of a horse and the torso and arms of a man. When Philyra saw him, she was so disgusted that she pleaded to be changed into anything other than what she was. The gods duly obliged by turning her into a linden-tree.[3] Thus Chiron was abandoned, later to be found by Apollo who became his foster-father and taught him many skills.

In the story of Chiron's birth we can already see some important psychological themes which are relevant to the meaning of the planet. He was rejected by his mother, and presumably never knew his father, Cronus. He was conceived while both his parents were in animal form, that is, from an instinctual union. I have found no account of any reconciliation between Chiron and Cronus, and Philyra rejected the product and expression of her own instinctual side to the point of preferring to be eternally imprisoned in a tree.

The wound of rejected instincts is one shared by countless people in our society. Many of us who have been primarily influenced by Judaeo-Christian Western culture and thought-forms were born to parents who repressed the instinctual side of themselves, having been carefully trained and 'educated' to do so. Such self-rejection has led to their being unable to acknowledge, much less to embrace and nurture, this aspect of their children. With later cultural developments expressing 'sexual liberation' the pendulum has swung the other way; however, we cannot relate to and respect a force by which we are possessed.

The loneliness and isolation that results from this combination of a negative, rejecting mother and an absent or weak father is a common psychological theme of our time, and sets the scene for the archetypal 'birth of a hero' scenario. Children of such parents often feel orphaned, that their earthly parents are not their true parents, and that one day the 'real' ones will come and rescue them – this seems to be a theme which emerges as a sense of individuality develops, especially as a self-protective response to a wounding early situation. When a child has no loving relationship with its parents or guardians, its psyche is left wide open to the imaginal realm, and ego-formation is hindered or prevented altogether. Positively, this can foster in us (just as Chiron was fostered) an early sense of destiny and the urgency to develop our own individuality; negatively, it may drive us to flee from the pain of our wounds into an increasing emphasis on the spiritual in a rarefied and one-sided way, where the instincts are suppressed in order to maintain a false sense of elevated consciousness. Needless to say, the instincts will eventually hit back in order to redress the imbalance, often by causing crises of physical or mental illness; these are among the more obvious manifestations of Chiron in the birth chart.

Another interesting point emerges at this stage. In the unfolding of the Greek story of the Creation, Chiron's birth is unique: it is the product of the first union that is not directly incestuous. All his ancestors on his father's side were conceived by unions of mother and son or sister and brother. Philyra was the niece of Cronus; therefore they are still related, but distantly. Thus Chiron also represents a breaking away from the original matrix, the primordial Earth Mother Gaia and her offspring. This symbolizes the assertion of individuality through a process of disruption of original unity and, in the story of Chiron, we see both the painful repercussions and also the resolution. At the moment of birth he encounters the Terrible Goddess in her destructive form, the rejecting face of his own mother; as we shall see, his eventual release from suffering occurs through voluntary surrender to death, returning again to the Earth Mother, this time to her healing embrace.

Apollo, the sun-god much revered by the Greeks, was Chiron's foster-father and teacher; in the absence of Cronus, he is significant as the primary masculine influence on Chiron's development. Apollo was god of music, prophecy, poetry and healing, a noble paragon of youth, beauty, wisdom and justice. He was never vengeful, but purified men of their guilt and transgressions.

He also offered divine protection against wild animals and disease, although he was god of the hunt and capable of sending plagues. His love affairs were mostly unfortunate; his ability to relate (Eros) seems to have given him difficulty, while the principle of reason and order (Logos) was much more developed. The archetypal energy represented by Apollo is the very opposite to the instinctual union of which Chiron was the result; their relationship, however, again depicts the theme of the juxtaposition of unbridled instinctuality with the controlling factors of reason and education.

In another version, Chiron gained his wisdom when Athene laid her hand on his forehead. Although Athene has her roots in ancient feminine wisdom figures, by the time her image had been filtered through Greek patriarchal thought, she was said to have been born fully armed from the head of Zeus. She is thus a powerful but somewhat disembodied image of the feminine, functioning mainly in service to the masculine principle, and dedicated to the processes of education and civilization.

Hence, although Chiron survives, he remains eternally wounded, divided against his instinctual self, which was humiliated and rejected; he becomes instead the mediator of Apollonian ideals in a kind of harmony, culture, order and creativity which sets itself *against* the instinctual. This is his first wound, and one which many of us share. Robert Stein describes this situation very clearly:

The development of the individual ego certainly involves a process of restricting and taming one's own nature, so it follows that the development of civilization may very well have necessitated the differentiation and separation between the spiritual and animal natures of man. But once the horse has been tamed and bridled, it is destructive to try forcefully and brutally to gain complete mastery over it. The relationship between man and horse must become harmonious and loving; the true Master is so in tune with his horse that he needs no bridle. Simply put, Western man has not been willing to relinquish any of the power he has gained in his conquest over Nature. Out of fear of losing his power, he continues to abuse and neglect his horse. The difficulty is that the power of consciousness lies in individuality, while Mother Nature cherishes all of her children equally and indiscriminately. Thus modern man regards the giving up or giving back of any of his power to Nature as a loss of individuality. Furthermore, the repressive measures which man has taken against Nature have resulted in a tremendous building up of dark and violent powers in his own soul which threaten to erupt at any moment.[4]

Chiron became a wise man, prophet, physician, teacher and musician. His ministry included the unruly Centaurs themselves, and various small kingdoms in Northern Greece. Local kings would entrust their sons to him to be educated in the skills of leadership appropriate for their future roles. He was the mentor of many famous Greek heroes, including Jason, Achilles, Hercules and Asclepius, who was eventually immortalized because of his own great healing powers. Chiron taught them everything from riding, archery, hunting, the arts of war and medicine (all survival skills), to ethics, music, religious rituals and the beginnings of natural science. Chiron is sometimes credited with the invention of the musical pipe and the spear, and also with having discovered several constellations as he began to map the heavens. He is also said to have originated the medicinal use of plants, although, as we have seen in the last chapter, this is an association with the archetypal figure of the Wounded Healer, rather than with Chiron himself; shamans were skilled in the use of plants long before the myth of Chiron was formulated by the Greeks.

There are numerous accounts of healings and divinations performed by Chiron, but perhaps the most relevant for our purposes is the healing of Telephus. He was wounded by a spear which Chiron had given to Peleus. When Telephus consulted the oracle of Apollo after his wound would not heal, he was told that 'the wound could only be healed by its cause'. Thus Chiron is associated with the principle of homoeopathic healing, where 'like cures like'; for example, minute quantities of snake venom can be used to cure snake bites. We can observe this principle at work when important transits of Chiron occur, and also in relationships involving significant aspects between Chiron and other planets. In psychological terms we can liken this to the 'repetition compulsion'. The memory of a painful feeling, stored in the unconscious, will tend to attract to it situations in the present which repeat the same ingredients and thus reactivate the old wound. However, these cycles of repetition occur because a wound is still seeking healing, and/or because some change of attitude or expansion of consciousness is trying to occur. At these times healing is possible, but if the dose of repetition becomes too large, the person may be overwhelmed, and the wound may deepen instead or turn into a fatal illness.

Chiron's Own Wounding

The episode which earned Chiron the title of Wounded Healer is central to his story. In the most widely known version, Hercules was invited to dinner by the Centaurs; a row erupted, and Hercules began to fight them. The Centaurs fled in all directions, pursued by Hercules, and one of his arrows struck Chiron in the leg; it created an unhealable wound from which Chiron suffered for the rest of his long life. In a variation on this theme, a wounded Centaur crawled into Chiron's cave for refuge. While trying to help him, Chiron was himself cut by the poisoned arrow and overcome with unceasing agony.[5] In yet another version, Chiron was wounded in a battle between the Lapiths and the Centaurs, caused by the Centaurs becoming drunk and attempting to rape a Lapith bride.

When we pause to consider the implications of this story, several significant points emerge. The battle during which Chiron is wounded involves the Centaurs against either Hercules or the Lapiths. Thus, the fighting factions symbolize the conflict embodied in Chiron's form: the Centaurs represent Chiron's lower half, the rejected animal part of him, while the Lapiths and Hercules represent his top, human half. This wound is the heritage of centuries of repressing and persecuting our instinctual selves, and it is the condition in which much of the so-called civilized world finds itself today. The conflict comes home to roost in Chiron's own wounding, and heralds his unique destiny as an image of the potential reconciliation of these painful opposites.

Hercules is a well-known and typical example of the Greek

hero-figure, and is an image of the drive for achievement and perfection; this aspect of the masculine principle has dominated much of Western culture over the last few centuries. Although on the positive side Hercules represents the noble virtues of strength, endurance and individuality, which are necessary for the ego emerging from unconsciousness, his negative side is unpleasant and destructive, and may be characterized by conquest and domination for no purpose, a 'might is right' psychology, a devaluation of the instinctual and the feminine, and an over-valuation of heroism at the cost of much human suffering. The manifestations of this in history and in the world today hardly need pointing out, and warrant a closer look at Hercules.

Hercules and the Heroic

In pre-classical Greece, the hero cult, like the cult of the dead, was the chthonic counterpart to the worship of the gods. It represented a progression from the cults of ancestor worship, but was still a local affair. The tomb of someone who had been heroicized was often the scene of blood sacrifice and elaborate rituals of mourning. Great ills could flow from the wrath of an unappeased spirit, who, equally, could bestow boons upon the suppliant at his tomb. The accomplishments of hero-figures, embellished over time, created a composite figure which subsequent generations sought to emulate. Thus, the hero originally had a religious function, as intermediary between the living and the dead, almost 'shamanic' in this respect. However, this image gradually became literalized and cultivated into an ideal way of being in the world, an attempt to attain immortality and to avoid oblivion.

Hercules was one of a pair of twins; his brother Iphicles was as fearful and timid as Hercules was tough, bold and heroic. Iphicles fades into insignificance, dies unheroically in battle and, by his absence, increases the one-sidedness of the figure of Hercules, who does not appear to incorporate any of Iphicles' qualities; his appetite for conquest breaks loose, untempered by the fear, frailty and moderation represented by his twin.

Hercules was one of Chiron's students, and this adds poignancy to the fact that it was he who caused the fateful wound. The arrow which struck Chiron was poisoned with the blood of the Hydra, a monster which Hercules encountered during one of his famous labours. Every time he cut off one of its heads, nine more would grow, suggesting the devouring destructive power of the feminine; it is also an image of the clutching and entangling beast which the underworld of our own instincts becomes when ignored and repressed, or if approached aggressively and 'confronted'. Hercules eventually overcame the Hydra by kneeling down before it and raising it into the air. I would understand this to describe how any attempt to cut off or eradicate our own instincts will cause them to multiply, dominate and seek vengeance. We may instead need to pay humble respect to the numinous instinctual power that the Hydra represents, protecting ourselves with consciousness from being overcome by it.

Significantly, Hercules eventually met his demise through a Centaur, Nessus, who wanted to avenge the devastation Hercules had wrought upon his race. Hercules killed Nessus for trying to rape his wife; the dying Nessus told her to use some of his blood as a charm against Hercules' frequent unfaithfulness. The blood was poisoned, however, and Hercules later met an agonizing death, wrapped in a tunic immersed in burning poison.

So we see Chiron in a curiously ambivalent relationship with the heroic principle. His life is saved by Apollo, who himself taught Chiron many of the skills which he then passes on to his young disciples, and yet it is one of these very heroes who wounds him. We also see this wherever the planet Chiron is in the chart: often it represents things we can do well for others, but cannot do for ourselves, qualities which others perceive strongly in us but which we do not see. Often these are the very things which we urgently need for our own growth and healing, but they 'slip through' and are passed on to others.

In the mythologem of Chiron there is also described a threesome of figures which constellates around the planet Chiron's position in the birth chart, in the areas of life suggested by its house and sign. These figures may be inner ones, conscious subpersonalities or unconscious shadow figures; or they may feature in projection, as actual people with whom the person interacts. Either way, there may be considerable conflict between them. The three figures are: the wounded one/victim, the wounder/persecutor, and the healer/saviour/rescuer. Just as in the myth, situations of psychological deadlock may sometimes be released by discovering this triad within. We will explore these themes in more detail later.

Chiron's Release from Suffering

Chiron suffered unceasingly from his wound. Being an immortal, he could not die from it; neither could he cure it, in spite of all his skills. Ironically, his ability to help others was increased by his continual search for relief from his own unhealable wound. This painful and humiliating situation is frequently met by people who work in the healing professions, whether orthodox or alternative. It also describes the repeating patterns which never seem to resolve, although one continually tries to 'make it better' and to search for healing and change, where one continues doggedly along a path leading to progressively worse disasters (like the repetition compulsion described earlier). At these times, the wisdom of the instincts could redirect us; if we could but listen, we would know immediately that we were on the wrong track. Yet, sadly, once that connection is broken, like Chiron, it may almost cost us our lives to learn humbly to listen again. Our righteous 'top halves' are only too eager to turn our dissociation into a philosophy, and even try and convince others of the rightness of it. This is one expression of the missionary zeal that is associated with Chiron. Wherever Chiron is in the chart, it is there that people are in danger of becoming 'possessed' – taken over by some idea, belief, purpose, which may perpetuate their own wounding and lead them to try and convince others of this 'truth', which may be no more than a desperate defence against their own inner pain. This is not to diminish the immense contributions to humanity that have been made by people motivated by their own wounds, but it does serve as a sobering image for our times, when a plethora of cures, philosophies and methods of growth continually seduce us into the sneaking feeling that 'If I could only just (scream it out, analyse it away, discover the meaning of it, understand the astrology of it, . . .) then everything would be all right.' Chiron's story underlines the need for acceptance of our woundedness as a precondition for any healing that may follow; it also shows how the wisdom of our own psyche may bring us healing in ways that we have difficulty receiving.

Chiron and Prometheus

Eventually, Chiron was released from his torment through a curious destiny swap with Prometheus, who thus represents a key figure in the resolution of Chiron's story, and may perhaps also hold for us a guiding image of the appropriate resolution to our own conflicts and the healing of our wounds. Prometheus had been bound to a rock by Zeus as a punishment for mocking him, and for his subsequent theft of fire. Every day a griffon, a huge vulture-like bird, would peck out his liver (ruled by Jupiter); because his liver would grow again each night, Prometheus suffered continual torture. Zeus decreed that Prometheus could only be released if an immortal agreed to go to Tartarus in his place, thus relinquishing his immortality, and on condition that Prometheus wear forever afterwards a crown of willow leaves on his head and a ring on his finger.

Hercules pleaded Chiron's case, and Zeus eventually agreed to the exchange. This resonates with the meaning of Chiron in the chart: the one who wounded Chiron is also the one who facilitated his healing. Here again, Chiron (the healer/saviour) did not act for himself; eventually it is *that within us which wounds us* which must repent and come to our aid, or we remain victims of our own fate and oblivious to our own destructiveness. Chiron took Prometheus' place and eventually died; after nine days Zeus immortalized him as the constellation Centaurus. Hercules, invoking Apollo, shot the griffon through the heart. This is also an evocative image. Rapacious monster-birds are often associated with the destructive side of the masculine spirit – negative thoughts which devour and prey upon our creativity and sense of meaning, and turn us against the life of the body. These lofty monsters within the mind can often only be stilled by the opening of the heart, by acceptance and compassion for ourselves and others.

Let us take a closer look at the story of Prometheus. The son of Iapetus (a Titan) and Clymene, he is said to have created the first mortals from clay and water, after which the goddess Athene breathed into them and brought them to life. Prometheus was originally portrayed as a primitive trickster-figure bent on out-witting the gods. Later, however, Aeschylus developed him into a culture hero, a figure who endures suffering for a noble cause, the champion and saviour of humanity, to whom he was teaching skills to help them develop. Zeus was contemptuous and dis-gusted with the human race; he wanted to eliminate them and create something better, perhaps jealous of Prometheus' role in their creation. He only spared them because Prometheus pleaded their cause. This lament from the chorus in Aeschylus'[1] *Prometheus Bound* expresses his dilemma:

> You defiant, Prometheus, and your spirit
> In spite of all your pain, yields not an inch.
> But there is too much freedom in your words.

Prometheus later responds:

> Oh, it is easy for the one who stands outside
> The prison wall of pain to exhort and teach the one who
>   suffers.[6]

Prometheus was once asked to mediate in a dispute about which parts of a sacrificed bull should be reserved for the gods, and which parts man should be permitted to eat. He skinned the bull and made two bags from its hide. In one he put the best flesh, but hidden beneath the stomach. In the other, he put the bones and offal, hidden underneath a juicy layer of fat. Prometheus laughed heartily when Zeus fell for the trick. Zeus was very angry, and punished Prometheus by withholding fire from humanity. Prometheus then felt obliged to retrieve it for hu-manity, who were, after all, of his making. He went secretly to

Olympus, stole back the precious glowing coal, hid it in a fennel-stalk and crept away to return fire to mankind.

When he discovered what Prometheus had done, Zeus retaliated by making from clay a beautiful woman named Pandora, complete with her famous box full of woes for mankind. He sent her to Prometheus' brother Epimetheus, who refused her, as Prometheus had already warned him against accepting gifts from Zeus. Foiled yet again, Zeus became even angrier; he made a final gesture of his supremacy by chaining Prometheus to a rock, and setting the tormenting griffon upon him. Prometheus stayed there unrelenting, until Chiron changed places with him.

Although the theft of fire is a famous mythological theme, the first part of the story is perhaps not as well known. Prometheus is often simplistically thought of as 'the one who brought the enlightenment of consciousness to the human race'. However, as the first part of the story shows, he is a figure somewhat more complex in meaning. As well as a healthy rebellion against inhuman or superpersonal authority, he also represents a lack of respect for the gods, and a dangerous attempt to cheat and humiliate them, to refuse to give them their due. His story illustrates the paradoxical fact that although it would seem to be in man's nature to strive for self-development and consciousness, and thus to try and get the best part of the bull for himself, as it were, if he does so without paying due respect to the gods from whom he is stealing, he may suffer 'punishment' in the form of physical or mental illness.

That is why in seeking for the meaning of your suffering you seek for the meaning of your life. You are searching for the greater pattern of your own life, which indicates why the wounded healer is the archetype of the Self – one of its most widespread features – and is at the bottom of all genuine healing procedures.[7]

Prometheus also represents that process of soul growth which unfolds as we courageously debunk our own false godlikeness, discovering and giving up our inflations and identification with archetypal images. The pain we inevitably experience during this process makes us more humble, and also more compassionate towards our own suffering and that of others – it makes us human. At one time or another, we may fall into inflation and hubris and have to 'fight the gods' in order to honour our human needs and feelings, limitations and frailty. We may also have to fight the values of parents and society in order to honour our humanness and our own soul.

The act of perceiving astrological archetypes and thus freeing oneself from the bondage of unconsciousness is, on one level, an extraordinary feat of human rebellion against archetypal manipulation; it is, in essence, stealing fire from the Gods. On a higher level, that theft itself is archetypally ordained, and that archetype is Prometheus. Astrology is Prometheus' fire.[8]

The story of Prometheus has been linked by some astrologers[9] to the sign of Aquarius, and, as we are now on the threshold of the Age of Aquarius, it is of course no accident that the planet Chiron has been discovered, and that resolution of Chiron's fate in the myth should be intimately connected with Prometheus. The archetypal pattern of the Wounded Healer has constellated, and Prometheus may indeed be seen as a guiding spirit for our age: he represents the clear recognition of the need to uphold our human values whatever the cost, and a parallel warning to give the gods their due. He represents the struggle of individuality emerging from enchainment by the forces of oppression which do not value human life, whether these forces be political or transpersonal. Joseph Campbell draws an analogy between the shamanic spirit of individualism and the Titan Prometheus:

[This spirit] . . . is now coming unbound within us – for the next world age. And the priests of Zeus may well tremble; for the bonds are disintegrating of themselves.[10]

To put this impassioned prediction within the context of the story of Chiron and Prometheus, let us conclude by looking at what happened to each of them after the exchange. Prometheus was freed, on condition that he would always wear a ring and a crown of willow leaves.

The ring may be seen as a symbolic reminder of his tormented period of enchainment; as a condition for his release it would seem to signify the need for humility. None of us can be free if we defy the gods for too long, unless we can substitute our own limits which include respect for them. As long we are not able or willing both to honour the gods and also to consider the limits appropriate to our own individual make-up, the society we live in, the relationships we form and the life we lead, we will never be free, but will always be answering to an external authority, often in a negative form. Chiron's astronomical position between Saturn and Uranus speaks of this, where Saturn represents form and tradition, the structures of society, and the urge to conserve and maintain, and Uranus represents the desire to destroy or rebel against structure and the status quo in the name of freedom, progress and individuality. In this context Chiron represents an *internalized* authority which is socially responsible and aware of the limits of human mortality, yet also committed to individual growth.

The willow crown is also significant, for the willow-tree is associated in general with the death-crone and in particular with Hecate, who lived on an island surrounded by willow-trees. Prometheus wearing her crown is thus an image of the acceptance of mortality. Equally, Chiron had to forgo his immortality, die and go to the Underworld, the realm of the death-crone, before being immortalized. Although in Greek mythology Hades is a male god, the land of the dead was previously the terrain of the great Earth Mother in her death aspect. Hence, the surrender and freeing of Prometheus and the death and resurrection of Chiron carry the same essential meaning. Both Zeus and Hades are Chiron's half-brothers: in the symbolic intersection of the Olympian realm of Zeus and the Underworld realm of Hades, the stories of Chiron and Prometheus come full circle. Prometheus regains his freedom and Chiron finds his long-sought healing: in this exchange both are released from their eternal suffering.

3 · The Wounded Healer Today

As we have seen, the shaman represents both a *historical* figure –
the healer/priest – and also an *archetypal* figure in the depths of the
collective psyche and thus in our own individual psyches as well:
he is part of both our psychological and our cultural pre-history.
However, we cannot turn back the clock of history and return
to the world-view within which shamanic societies operated.
Shamanic societies, past or present, are usually tribal in character,
living in much closer contact with nature and the world of the
instincts than most of us do today. Shamans become individualized through their initiatory illness and the disruption of their
normal life. Today, whole cultures are already in a state of
disruption, dissociated from harmony with nature and flounder-
ing in a profusion of broken religious, societal and family traditions. We could see in this the symptoms of a *collective* initiatory
illness.

As I have already suggested, the arrival and recognition of the
planet Chiron perhaps symbolize the need to work with and
consciously reintegrate the archetypal pattern of the Wounded
Healer, which has constellated in response to our present global
situation. This period of history also marks the end of the Age of
Pisces and the beginning of the Age of Aquarius, a theme to which
we will return in Chapter 6. However, the current importance of
the shamanic paradigm does not necessarily mean that 'shamanic'
experiences which may occur in the lives of individuals are signs
of a healing vocation. These psychological and spiritual events
accompany the process of *individualization*, just as they did for the
shaman, historically speaking.

Let us explore what this might mean in terms of individual
psychology. Our physical development within the womb, from

conception to birth, recapitulates many of the characteristics of our archaic evolutionary past, as 'ontogeny recreates phylogeny'.[1] The parallel in terms of consciousness is this: before we have begun to experience ourselves as separate individuals, our primary mode of consciousness is 'typhonic', as previously described. In the magic universe of which we are the centre, inner and outer are merged, emotions and sensations form a seamless web where vulnerability alternates with a sense of omnipotence. A baby still experiences life in its full archetypal intensity: it is peopled with primordial gods and demons, the imaginal counterparts to the 'real world' with which he or she gradually becomes familiar, in the form of first his or her mother and later others in his environment. For the purposes of this discussion, I will use the term 'typhonic' to refer to the mode of consciousness prevailing during the period from conception, through birth, until about age three. In Western cultures typhonic consciousness fades with the development of language; unlike 'primitive' cultures, we tend to emphasize differentiation and separation rather than the maintaining of unity.

Thus the shamanic paradigm with its archaic mode of consciousness often constellates in response to the wounds, traumas, conflicts and deprivations of this early period. However, even in the most loving and harmonious of early situations, our sense of individuality develops partly through 'wounding' encounters with an 'other' whom we must learn is not subject to our magical omnipotence. The frustrations of confronting a universe which we cannot control are endemic to the process of growing up, and the transition from an all-embracing unified field of consciousness to the more differentiated thought-forms from which our language develops is painful at the best of times. Specific difficulties or traumas during this early period leave very deep wounds, and often during transits of Chiron it is these early wounds which begin bleeding again, so to speak, crying out for attention and care. The re-emergence of pain which originates in the preverbal period of our past, whether or not we acknowledge it consciously, is frequently accompanied by an expansion of consciousness into vitalistic and/or archetypal realms, congruent with the earliest stages of our psychological development.

Transits of Chiron often accompany such expansions, but these transpersonal experiences are not just an expression, or avoidance, of our woundedness: to assume this would be a neo-Freudian idiocy. However, during periods of sickness, crisis, or states of expanded awareness, if we embrace one level to the exclusion of the other, we might misinterpret the signals of the psyche, and perhaps cut short a process of healing or 'whole-making' which is trying to take place.

Thus, to summarize, shamanic consciousness and its characteristic 'pre-personal immersion in nature and instinct'[2] may be the archetypal accompaniment of any inner journey evoked by our own woundedness, a journey which is the prelude to a new step of individualization and expression of personal destiny. However, the purpose and goal of the healing journey is unique to each traveller, but, Deo gratias, it can result both in the reclaiming of a lost sense of individual self, and its fulfilment through consecration to a larger purpose. The vocation of the shaman is to surrender to this process, whatever it entails. For some, the humbling experience of feeling like a helpless and suffering infant might become necessary as a counterpart to high-flown ideals and mental sophistication. For others, an experience of expanded awareness and a shift of philosophical perspective might be called forth to balance an ingrained but perhaps unconscious identification with suffering, helplessness and victimization.

Mircea Eliade defines shamanism as a 'technique of ecstasy'.[3] 'Ecstasy' means literally 'to be taken out of oneself, or to be in a condition that is off-centre', from the Greek word meaning 'displacement'. During periods of re-orientation such as often occur during transits involving Chiron, we may have ecstatic experiences; we become off-centre to varying degrees. What we previously took as the centre of our world-view, our life, or our self-concept, becomes inappropriate; while waiting for the new centre to be created and to emerge, we need to make allowances for the fact that we may be off-balance for a considerable period of time. Knowing that long-forgotten memories, repressed pain or traumatic memories may be reactivated can help us to determine when to act and when to remain reflective, when to speak and when to remain silent.

In *The Atman Project*, Ken Wilbur describes a mode of consciousness that he calls 'Centauric', which is relevant to the planet Chiron not just because of the name synchronously chosen! Wilbur clearly contrasts this more sophisticated Centauric mode with the 'older' typhonic mode, which is exclusively instinctually based:

The infantile body–ego was, recall, a stage wherein body and self or body and ego were undifferentiated. The mature Centaur or total body-mind is the point where body and ego begin to go into transdifferentiation and higher order integration – that is to say, body and ego-mind, once having been differentiated, are now integrated.[4]

Thus, the *reintegration* of mind and body is the key, and this indeed is one of the major themes associated with the planet Chiron. Centauric consciousness, then, is the capacity for *both/and* – for *both* differentiated rational thought *and* awareness of our connection to the unified force-field which lies beyond what our senses can perceive. To confuse these two would mean possibly leaving our own bleeding wounds unaddressed, with inevitable repercussions later on, for both ourselves and others, for: 'It is one thing to recontact the typhon and integrate it with the mind so as to eventually transcend both; quite another to recontact the typhon and stay there.'[5]

At the mature Centaur [level the] individual has completed the formation of language and conceptual thought; he has transformed the infantile wishes of the typhon to more social and consensual forms; he has moved out of the infantile embeddedness structures . . . The phantasy process is not now a way to regress to pre-verbal phantasies, but a way to contact transverbal realities.[6]

Let us take a wider perspective and explore the religious implications of all this. As we have seen, the shaman's role, historically, was essentially a religious one; the word 'religion' is derived from the Latin *religo*, a verb meaning to relink, unite, bind together, or reconnect. It is by virtue of his personal connection with the larger whole of life, visible and invisible, that the shaman is able to perform this function for his tribe or society. When laws, scriptures and dogma take precedence over personal experience of the divine, eventually all that remains is an institutionalized religion, which over time becomes increasingly ill adapted and therefore inappropriate to the religious needs of the collective; it may then become mainly an instrument of social control, an 'opiate of the people', to use Marx's famous phrase. Fundamentalism and dogmatism increase; scriptural law is literalized and enforced through guilt and fear of ostracism. People persecute or even kill in their desperation to convince others of their favoured position with God. History abounds with examples; however, in Chapter 11 we will examine the converse, where the unprecedented 'religious freedom' of the United States allowed the personal revelations of an ordained minister, one Reverend Jim Jones, to escalate into a catastrophe in which nearly 1000 people died.

Today we are witnessing the progressive disintegration of religious structures that once encouraged people to uphold the moral codes contributing to social cohesion. Somewhat like the shaman, a priest performing Holy Communion or any other ritual, is a mediator: he enacts, embodies and dramatizes powerful symbols which lie within the collective psyche of the group. Organized religion also protects individuals from unmediated encounters with the numinous which could be disorienting. On the other hand, it prescribes what they are 'allowed' to experience, and what is forbidden: personal revelation and individual numinous experience are discouraged unless they can be interpreted within the existing belief structure. Opening ourselves up to the inner dimensions of the individual psyche will usually set us swimming upstream, philosophically speaking; the current ferment is anyway prompting many people to seek direct ecstatic experience leading to *gnosis* or a deep sense of communion with an inner source of divine wisdom, strength and energy.

Notwithstanding the fundamentalism currently flowering within some Christian and Islamic sects, today we can also see occurring on a wide scale a religious cross-fertilization, a re-embracing of the discarded, 'primitive' elements represented within shamanism and also religions which have retained their shamanic heritage in one form or another (Tibetan Buddhism and Tantrism, for example). The proliferation of new cults, the intense questioning of hitherto unassailable issues of dogma, and the withdrawal of many people from overt religious affiliations are all symptoms of this urgent need for *personal* reconnection with the numinous. This is not without its dangers, as Wilbur points out:

In America (and Europe), where the New Age is most loudly announced, a significant majority of individuals are suffering from the stresses of these civilizations' failure to support truly rational and egoic structures, and thus these individuals are actually regressing to pre-personal, cultic and narcissistic pursuits . . . Often, however, the cults of Narcissus claim that this regression is actually a pursuit of transpersonal realities, or at least 'humanistic' freedom.[7]

Thus, the single greatest service that transpersonalists, as well as humanists, could perform is to champion, not just transreason, but an honest embrace of simple reason itself . . . if the Holocaust engulfs us all, it will not prove, to use the words of Jack Crittenden, 'that reason has failed, but that, for the most part, it has not yet been fully tried'.[8]

Thus, Chiron in the horoscope shows where this sometimes perilous search is likely to occur in a particularly intense way. Often, Chiron's house position represents an area of life that is initially blocked, wounded or functioning poorly, although it can also describe where we have a unique and individual contribution to make: Richard Nolle refers to Chiron's house position as the Chironian, or the cave where he dwelled. The pain and frustration we experience here may force us in upon ourselves, and thus begin our inner journey of healing, often qualitatively described by the sign position of Chiron. Planets in aspect to Chiron also tell us something about the type of terrain we may be required to cross, the helpers or foes we meet, and the monsters we may need to befriend, vanquish or be devoured by. They are like the various heroes under Chiron's tuition which depart from the Chironian in order to make their own journeys, thus symbolizing gifts and potentials we could express.

Chiron stimulates this process of initiation and leads towards a new beginning, a psychological rebirth. It breaks open our awareness, challenges us to transform our concepts of reality, and perhaps summons intense transpersonal experiences. If we cannot surrender and go gently, we may live a life of futile struggle like Chiron in the myth, forever trying to heal our wounds, and perhaps succumbing to serious illness or madness. The invitation for our inner journey may be presented via illness, crisis, chance encounters or other synchronous phenomena: Chiron follows us on our way, bringing opportunities for us to digest and process both the experience of our own suffering and also the expansion of consciousness that may accompany it.

Thus the astrological features surrounding Chiron in the horoscope represent our natural pathway of reconnection with the numinous dimensions of life, as well as an opportunity to re-embrace with compassion our own neglected suffering. Chiron may be heralding the dawn of a new kind of consciousness, as I have tried to describe above: one which is able both to embrace the dualism and pragmatism which is our Western heritage, and also to expand to a cosmology beyond it, including and permeating it. I would call it a 'biospiritual consciousness', neither exclusively material/psychological nor exclusively religious/spiritual, but both. Chironian consciousness does not seek to rise above or transcend human life, but rather to embrace it, acknowledging both divine immanence and also the reality of the unknowable beyond the forms which our senses perceive and our minds imagine.

Chiron's role in the transition from the Age of Pisces to the Age of Aquarius is discussed further in Chapter 6, and in Chapter 11 we will continue exploring how Chiron's themes have recently manifested themselves within the collective. Meanwhile, let us turn to a very important feature of the mythologem of Chiron which we have not so far addressed.

4 · The Feminine Journey

The Greek myths were formulated when many shrines and temples sacred to the various forms of the Great Goddess were being overrun and rededicated to Zeus and other Olympian gods. Hence, in many of these myths the female figures do not fare too well, and the story of Chiron is no exception. However, it does contain two particular archetypal patterns of the feminine which may be seen at work in the lives of women in whose horoscopes Chiron is prominent natally, or by transit. Toni Wolff, student and mistress of C. G. Jung, suggested there were four main 'types' within individual feminine psychology; each is represented by an archetypal pattern, but is also a 'basic instinctive and primary way of life'.[1] This model is useful for our purposes, although it should not be taken too rigidly and literally.

These four types consist of two pairs. The first pair is the Mother and the Hetaira. The Mother focuses on taking care of others, whether or not they need it. She may provide stability, security and instinctual wisdom, but may also devour, possess and destroy her children, unable to let them be individuals in their own right. The Hetaira, her opposite number, is mistress and erotic companion rather than wife and mother. With her scintillating charm and beauty she may inspire a man to fulfil his creativity; negatively, however, her flighty and deceptive qualities can seduce, flatter and hurt a man who expects commitment which she is unable to give. Toni Wolff goes on to observe that the second pair has become increasingly important in recent times:[2] the mediumistic type and the Amazon. Unlike the other two, neither centres herself around relationships with men; both are somewhat divorced from the instinctual side of life, which may create problems in relationships. These are the two which feature in the story of Chiron.

The mediumistic woman is permeated with the unconscious of others; she is sensitive to thoughts and feelings which lie beneath the surface, and may facilitate them into conscious expression, sometimes with disastrous results. She may appear rather formless, is often otherworldly and impractical, more focused on being than doing. She has a hysterical streak, often being drawn into complex and confusing emotional entanglements. With maturity, however, the mediumistic woman may show intuitive wisdom and visionary gifts, as well as the capacity for facilitating personal growth in others. Sometimes, it is when these gifts are denied that the mediumistic type will feel herself to be a helpless victim, especially of her own and others' emotions.

In contrast, the Amazon represents the principle of self-sufficiency. She fulfils herself by being independent and self-contained, and by striving to express her own talents and abilities. Her relationship to men may be one of rivalry, co-operation and challenge; dependence on a man is anathema to her. Practical activity and achievement in the world are important to her, and she is a personality in her own right, rather than taking her sense of identity from those whom she nurtures or to whom she relates. Her dark side, however, may be domineering, arrogant, castrating and unrelated.

The female characters in Chiron's story all show traces of the mediumistic type, but its shadow counterpart, the figure of the Amazon, is never far away. Chiron's wife Chariclo was a Naiad or fresh-water nymph who is barely mentioned in the story. Nymphs, as semi-divine nature spirits, were honoured with religious cults; although not immortal, having an approximate lifespan of a mere 9620 years,[3] they would occasionally visit Olympus. Originally, however, nymphs were not disembodied spirits, but women who served as priestesses in ancient temples of the goddess, especially in sexual ceremonies; they would heal and prophesy, perform oracles and sacred dances.[4] Their strong connection with sexuality is preserved in the word 'nymphomania'. By the time of the Greek myths, however, the nymphs had lost most of their original instinctual vitality and dignity, and were reduced to benevolent nature spirits whose functions were to prophesy, heal, act as oracles and watch over plants and livestock. Shades of their former nature can be seen in myths where nymphs occasionally become dangerous to mortal men whom they favoured: like the Sirens, or the Slavonic Rusalki, they could seduce and lure them to a watery death at the bottom of their domain.

Chariclo is not developed as a character, and so we may perhaps assume she conforms with this image of the nymph, which has obvious resonance with the mediumistic type. As a nature spirit, we do not know whether Chariclo remained to fulfil the ongoing role of wife, mother and helpmate. She and Chiron had no sons, but only one daughter known variously as Endeis, Thea, Thetis or, most commonly, Euippe. She displeased Chiron by prophesying that he would one day renounce his immortality. Euippe was a hunting-companion of the goddess Artemis, a seer and prophetess in her own right, and thus a challenge to her father's authority. Clement of Alexandria regards her as an important early natural scientist and astrologer.[5] Euippe became pregnant by one Aeolus,[6] and so feared the wrath of her father Chiron and her patron goddess Artemis, that she sought refuge with her uncle Poseidon (Neptune). When her daughter Melanippe was born, Euippe was changed into the constellation now called Pegasus after the famous flying horse. Melanippe had an adventurous career: she was seduced by Poseidon, had her name changed to Arne, was blinded by her jealous guardian Desmontes and walled up alive in a tomb. She gave birth to twins who were taken away and left exposed on a hillside to die, but like their grandfather Chiron, and in the time-honoured manner of myth and legend, were found and fostered by a shepherd. They eventually returned to free their mother, after Poseidon had divulged their divine parentage and restored her sight.

Elsewhere, however, we find an Amazon queen of disputed parentage, also named Melanippe; she is sometimes equated with Hippolyte, perhaps the most famous of the Amazons, who was accidentally killed by her sister Penthesilea, another Amazon queen – just as Chiron was wounded by Hercules. In another version, Hercules was said to have killed Melanippe as his sixth or ninth labour.[7] Chiron has a strong connection with the sixth and ninth signs of the zodiac, and Hercules met his own death at the hands of a Centaur. This network of interconnections between the Amazons, the Centaurs, and the gods of healing[8] is preserved for posterity at the site of the Greek temple of Epidaurus, the healing sanctuary of the god Asclepius, pupil of Chiron: the east pediment depicts warring Centaurs, while Amazons adorn the western one. Within its precincts is a shrine sacred to Artemis, the goddess to whom the Amazons paid allegiance.[9] Artemis killed the mother of Asclepius, whose father was Apollo; Asclepius, his son, was then fostered by Chiron, just as Apollo had fostered him.

The Amazons were closely associated with Artemis, who was also the patron goddess of Euippe; Artemis is usually considered to be the twin sister of Apollo, Chiron's foster-father. Amazon names often include the syllable 'ippe' or 'ippo', from the Greek word for horse, thus underlining their connection with horses: Euippe means 'goodly mare', and Melanippe 'black mare'. Their misfortunes, seductions and persecutions present them as 'victim' – a distortion of the mediumistic type, providing a sharp contrast with the figure of the Amazon who worshipped Artemis, and to whom horses were sacrificed by the Taurians.

The Greek imagination was fired by descriptions of wild women warriors dressed in animal skins, carrying shields shaped like half-moons. They used spears, bows and arrows; their insignia was the labyris or double-headed axe sacred to the moon-goddess. Although there is no existing representation of this in Greek art, the Amazons were said to burn or cut off their right breasts in order to be able to draw their bows more easily.[10] Significantly, they were also reputedly the first to tame and breed horses, which they rode in battle – a compelling image of the harnessing of instinctual energy. The Amazons excluded men from their settlements except during a yearly spring festival of love-making held in the dark of night, so that the fathers of any children conceived would remain unknown. Male children were supposedly crippled and kept in servitude. The figure of Artemis looms large behind their cult:

She whom Homer calls the 'cheerful archer' storms drunkenly about with her golden bow and deadly arrows, her whole appearance fiercely aglow. The peaks of lofty mountains tremble and gloomy forests crash with frightful sounds when the hunt rages; the earth and sea shiver; all about her swarm the fleet-footed nymphs, the howling hounds and the shrill cries of the chase.[11]

Artemis is fiercely virgin, unmarried and whole in herself. Although she presides over the loss of virginity, pregnancy and childbirth, the priestesses and young girls in her entourage were supposed to be physically chaste and forbidden to bear children themselves. Hence, Artemis is midwife rather than child-bearer, foster-mother to the process of becoming on all levels, the Mother of mothers. Her energy is active, powerful and trans-formative – the unrelenting fertility of nature unbound by con-vention, society or marriage. One of her most well-known animal representations is the Great She-bear, *Ursa Major*, ruler of stars and protectress of the *axis mundi*. According to Ptolemy, this constellation is of the nature of Mars,[12] echoing the psychological characteristics of the Amazon type.

Historically, the Amazon legends compensated for the actual situation of women in classical Greece, where they mostly lived under virtual house arrest, and were sold as slaves if considered unmarriageable.[13] Before birth-control, women were inescap-ably tied to the process of procreation, whether or not they were individually suited to motherhood. Now that there is choice in the matter, many women find themselves searching for a new feminine identity, for new forms through which to express their innate feminine natures in ways rooted in the depth of their instinctual beings. As René Malamud has said, '. . . we can understand the divine Amazon, Artemis, as a new leading-image in a woman's process of becoming conscious.'[14]

In our century, since the suffragettes, the archetypal figure of the Amazon may be seen empowering the women's liberation movement. Like any collective movement, however, its attitudes and beliefs may subsume the individuals within it. Here, the shadow side includes destructive aggression towards men and the masculine principle, hunger for power, obsession with self-sufficiency to the point of inability to relate, and thus eventually emotional and perhaps physical sterility. Positively, some of Artemis' epithets reflect the qualities she may bestow upon those who serve her: she is known as 'Lady of the Wild Things', 'She Who Strikes at a Distance', or 'Mistress of the Animals', these titles referring to her contained wildness, her ability to aim true, to enlist her instinctual energy into formulating and achieving ambitions.

The Amazon is the 'heroic feminine'. Just as male heroes must slay the dragon of their regressive desires to dwell unconsciously within the embrace of the Mother, so feminine heroines may need to come to terms with the attraction of incest with the spiritual Father if they are to progress into full womanhood. There exists a series of half-relief marble metopes from the Parthenon, now in the British Museum, depicting the fierce battles between the Amazons and the Heroes, which attest to this struggle. To make this transition, a woman may need to draw upon her Amazon qualities, rather than meekly taking her values and attitudes from her father and the men in her life, or relying on them to express vicariously her own masculine side. On the other hand, if a woman does not progress into loving relatedness to the masculine principle, both inner and outer, emotional and/or creative sterility may well be the result. As the Amazon type has a tendency to reject the feminine instincts lest they make her subservient to a man, her sexuality may remain dormant or become obsessive and power-driven; either way men are overtly or unconsciously seen as enemies to be conquered, exploited and dominated by sexual or other means.

Developmentally, the threshold of puberty and the blood initiation of the first menstruation herald the momentous event of biological fertility, and the meeting of the 'other'. However, this metaphor operates at all levels of feminine psychology where fertility and creativity are seeking expression. This transition, whether developmental and biological, or artistic and cultural, means leaving behind the retinue of Artemis, the wild untamed virgin and the circumscribed world of women, and submitting to the limitations imposed by fertility and relatedness to the masculine principle. The consequences of fertility on any level imply the responsibility of maturing, nurturing and taking our place in the world, which a woman still under the sway of Artemis will refuse. The Amazon is the shadow counterpart to the shy nymph, the ethereal and mediumistic 'father's daughter', who may be no less a devotee of the awesome Artemis, 'lion to men' and demander of blood sacrifice.

As we can see from the stories of Euippe and Melanippe, their transition into fertility was at best fraught with peril and at worst fatal. Euippe had creative spiritual gifts of her own, but when she became pregnant in violation of her allegiance to Artemis she suffered dire consequences: her encounter with the biological realm and motherhood turned her into a flying horse, and her daughter Melanippe fared little better. Euippe took refuge in the sea (with Poseidon), and Melanippe lost her sight and her name and suffered a period of imprisonment in a tomb. Both Chiron's parents were descendants of the Titans, the earthy offspring so despised and reviled by their father, the sky-god Uranus. Chiron's female descendants seem to lack this earthiness and indeed fall foul of the elements of water and earth, like their male ancestors. These images of the sea-womb, and isolation in an earthy tomb, speak of the primordial feminine, and suggest here a difficulty with the instinctual realm. One way or another, however, we must come to terms with it, if need be by means of a journey into the depths of the unconscious.

Let us explore what this might mean in terms of the individual feminine journey. In the horoscope, Chiron seems to represent where some *non-biological* expression of a woman's own uniqueness is seeking form. There are several ways in which this may be seen working out in life. A woman is often fatally, or rather fatedly, attracted to men who embody the qualities suggested by her Chiron. They may be 'Chironian' figures: gurus, mentors, teachers, wise men, or even wounded men. She may bear a child on to whom the qualities, gifts, wounds and possibilities suggested by her own Chiron placement will be projected, and these may or may not be congruent with the child's individual nature. These relationships are likely to be highly charged, often characterized by mutual wounding and disappointment. Should such a relationship break down, the emotional suffering which follows may initiate an important period of psychological growth. If the woman is eventually able to recognize her own Chiron qualities by regarding the situation symbolically, and by reflecting upon what might be the inner meaning of the relationship, she may be reborn into a new sense of independence and creativity. On a wider scale too, a woman may have the ability to foster, encourage and develop her own Chiron qualities in others; some women may spend much of their life invisibly doing this for others, and may need to learn quietly to value it without recognition. However, if a woman is fated to struggle to express her individuality in some form uniquely her own, a journey into her own inner depths is usually precipitated at some point in her life, often while Chiron is active by transit.

Chiron in the horoscopes of women also shows where and how their instinctual nature is wounded and/or wounding. The areas of sexual attraction and exchange, the ability to bear and nurture children and to promote relatedness between people may be affected. Such a woman may have a profound mistrust of life and hold herself away from it, taking refuge in masculine attitudes and aspirations. The archetypal pattern of the Amazon may take her over: aided and abetted by collective 'feminist' attitudes, she may ignore her own woundedness in relationships with men. Such a woman may have gifts of her own but be unable to enjoy them or allow them to bear fruit unless she has come to terms with the instinctual side of her nature and has a positive relationship with the masculine principle. On the other hand, preoccupation with mothering and relatedness to others can be overdeveloped to the point of stifling her intellect and other creative potentials within her which need the inner masculine in order to be expressed in life. A woman who lives only to serve the men in her life may fulfil part of her nature, but if her own creative spirit remains entirely outside herself and unclaimed, she may be unable to honour her own inner creative potential, and suffer pain in consequence.

Chiron's father Saturn castrated his own father Uranus, whose bleeding genitals were cast into the sea, which was thus fertilized; from this union was born Aphrodite, the goddess of sensual love – an important figure to whom we shall return. Saturn ended his days in Tartarus, the deepest region of the subterranean world, while Uranus' death is associated with the sea. Thus, in the creation sequence as described by Hesiod, the transition to the next stage of incarnation is made through the portals of water and earth. As we have seen, this motif is repeated in the fates of Chiron's descendants: his daughter took refuge and met her death in the sea, while his granddaughter suffered imprisonment in a cave.

I understand this to be alluding to the need for a woman's non-biological creativity to be rooted in feeling values and relatedness (water), and grounded in her body and instinctuality (earth). Without this, she risks being taken over by her masculine side, the animus, in the form of duty-bound conventionality, pseudo-spiritual aspirations, premature action and abstraction, which effectively cut her off from life and may eventually provoke reaction from her own outraged feminine instincts in the form of emotional and physical crisis. As a result of his early work with hysteria, Freud claimed that most symptoms had their origins in sexual issues. Although this theory is no longer fashionable, it is worth reflecting upon where Chiron is at work. Hysteria means 'wandering womb'; both Euippe and Melanippe would appear to have ambivalent attitudes to their physical fertility, as witnessed by the tragedies which befall them and result in their being enwombed within the elements.

For the woman whose instincts have been severely wounded early in life, it may not be possible to express and ground her instinctual nature through enacting the traditional roles of wife and mother; or, these roles may simply not suit her individual nature. Instead her rootedness may have to be developed inwardly, through consciously suffering the pain of these wounded areas. Instead of feeling cast out from the traditional world of feminine activity, she may then be reborn from the bitter womb of self-blame and envy into compassion for herself, and her own creativity may re-emerge at another level. Transits of Chiron frequently open up the possibility for this process to begin. Rebirth of an inner sense of fertility may follow a period of psychological re-enwombment; the winged horse of our creativy and intuition may be released into life, and we may rejoice in it rather than fearing it or projecting it on to others.

Chiron promotes the *both/and*, and seeks to heal the *either/or*; here the figure of Aphrodite (Venus) becomes important. As ruler of Taurus and Libra, she encompasses both the realm of ideas (artistic and cultural activities), and also that of the senses (the body and material resources). She was notoriously beautiful and desired by many men, but was made the reluctant wife of Hephaestus, a Chironian figure whom we shall meet again in the section on Chiron in Taurus. One of her consuming passions was for Ares, the god of war; unlike the Amazons, who worshipped Ares, Aphrodite's powerful sensuality makes her the appropriate counterpart to his warlike and Martian qualities. In contrast to wild Artemis, Aphrodite is cultivated and refined, but her delight in earthly sensuality and beauty also provides a feminine image of progressing beyond the unfortunate and somewhat disembodied images of Euippe, turned into a flying horse, and Melanippe, imprisoned in a tomb. The Chironian preoccupations of questing for consciousness and expressing something uniquely our own in a creative sense may become a destructive and isolating pressure for women who have a legacy of rejection of the instinctual life; this makes it difficult for new directions or creative ideas to take form in real life, and may also play havoc in relationships. However, when Chiron is strong by transit or in the natal chart, it may also bring reconnection with the body and the instincts. A healthy dose of pleasure and Venusian self-indulgence may provide enough grounding in positive life-experience to enable us to embrace the acceleration of the psychological growth and shift in perspective which frequently accompany these transmits. In the figure of Aphrodite, the disembodied nymph comes full circle, reconnected with her original sexual vitality and delighting in both the world of the senses and the world of the spirit.

PART TWO

THE INDIVIDUAL
JOURNEY

Chiron's themes – a word picture

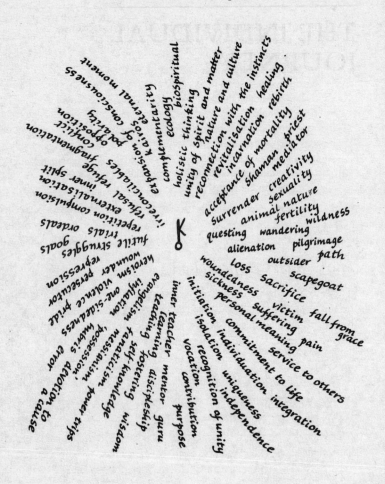

5 · Chironian Themes

I am not a mechanism, an assembly of various sections.
And it is not because the mechanism is working
    wrongly, that I am ill.
I am ill because of wounds to the soul, to the deep
    emotional self
and the wounds to the soul take a long, long time, only
    time can help
and patience, and a certain difficult repentance
long difficult repentance, realisations of life's mistake,
    and the freeing oneself
from the endless repetition of the mistake
which mankind at large has chosen to sanctify.

                    D. H. Lawrence, 'Healing'

The Chiron Configuration

In the forthcoming chapters on the meaning of Chiron within
the individual chart, I will use the phrase 'Chiron configuration'
for simplicity, to describe all the astrological factors connected
with the planet. The following ingredients comprise the Chiron
configuration:

i) The sign in which Chiron is placed

ii) The planet which rules the sign in which Chiron is placed
For example, if Chiron is in Aries, then it is likely that Mars will in
turn show Chironian themes. If Mars is already beset with
difficult aspects, these may be of a Chironian nature, and you may
want to refer to the section on Chiron in aspect to Mars.

iii) All planets or angles in aspect to Chiron

iv) The house in which Chiron is placed
All matters to do with this house will be affected by Chironian

themes, but different themes may apply to different levels of meaning within the house. On closer inspection, however, these apparently different manifestations will often resolve into a single theme.

For example, one client with Chiron in the 8th house was always in debt, and found having to borrow money humiliating and wounding (the 8th house concerns other people's resources on a mundane level). In the Scorpionic area of sexuality, however, this person experienced herself as very free, even to the point of promiscuity. When Pluto transited her Chiron in Scorpio, she realized that both these prominent areas of her life were connected with her anger against her mother: the debts were an expression of the feeling that someone else (mother) should be taking care of her, while her promiscuity reflected, on the one hand, a desire for physical closeness and substitute mothering and, on the other, an attempt to outdo her mother, whom she saw as sexually repressed.

As another example, a client with Chiron in Aries in the 6th house appeared to have plenty of will-power and initiative in work situations, but found she was terrified of learning to drive a car. In discussing this, she discovered that she was only able to show initiative *on behalf of someone else*; she longed to be able to have this quality for herself, and driving symbolized this for her.

v) The sign on the cusp of the house in which Chiron is placed, and the planet which rules it
For example, if Chiron is in the 6th house with a Capricornian cusp, then the condition surrounding that person's Saturn may also show Chironian themes.

vi) The planetary pairs drawn together by having Chiron at their midpoint
For example, even if the Moon and Mars are not in aspect, when Chiron is at the direct or indirect midpoint, they will be drawn together and will be likely to show Chironian themes. Likely manifestations of this would include: conflicts (Mars) with the mother or other female figures (Moon); a military attitude (Mars) to feeling vulnerability (Moon); emotional moodiness (Moon) interfering with the ability to take action (Mars).

★

Having explored in some detail the origins and archetypal background to the story of Chiron, we can now describe the major themes it represents within the lives of individuals, as reflected in their horoscopes. Obviously, not every theme mentioned here will manifest itself in any given life. However, should any of the following themes dominate an area of our own life, or that of a client, then behind this difficulty we are likely to find the archetypal pattern of the Wounded Healer. Knowing this may be helpful, as an in–depth look at the Chiron configuration might then enable us to intuit the underlying meaning of a life-pattern, a transpersonal experience, or a repeated cycle of suffering and illness.

Chiron's Position in the Solar System

Chiron is found between Saturn and Uranus; however, on its way to perihelion it crosses Saturn's orbit and spends some time between Jupiter and Saturn (see Appendix 1 for further detail). In mythology, the primordial sky-god Uranus was castrated by his son Cronus (Saturn). Cronus was subsequently informed by an oracle that one of his own sons in turn would overthrow him. Determined to prevent this, Cronus swallowed all his offspring as they appeared. As we saw in Chapter 2, it was while searching for his new baby Zeus that Cronus was first enamoured of Philyra, who became the mother of Chiron. Cronus never did find Zeus, who had been well hidden by Rhea, and was safely fostered by three nymphs, including the kindly goat-nymph Amaltheia. Zeus grew up to fulfil the prophecy and to overthrow his father with the assistance of Poseidon and Hades; he struck Cronus dead with a thunderbolt.

Thus Chiron was conceived during a period of time when his father Cronus was trying to pre-empt his fate as foretold by the oracle. Cronus was trying to 'stop the process', to avoid the inevitable, and was forcibly overthrown by those whom he had previously confined to Tartarus; he in turn was consigned to the nether regions of Tartarus. Chiron, however, of his own will surrendered his immortality; in psychological terms this 'death' is our rebirth into life. Chiron in the individual chart may indicate an inheritance that we are carrying forward from our parents, which is both a burden and an affliction (Saturn) but also the opportunity to incorporate its ingredients into our life in a new and creative way (Uranus). The theme of ancestral inheritance is especially strong when Chiron is in aspect to Saturn, as we will see in Chapter 8. This inheritance may be unconscious, consisting of unfulfilled hopes or dreams; it may also be a build-up of psychological pressure where for generations certain personal characteristics have been developed at the expense of others; this one-sidedness may seek release and rebalancing, and create a 'black sheep' or outsider in the family, positive or negative. Similarly, Chiron's house position often indicates a blockage of energy, a refusal to incarnate a 'no' to life in that area; however, it also opens up the possibility for a creative outcome to the suffering that results from this.

For example, one woman, with Chiron in Libra in the 2nd house opposite both Sun and Moon in Aries in the 8th house, was conceived during a time when her parents were in severe conflict, overtly about money (2nd house). Later on, her corresponding inner pattern became one of sabotage, interference and warfare between her masculine and feminine sides, and she was for a long time unable to achieve financial independence from her parents. Her obvious blockage was an inability or refusal to draw on her own resources (Chiron in the 2nd house). Whenever the Aries Sun would want to initiate something new, to take on a challenge, the Moon would respond by tearing it down with self-criticism and destructive emotionality. Hence, initially, both the solar and lunar principles were operating in a negative way. Congruent with Aries ruling the head, she was prone to migraine headaches. However, when Chiron opposed its natal place, she began studying martial arts, and eventually started teaching classes herself. This discipline gave her an opportunity to balance the warring aspects within herself, and to express them in a focused (Chiron/Aries Sun) and aesthetic way (Chiron in Libra), involving both her physical body (Chiron in the 2nd house, opposite Moon) and also balancing the currents of subtle energy within her (8th house). Teaching that promotes personal well-being and harmony between mind and body, is a typically Chironian profession.

Chiron symbolizes a unique combination of the potential creativity and vision of Uranus with the Saturnian respect for the past, personal limits and the laws of society and the material world. Further, there is the opportunity to bring it into our lives, to socialize this impulse in the Jupiterian realm. We do not need to betray our individuality by believing that we are blocked and frustrated by the negative Saturnian aspects of the collective, such as apathy, conformism and preoccupation with status and un-thinking conservatism. Nor do we need to be out on a limb, alienated from the rest of society by iconoclastic, anti-social and unrealistic Uranian ideals. With Chiron, we have the opportunity for a creative combination of both, which provides the possibility of meaning, release and expansion (Jupiter) in the process of being true to ourselves. Standing at the threshold, Chiron relates us on the one hand to the Saturnian world of form and structure, and on the other to the Uranian desire to break these established structures and release the energy potential held within them. Thus we are challenged to create new forms, inner and outer, expressive of this new order of being.

Several researchers, including Zane Stein who first suggested this principle, have found that the midpoint between Saturn and Uranus is a 'Chiron-sensitive' point on the chart. This means several things. First, should a planet or angle be found on that midpoint, it will behave as if it is aspected by Chiron. For example, someone with the MC at the midpoint of Saturn and Uranus was told by a clairvoyant that she should work as a healer; this happened on her first Chiron/Chiron square, at the age of fourteen. She spent the next twenty years or so, until her Chiron/Chiron opposition, struggling to come to terms with this issue, which initially she felt burdened by (Saturn) and rebellious towards (Uranus). Secondly, if a planet should transit that midpoint, especially by conjunction but also by any hard aspect, Chironian themes will be set in motion in the person's life. When Chiron itself activates that point by transit, the issues represented by Chiron in the horoscope often come to a head; however, in addition to the possible unleashing of destructiveness and suffering, there also appears to be a special opportunity for the healing of these issues. If someone has the midpoint configuration Chiron = Saturn/Uranus in the natal chart, the same applies and his or her life may be strongly coloured by typically Chironian themes.

In our times, Saturnian structures of all kinds are breaking down, and the reactionary Uranian individualism unleashed – most notably during the 1960s – is foundering on the rocks of isolation, meaninglessness and fragmentation. Chiron's discovery during this period of disorientation may offer us the possibility of a new synthesis which respects both. In psychological terms, Chiron stands at the doorway between the personal and transpersonal realms. He represents the interface between the confines of the ego and the structures of the known world and the vast force-field of archetypal and transpersonal energies that lie beyond, and indeed within, the world of form. Chiron's dimension and way of thinking is that of both/and, rather than either/or. If we are identified with the Saturnian principle, we may become rigid and fear to express our individuality. Any change of external situation or inner attitude may be felt to be a threat against which we must protect ourselves, and we may limit ourselves in this way. On the other hand, if the Uranian perspective is dominant in our lives, we may be subjected willy-nilly to change without being able to integrate it; we may compulsively embrace the future, new insights and new ideas, but at great cost to our feeling lives and human needs.

Between 1952 and 1989, Chiron made about forty-one exact oppositions to Uranus; it was within orb for almost the entire period, and strongly Uranian influences can indeed be seen at work within the collective. By contrast, Saturn has made only two exact conjunctions with Chiron over the last hundred years: April 1883 and April 1966. The Sabian Symbols for the degrees in which they occurred are interesting, as they form a sequence which has meaning in the light of Chiron's themes. The first was at 27° Taurus, for which the symbol is: 'An old Indian woman selling the artefacts of her tribe to passers-by.' Rudhyar's interpretation speaks of peaceful acceptance and reintegration of the individual into the psychic matrix of his group and culture:

'In old age, the power of the collectivity once more reasserts itself, overcoming the perhaps wearying effort man makes to assert his unique-ness and individual character.'[1]

The second conjunction was at 24° Pisces; the symbol is: 'On a small island surrounded by the vast expanse of the sea, people are seen living in close interaction.' In the interpretation Rudhyar emphasizes the 'need to consciously accept one's own personal limitations in order to concentrate one's energies and live a centred and fulfilled life'.[2] He goes on to point out that the ego is necessary to 'set boundaries and give a specific character to the consciousness', and although our duty is to be what we are as individuals, we also have 'a particular dharma or place and function within the vaster whole'.[3]

Let us consider the possible meaning of these two symbols with regard to the last two Chiron/Saturn conjunctions. In the first, we are not told whether the passers-by are Indians or American tourists, but the image of buying and selling (typically Taurean) symbolizes something changing hands. The old woman offers artefacts which symbolically contain her cultural and perhaps religious heritage. The wisdom of an indigenous culture which lived in closer harmony with nature (Taurus) is being offered; it is recognized as being of value and thus money is given in exchange.

The second symbol depicts an island upon which people live in close interaction, surrounded by a vast sea. Here the emphasis is on relatedness, both of man to man, and also of the community to the larger whole represented by the sea (Chiron/Saturn in Pisces). In order for this relatedness to develop, the instinctual and feminine wisdom represented by the old Indian woman of the previous symbol is necessary. In Rudhyar's interpretations, we see the development of a both/and perspective which is typical of Chiron: in the first, separate individuality is peacefully relin-quished, while in the second the need for both individuality and relatedness to the larger whole is acknowledged.

Juxtaposing the two Chiron/Saturn conjunctions with the many Chiron/Uranus oppositions, we see that Chiron has sym-bolically pierced the Saturnian principle by crossing its orbit, in order for the feminine and instinctual earthy energy to be absorbed. Chiron also balances the unworkable nature of a one-sidedly Uranian attitude to life.

Individuation, Immortality and the Inner Teacher

We can describe the term 'individuation' as meaning the *unfolding* of who we innately are, just as a kitten will grow up to become a cat, and not a dog or a kangaroo. No single astrological factor signifies this process, but rather the entire horoscope is as a reflection of who we are, a mirror of the psyche in both its conscious and unconscious aspects. However, the urge to individuate takes on particular urgency for those factors affected by Chiron. There the arrow of the Centaur infuses us with an intensity which often means great suffering, but also indicates the possibility of creating something individual and uniquely our own, based on acceptance of our true inner nature and our relationship with this mysterious self which both contains and is greater than all our multiple facets, positive and negative.

This pressure towards inner self-discovery and its outer expression provides gifts and opportunities, but also has its pitfalls. For as we shall see, wherever Chiron is found there is a tendency to *externalize* things which perhaps need to be taken inwardly and symbolically, and there is a relentless struggle to achieve, which may actually be an enactment of an attempt to heal ourselves, to 'get' something which we misguidedly imagine will assuage our pain. The balance of inner/outer or literal/symbolic is ultimately particular to each person's unique destiny; however, if we notice that our own Chiron configuration seems repeatedly to be expressing itself in illness or catastrophe, it may be worth considering whether this principle is at work, and whether there is something which needs to be internalized or de-literalized, taken symbolically rather than acted upon. Social, professional or political preoccupations may contain a strong element of this: struggling to resolve and to heal collective issues may be a vicarious attempt to heal our inner suffering.

The Chiron configuration describes the person's 'path', as expressed by the Arabic word *tariqa*. In traditional Sufism, a group of disciples collects around a teacher who embodies certain qualities representing the particular *tariqa* or 'path to the divine' which they will follow, through his instruction and example. For some, a relationship with God is sought through music, for others through philosophy, for yet others through action, and so on. If an individual is devoted to a particular guru or spiritual tradition, often the individual projects onto the teacher or group the qualities described by his or her Chiron configuration, which will in turn describe the kinds of experience he or she has in this connection. An example that is not specifically religious will illustrate this: a man who had Chiron in Scorpio, squaring Saturn and Pluto in Leo was a member of an underground political movement in Africa which demanded secrecy (Pluto) and strict discipline (Saturn), and whose members participated in dangerous guerrilla activities. Although he was a professed atheist, his *tariqa* or path is obviously Plutonian: his total allegiance to the revolution aiming to precipitate the rebirth of his country included the possibility of experiencing violence or even losing his own life.

In psychological terms, Chiron is the *Inner Teacher* to whom we owe our allegiance. The cluster of astrological ingredients surrounding it may symbolize the tests, tasks, disciplines and ordeals which unfold under the tutelage of this Inner Teacher, whose path or *tariqa* is life itself, whether or not this includes following a particular spiritual tradition. Major crises or learning–experiences can be reflected by any factor within the horoscope, but they are likely to be *interpreted and processed* in a manner congruent with the Chiron configuration: Chiron describes the nature of what we learn from our life-experiences. For example, those with Chiron in Sagittarius may experience many twists and turns on their search for the meaning of life. Their enthusiasms, 'trips' and disappointments may irritate both themselves and others, but search they must. After 'failing' to find enduring meaning in anything external, all the questing and questioning may yield the thought that perhaps there is no ultimate final meaning to be sought, as meaning is a subjective quality infused into an experience, not something intrinsic to it that has to be hunted down and 'got'. However, wisdom and understanding may have thus been gained, of benefit to themselves and others. As another example, those with Chiron in Scorpio often interpret experience in terms of life-and-death struggles, where one wins and the other dies, one is all good and the other is positively evil. They may spend much energy trying to disprove their conviction that life is out to get them, or that they are too destructive to be safe around the things that matter to them. With a Plutonian Inner Teacher, so to speak, such a person will surely confront the reality of death as well as the mysteries of transformation, negativity and destructiveness, neither disowning it in his or herself nor feeling responsible for it in others, thus developing an acceptance of death in life and life in death. If we are unable or unwilling to listen to this Inner Teacher, he or she may creep up from behind. We may then become someone who is compelled to give unsolicited advice; we may be unable to listen without feeling compelled to 'fix things', suggest psychological techniques, healers to see, and so on! This is a 'blocked Chiron', like Cronus trying to prevent his fate.

With regard to the question of immortality, we have seen that following Chiron's death in the Underworld he was immortalized in the constellation Centaurus, or, in other versions, Sagittarius. People frequently develop preoccupations or obsessions that are graphically described by their Chiron position: they want to *do* something or *become* something which will make them wise, rich, famous, well-respected, loved by everyone – make them immortal, in other words. Searching through the horoscopes of well-known people reveals how often Chiron describes with sometimes amusing accuracy the very thing for which the person was famous or infamous, renowned or feared. There are many examples of this in the following chapters, but let us look at a few here.

Rudolph Valentino has Chiron conjunct Moon in Libra, both in the 7th house; it is sesquiquadrate Mercury in Taurus in the 2nd house, trine Pluto in Gemini in the 3rd house and square Jupiter conjunct Mars in Cancer in the 4th house. He was hailed as 'the greatest lover (Chiron in Libra) of the silent screen'. Chiron aspects Mercury, and also Pluto in Gemini, here representing power through silence. His sexuality (Chiron/Pluto) was both refined and exotic (Chiron in Libra, Venus-ruled); it provoked hysteria in women (Chiron/Moon in the 7th – *others* went hysterical!), and he was idolized also after his death, becoming a kind of cult figure typical of Chiron/Jupiter.

Alfred Hitchcock has Chiron conjunct Uranus in Sagittarius, square Mercury in Virgo. He is famous for cold-blooded (Chiron/Uranus) thrillers, often with frightening and twisted mental dimensions (Chiron square Mercury); his plots are clever and calculating (Chiron/Mercury in Virgo); he is a master of suspense, able to conjure up (Chiron/Mercury as the Trickster) intense fear in his audience by hinting at violent possibilities (Chiron in Sagittarius often focuses on negative possibilities).

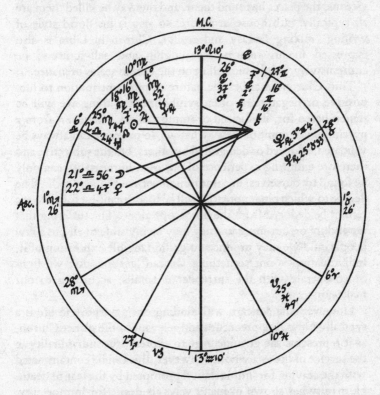

D. H. Lawrence

D. H. Lawrence has Chiron in the 8th house in Gemini, and we shall explore his horoscope further in Chapters 7 and 8. He has. been called the 'prophet of sexual liberation', although his books were initially censored and even burned. He was able to articulate (Gemini) a sense of the sacredness of sexual communion (8th house) in both its personal and transpersonal dimensions (Chiron in Gemini).

Dennis Nilsen has Chiron in Libra in the 12th house; he murdered fifteen people, usually by strangulation, and dismembered their bodies. All but one were not missed by anyone, as they were often lonely rootless people picked up in bars; Nilsen's biography is called *Killing for Company* (Chiron in Libra). His victims, the places he found them, and the way he killed them are all typically 12th house in nature; so also is his florid style of writing, mixing fantasy and reality. Chiron in Libra is also expressed in his remorseless judging and self-scrutiny; he compulsively weighs himself upon the Libran scales of justice.

Thus Chiron describes the nature of our contribution to life, positive or negative; it often symbolizes the thing we will be remembered for, heroicized or immortalized. However, from a psychological point of view, what we do or create can always be validated, admired or denigrated by others, but the subjective and therefore enduring experience of our own immortality can only be found by ourselves, in communion with our inner depths. The degree to which inner potential will be made manifest for all to see cannot be deduced from the horoscope alone. The suffering that we endure on our inner journey may be invisible to all but a few people, and we may produce no grand tangible expression of it. Individuation is not something we can 'get' or 'do'; we fight or co-operate with the surrender it entails, according to our make-up.

However, the concern with finding one's purpose in life is a typically New Age preoccupation relevant to the planet Chiron, as it represents the genuine urge to express true individuality in the service of life as a whole. However, this can be contaminated with the craving for 'immortality' prompted by the fear of death. Humanity has shown in many ways its desire for immortality; the hero cult mentioned in Chapter 3 is an example. The procreation of children to carry our name, the building of large tombs and mausoleums, the creation of works of art that live on after our death all testify to the difficulty we feel in accepting the finality of physical death. However, all this is also an expression of the Promethean creative impulse, the urge to find *within oneself* that invisible spark of divinity, that void, that immortal soul which persists and which is not bound by the laws of linear time and physical decay.

In this context, then, Chiron often describes a concretization of a quality of being or a transformation of consciousness which is trying to develop and be born for the sake of our wholeness; it may be inappropriately or compulsively translated into something that must be done, achieved or pursued. Hence the theme of the quest, which is so important to Chiron. The goal of the quest is the self, which is not to be found in other places or with other people, although they may provide a reflection; it is not in books, nor can it be achieved, bought, borrowed or stolen. Yet, when we have learned how to listen to the Inner Teacher, any experience can be enriching and is part of the journey which is our life, which we cannot but travel, even in death.

> We shall not cease from exploration
> And the end of all our exploring
> Will be to arrive where we started
> And to know the place for the first time.[4]

The Healer, the Wounded One and the Wounder

The image of the Wounded Healer is an evocative one which can easily be associated with the Chiron configuration in the horoscope. However, there is a further ingredient to consider if this image is truly to represent what we find when we observe how Chiron's themes are expressed in real life. Jung points out 'the mythological truth that the wounded wounder is the agent of healing, and that the sufferer takes away suffering'.[5] Adding the 'one who wounds' to the image often makes sense of otherwise puzzling manifestations of Chiron. For example, we see Chiron closely conjunct the Ascendant in the 12th house in the horoscope of

Dennis Nilsen. In his case, the figure of the wounder, the murderer, is the most obvious one, but his biography also reveals in poignant detail his own woundedness and increasing identification with the 'one who suffers', both in the specific sense of identifying with his dead victims, and also as a role within the collective. During his trial he wrote, 'I want others to see that I suffer. I do not like suffering, but it seems now to be expected of me.'[6]

This threesome of figures – the Healer, the Wounded One and the Wounder – is also clearly depicted in the myth, as Chiron is wounded firstly by his mother, and secondly by his pupil Hercules. As new-born babies, we are literally wounded as blood is drawn to cut the umbilical cord; and later stages of psychological separation from the mother may in different ways be as painful. We can often look back on events initially experienced as wounding and see that we matured in understanding through them. When Chiron decides to renounce his immortality and chooses death, he makes a heroic decision which takes him into the realm of the Death Goddess. In this act, he symbolically embraces the two agents of his own wounding, consciously taking them into his life. On a psychological level, when we are aware of *that within us* which wounds both ourselves and others and have fully accepted it as a part of our make-up, it may sometimes unexpectedly come to our aid. As long as we are trying to get rid of it, the 'one who wounds' is likely to rebound on us and those closest to us.

Chiron in the horoscope describes the nature of wounds that we have received in the very early stages of our life, and of major influences upon us during these formative years. For example, when Chiron is in aspect to Jupiter, it usually indicates that the religious influences within the person's early life are not mere background music, but may embody strong conflicts and issues which clamour for resolution, and are often suffused with psychological ingredients belonging to the wounded parent–child relationship. One woman, who had Jupiter conjunct the Moon in Sagittarius, square Chiron in Pisces in the 2nd house, had great difficulty separating herself from her close relationship with her mother (Chiron/Moon). The mother had strong spiritual longings which she had not honoured for herself. She introduced her daughter in childhood to Eastern religion, and encouraged her in this direction. Later, the daughter rebelled by rejecting everything to do with spirituality. However, at her first Chiron/Chiron square, she became ill and realized that she had to find another way of embracing this inheritance of spiritual longing (Chiron in Pisces) and philosophical confusion (Chiron square Jupiter in Sagittarius).

The Chiron configuration often describes what connects an individual with his or her inner suffering, and also a route through this to healing. For example, those with Chiron in Gemini or the 3rd house, or a Chiron/Mercury aspect, can find words, both written and spoken, very healing; kind words may quickly open them up to tears and vulnerability. Equally, in childhood, they may have been repeatedly wounded by hostile and angry words, such as destructive criticism or arguments with brothers and sisters. Those with Chiron in Taurus or the 2nd house often respond very well to massage or bodywork, while those with Chiron in aspect to Venus experience both wounding and healing through relationships with others.

By the same token, the Chiron configuration also describes the nature of the healing that people may have to offer to others. This applies whether or not they work professionally in the field of healing, as it is a natural quality, an emanation rather than a learned technique. For example, those with Chiron in Cancer have a strong capacity for quiet empathy. The person with Chiron in Virgo may excel at simple practical gestures which show great kindness: for example, he or she may arrive with a bag of groceries when a friend is ill, rather than sending a get-well card. A woman with Chiron aspecting Saturn in the 10th house felt wounded by the strict and repressive attitudes in her early environment, especially those expressed by her mother. She left home very young, rebelling and rejecting society to the point of getting arrested for shop-lifting. She felt wounded by the Saturnian principle, and then sought to wound it in turn. At her Chiron opposition, she began working with juvenile probationers in a day centre and, from what she told me, her approach to them was typically Saturnian in a positive way. She spoke of the need to set limits, to be direct, and so to provide appropriate boundaries for the young people in her care. Having once been wounded by the Saturnian principle, she had become able to enlist these qualities in the service of healing.

As Chiron also symbolizes the Inner Wounder, it may show how we inadvertently inflict pain on others or carry suppressed aggression towards them. A man with Chiron in the 1st house realized that he demonstrated passive aggression towards others, never asserting himself; he would wait for others to take the initiative so that he could then fight them! A woman with Chiron in Gemini in the 8th house realized she spoiled her relationships by thinking negative thoughts which she neither expressed nor admitted; a negative emotional atmosphere would build up and make her unreachable. As a final example, let us consider Dennis Nilsen's horoscope. With his Chiron in Libra in the 12th house he longed for total union of experience with another to the point of extinguishing separate personalities – a typically 12th house fantasy which he literally achieved. At his trial were witnesses who had survived the attempts made on their lives. They described him as initially charming and companionable (Chiron in Libra), even consoling them in their distress after the failed murder attempt.

Repetition and Futile Struggles

Areas of the psyche indicated by the Chiron configuration may be very vulnerable, as they show where we are wounded, even though these wounds may be unconscious. Later a sequence of synchronous inner and/or outer events and emotions may occur, which actually represents a replay of an earlier wounding situation, the repetition compulsion as described in Chapter 2. Just as Chiron shows where we are already wounded, so it also shows where we may attract further wounding situations; however, this can also be like the 'sword which heals the wound it inflicted', whereby what we dread and fear may also be the very thing through which healing comes our way.

For example, someone with Chiron in Virgo in the 11th house had a horror of being in groups of people: workshops, study groups, and eventually even social groups became increasingly frightening and distasteful to her. She would either withdraw or fall into the role of the outsider, the one who always said: 'But what about . . .' Because of her innate need to challenge authority (Chiron in the 11th house) she would compulsively do so in groups, despite her vulnerability and fear, and then end up feeling unaccepted and unacceptable. During a period of therapy, it became obvious that she felt the same with her family: unseen and unacceptable in her deepest self, but having to conform with rather negatively Virgoan family values of emotional control and proper 'standards'. She rebelled in the same way, and got the same response. This pattern recapitulated every time she became involved in groups of people, especially those with a common intent. Eventually, a memory of a 'past-life experience' emerged of meeting death at the hands of an angry mob. Distressing though this was to encounter, it contributed to her gradually releasing the fear. It connected her with the deep anger she felt at her role in her family and also with her need to feel accepted, and gradually the repetition stopped. As transiting Chiron reached the waning square to her natal Chiron, she began training to work with groups of people, teaching craft skills (Chiron in Virgo) as rehabilitation for people in hospital.

Another pattern we can observe at work in connection with the Chiron configuration is a cycle of apparently futile struggle and failure, where we can neither succeed nor give up. Sisyphus, who was a remote descendant of Chiron, was foolish enough to imprison Hades above the ground, so that nobody could die until Ares intervened and delivered him in turn to Hades. His hubris was curbed by another famous eternal punishment. He had to roll an enormous stone up a hill. However, when he reached the top it would roll down, and he would have to start all over again at the bottom, pushing upwards. As a descendant of Chiron, Sisyphus perhaps is an image of the result of an accumulated refusal to face mortality and death: the conviction that life is a round of meaningless struggle in which nothing can be achieved and nothing goes anywhere and all effort bears no fruit. Sometimes the apparently futile struggles which we endure in connection with our Chiron configuration are a way of protecting something that is actually already dead, existing only in an empty form, a cherished dream or pet nightmare. Perhaps an ideal, a belief or an ambition has outlived its relevance, a relationship or career may have gone full cycle and died. If we are unable to let go and mourn, other areas of our life may seem to 'die' on us.

The Chiron configuration often describes a cluster of events, patterns and circumstances which repeat *ad nauseam*, in spite of our efforts to change things. It is those things which do not go away, and which cannot be worked through in the sense of being sorted out and left behind. They can, however, be worked *with* and once truly accepted with compassion they can sometimes be healed. Like old war wounds, however, they may still hurt from time to time: Jung has said that we cannot cure complexes, but we can outgrow them. Attempts to cut loose from our pain using strong-arm techniques to deal with the limitations that it creates will activate this unceasing struggle. Like Chiron in the myth, the Chiron configuration shows where we may try unsuccessfully to make something better, and may eventually be forced to give up.

Anything in our lives can be a 'symptom'; for example, the ancient Greeks regarded poverty as a curable disease, a legitimate illness that could be taken to the temple of Asclepius for healing. One client with Chiron in the 1st house square Saturn conjunct the Moon in the 4th house could not keep control of her domestic situation; she had five children, and her house was always messy and untidy, causing a great deal of irritation, frustration, guilt and lost energy. She struggled for years to regain control over it, and when she finally admitted that she found it overwhelming, she realized that what she needed was to pay someone to help her! She had enough money to do this, but never thought of it: her stubborn independence (Chiron in the 1st) blocked her from acknowledging that she could not cope alone. Saturn conjunct the Moon, both aspecting Chiron, here suggests denial of her own needs, and also represents burdensome 'shoulds' inherited from her original family, making her feel that it was her duty to manage her family efficiently and single-handedly, and that anything less would be failure. Once she could admit this 'failure', the obvious solution presented itself. Moreover, she realized that the true source of her frustration was actually her anger at these unnecessarily self-repressive *inner* attitudes, which kept her duty-bound in an unfulfilling way. Her guilt was really about spending so much time trying to keep control of the home environment that she did not have enough time and energy left to spend creatively with her children.

It remains an open question as to whether these struggles are really futile, however, as this depends on how we define our goals in life. The life-and-death struggle of birth is preceded by a period of intense pressure and increasing confinement: the experience of a 'no exit' situation. Later in life, the birth of new awareness is often preceded by intense struggles, inner and/or outer. As onlookers, we do not know whether another's struggles are in fact futile, because we cannot know what purpose the self or Inner Teacher of that person has in mind, or what is trying to be born in its own time.

Do Unto Others

Often Chiron symbolizes things we can do for others, but which we cannot do for ourselves. The mythological parallel for this is clear, as Chiron could not heal his own wounds in spite of being able to heal others; he was initially unable to benefit himself from what he offered others. For example, sometimes individuals with Chiron in aspect to Mercury can bring order and clarity into any situation except their own lives or their own thought-processes; they may be considered as intelligent and original in their thinking by everyone except themselves. Those with Chiron in the 1st house often feel they lack personal will-power, not realizing how strong they appear to others. A woman with Chiron conjunct Venus had always felt she was ugly, although admired by others for her beauty.

We often find these strange discrepancies and blind spots where Chiron is. Sometimes they conceal a form of false omnipotence, as we try to 'do out there' to others the healing which we need within ourselves, but cannot make the necessary inner surrender to receive. On the other hand, these imbalances and eccentricities present opportunities for creative and conscious choices made with full awareness of one's own unhealable wound. For example, a woman who had Chiron opposite the Moon was unable to conceive a child, which caused her much anguish. She and her husband decided to accept this rather than try various medical treatments suggested by her doctor, such as fertility drugs. They eventually decided to foster children taken into care from broken homes, and were able to give compassionate parenting to many children. This example recalls the Chironian theme of fostering qualities in others and nurturing their growth: Chiron was the foster-child of Apollo and was in turn foster-father to many Greek heroes.

Shadow and Polarity

In psychological terms the shadow represents what lies 'behind' or 'underneath' our conscious awareness, often in opposition to our usual mode of behaviour or self-concept. It may be positive or negative in quality, and usually contains ingredients from the past such as unresolved parental issues. However, it can also contain potentials that have remained undeveloped and are not present in our life. Because the shadow initially represents a threat to the ego or our current knowledge and experience of ourselves, its appearance is often accompanied by fear, anger and an attempt to eliminate it from our life. The shadow, initially an unknown quantity, will often be projected on to others, and is revealed by a strong emotional 'charge' or uncontrollable reaction to a certain person, belief system or racial group. There is no single astrological factor which represents the shadow; any part of the horoscope may represent qualities that are repressed or unconscious, and therefore apparently absent.

Where Chiron is involved, as we have seen above, there is a group of three figures – the Healer, the Wounded One and the Wounder. In an individual life, one of these will usually be more obvious than the other two, which will be unconscious or part of the shadow. Often, the figure of the Healer is the more developed. This figure of course not only represents someone who works in the healing professions or who enjoys being of service to others. Chiron in the myth was also a wise man, a kindly mentor and guide – and an eminently civilized one at that. Through the process of education and becoming socialized, we are usually encouraged to develop these qualities; our deep pain and our capacity for wounding are likely to get left behind and remain buried – although there are exceptions to this, as we shall see. In order to contain and survive our pain, we may develop our 'top half' at the expense of our 'bottom half' – to use Chiron's image in which his top half was a wise healer, and his bottom half a wounded animal. We may become urbane, sophisticated and well-groomed, or idealistic and full of noble aspirations, and yet ignore the wounded animal on which we stand, until an illness or crisis forces us to take our pain into account.

In some horoscopes, Chiron represents the figure of the Wounded One. Those for whom this is the case identify with the wounded, undeveloped and outcast aspects of their psyche, or are born with unfortunate mental or physical abormalities. Some may be outsiders, victims or scapegoats who spend much of their life in institutions or hospitals. In an ancient custom, which still survives in psychological terms, societies would rid themselves of evil by projecting it on to a scapegoat – an animal, or even a person, which was then either ritually killed or banished into the wilderness to fend for itself. Horses were used in this way in northern India and possibly elsewhere, and this provides an anthropological association with Chiron.

Sometimes the 'one who wounds' will be dominant, and the person may spend much energy suppressing this or, tragically, acting it out. In the horoscopes of Hitler, and mass murderers Dennis Nilsen and Jim Jones we can see this side expressed; we shall refer to these horoscopes again in subsequent chapters. It is seldom possible from the horoscope alone to determine which of these three faces of Chiron will be dominant, especially as the balance may shift over time. For example, Jim Jones began his career as a saviour/healer, and ended it as both killer and victim. Those who commit atrocities and are punished become scapegoats for the collective; we read about the horror in the newspaper, relieved that evil has been brought to justice, feeling confirmed in our on purity.

From a psychological point of view, Chiron embodies an image which suggests an urgent need for reconciliation and healing of deep splits within us. When considering Chiron by sign and house within the horoscope, it is useful to include the opposite sign and house. This may be especially revealing where the wise, civilized and educated qualities of Chiron appear to be more developed, or where Chiron appears to be a 'dumb note' in the horoscope. In such a case, we may take refuge from our pain in activities described by the opposite sign or house. Sadly, we may also forgo the creative possibilities of the Chiron placement by doing this. Sometimes, in order to gather enough personal stability and strength to face our deepest pain, we need to hide for a while. However, if our refuge should become an entrenched position, it will not usually bring continuing growth; instead we may suffer subtle feelings of guilt, of having cheated ourselves or of being somehow phoney.

Some examples will clarify this. A woman had Chiron in the 4th house in Libra, which suggests wounds received within the context of family relationships, perhaps especially with her father. She decided she did not want a family herself, and put all her energy into her career (10th house). Although she achieved a high managerial position in the competitive world of commerce, as transiting Chiron approached the waxing square to its own place, she realized how unfulfilled she really felt, and that a great deal of the emotional energy which took her to the top of her profession was actually fuelled by unexpressed anger towards her father. She decided to change direction and train instead in personnel work – which suited her Chiron-in-Libra placement very well – relating to people in a more equal and caring way, rather than competing in the 10th house/Aries sense, which here expresses the shadow side of Chiron in Libra. She also took classes in pattern-cutting and dress-making; this was something she had always wanted to do, and making clothes which were beautiful and also original fulfilled the artistic side of Chiron in Libra.

Those with Chiron in the 1st house may flee into relationships, forming their sense of identity and values around other people. First-house activities such as taking initiative may open up their deepest pain, where they are confronted with extremes of either wilfulness or lack of will. Another example can be seen in the life of a woman who had Chiron conjunct the Sun in Scorpio in the 5th house, a placement which suggests a possible wound in the area of sexual self-expression. When transiting Pluto was conjuncting this combination, she joined a New Age group (11th house) focused around personal growth, and, although married, decided to become celibate. She recognized that she was avoiding a confrontation with the difficulties in her marriage, but also hoped that, with the support and personal growth that she was experiencing in the group, she would in time find enough strength to do so.

Possession and Inflation

In traditional shamanism, across many different cultures, the phenomenon of possession was often central to the shaman's sickness and initiation, and later an intrinsic part of his skills in shamanic healing and divination. In ancient-Greek times, symptoms were considered to be the touch of a god or goddess; in order for healing to occur, it was necessary to discover and encounter the deity which lay behind the symptom, and then to perform the appropriate sacrifices and oblations, setting up an altar in honour of the god or goddess, or perhaps dedicating oneself to his or her service. This is not the same as an exorcism, where we attempt to get rid of something, but rather describes the creation of a *relationship* with an archetypal energy that impinges strongly on our lives, and which may cause sickness or disaster if unacknowledged or allowed to take control.

When we look at Chiron in the natal horoscope, we often see a curious phenomenon which is symbolized by these ancient images and principles. Sometimes, a planet in aspect to Chiron will appear dominant in the life of an individual, whether or not that planet is in emphasis owing to other factors. The nature of the aspect seems less important here than the closeness of the orb. Given that Chiron represents where we are wounded, where the membrane that separates us from the collective unconscious and the realm of the archetypes is very thin, or is damaged, it is here that the most potent archetypal levels of the other planet pour through into our personal lives, often in a one-sided and inflated way until we have embraced our own woundedness.

For example, Marilyn Monroe had Chiron conjunct the MC, both in Taurus and also conjunct Venus in Aries in the 9th house; this is the only personal planet aspected by Chiron, the others being a trine to Neptune in Leo in the 1st house and a quintile to Pluto in Cancer in the 11th house. Monroe became virtually subsumed by the larger-than-life Venusian stereotype developed around her by the film industry (Chiron/Neptune), which served to mask her inner pain. She portrayed for the world (Chiron/MC) the beautiful goddess (Chiron in the 9th) of love (Chiron/Venus), but suffered great unhappiness in her personal relationships; there has even been speculation that she was murdered because of her sexual involvement with key political figures (Chiron/Pluto). She spent much of her childhood in orphanages, suffering continually fragmented relationships (Chiron/Venus); later she was mercilessly exploited by the studios who built her image – another Chiron/Venus hazard. In 1987, when transiting Chiron was posthumously conjunct Marilyn's Gemini Sun, Gloria Steinem, author of a recent biography, announced that proceeds from the book would go towards the creation of a fund to help 'profoundly damaged children'. This is a poignant counterpart to the archetypal image of the celluloid Goddess of Love, which indeed concealed the wounded child beneath, now finally being seen with compassion by the public.

So the individual may be driven or seem 'possessed' by a larger-than-life version of the planet which is in aspect to Chiron. Often he or she is not aware that these qualities are obvious to others. The well-known Nazi-hunter Simon Wiesenthal has Chiron in the 5th house in Aquarius, square Mars in Scorpio in the 2nd and trine Pluto in Gemini in the 9th. Wiesenthal has become an agent of collective retribution and vengeance (Chiron/Mars/Pluto); although his personal anger and pain cannot but provide motivation for his actions (Chiron/Mars), he describes feeling personally detached from his role (Chiron in Aquarius), pointing out that, if it were not so, he would long ago have been destroyed by the intensity of negative emotion.

By the same token, Chiron in the horoscope may show where we harbour hidden or overt inflations – our extremes, grandiosities or unconscious identification with mythic figures. We may tenaciously cling to these, for they often conceal the pain of our deepest wounds. Transits involving the Chiron configuration sometimes bring the experience of a crash from this spurious inviolability into the humbling experience of human frailty and dependence.

For example, a woman with Chiron conjunct the Moon in Scorpio in the 4th house believed that she once had a great deal of power and charisma in a previous incarnation (Chiron in the 4th), both overtly within society (echoes of the 10th house) and also by way of personal influence, having been the centre of a circle of influential people (Chiron/Moon in the 4th). In her present life, however, she was trapped in work which she hated, with neither power nor influence, and was very angry about it. Here Chiron in Scorpio indicated the sense of having fallen from grace, from power to powerlessness. On the day of her chart-reading, transiting Mercury was exactly opposite her natal Chiron. She was very upset, and expressed for the first time this conviction about her past life; she said that she couldn't understand the discrepancy between her former position of power and her current situation, although she feared that she may also have done something terrible and was now being punished: this is a belief frequently expressed by those with Chiron in Scorpio. The energy invested in this repressed image (Chiron in the 4th) prevented her from facing her present situation and proceeding creatively; it was easier to hold on to the fantasy of her former glory. Having voiced this fantasy, she soon began to feel the vulnerability and anger from her early relationship with her mother, whom she described as a powerful and emotionally manipulative woman – a negative version of the figure whom she believed she had been in a past life. The past-life fantasy was shielding her from the impact of these painful feelings. Although this does not mean that there was no truth in her belief, her exclusively literal interpretation had frozen much energy; allowing the symbolic aspect of the fantasy gave room for her personal feelings to emerge.

Incarnation and Reincarnation

Several researchers have suggested that Chiron may have something to do with the process of incarnation and reincarnation. Although there are many differing views as to what this means, I would like briefly to explore this theme with a working model which I hope will be of use to the astrologer working with clients in a psychological context. There is a mythological parallel in considering this theme: the ghandarvas, the Vedic equivalent of the Centaurs, are said to represent that part of the individual soul which continues on its journey through different incarnations.

A view commonly held is that the soul either chooses or is drawn to its parents at the moment of conception, having spent time on other levels preparing for another incarnation. The soul brings its karma: fragments of personal experience which relate to other times and places, and which may include karmic debts to be paid; it also brings gifts and wisdom gained during these other lives. This concept implies the idea of linear time, and the continuance of the same individual soul through it. There is another view of reincarnation, however, in which time is considered as non-linear. In this model all moments of time are eternally present, and there is no continuity of the individual soul through it. There is rather a universe eternally unfolding with our temporary participation; individuality does not continue, but melts back into the totality which continually recoagulates, forming new 'individuals'. At the deeper levels of the psyche, we all join with the timeless accumulation of human experience, the collective unconscious, and we are all 'Everyman' on his journey.[7]

Transits of Chiron frequently bring to light dreams, thoughts and fantasies about past lives. From a psychological point of view, it is useful to consider 'past-life' material as symbolic, regardless of which model makes more sense to us personally, or to a client who may have brought the material. This approach does not deny or take issue with the metaphysics involved, but rather provides the opportunity to understand and integrate the meaning of the experience. Whatever is brought from other planes of existence will often be fragments of unresolved experience, which then reconstellate in this life in exactly the same way as do traumatic experiences from our early childhood. This process can be seen as an extension of Freud's concept of the repetition compulsion, where the events in this life which set in motion the repetition are themselves set in motion 'before this life', a process which likewise may continue with increasing intensity until some healing or resolution is possible.

Recollections of past lives may be very dramatic, very alien; often they are upsetting and difficult to integrate. Explaining away experiences as coming from a past life may leave us caught up in the glamour of the experience without grounding it in this life. When an emotional pain is at first too great for us to bear, frequently the psyche compensates by producing a florid inner experience that protects us from the feelings for a while. However, that is not the end of the process, and I believe we may rob ourselves to regard it as such. If past-life experiences can be viewed symbolically, they may often herald something important which relates to our human vulnerability in this life.

I am by no means suggesting that all past-life material may be elucidated by reductive analysis. There are more things in heaven and earth than psychotherapists and astrologers can know about! However, as a working astrologer, one may encounter clients bringing this kind of material for discussion, validation and clarification. From a practical point of view, the symbolic approach may enable one to approach the area of suffering relevant to *this life* which lies concealed in such material. This can bring enormous relief and even set a process of healing in motion.

Sacrifice

The theme of sacrifice is frequently seen in connection with the house and sign placement of Chiron: we may be forcibly separated from something which we feel we cannot live without, and thus be precipitated, willingly or unwillingly, on our inner journey. For example, the theme of loss of a position of power, by accident or by choice, is common in the lives of those with Chiron in Scorpio. With Chiron in the 7th house, the loss of an important relationship may begin the inner journey. For one woman with Chiron in Gemini, failing to get a scholarship to continue at university, after her parents had become unable to afford the fees, felt like the end of her world; after a long period of confusion, however, she studied sign language and worked with deaf and dumb people, thus expressing her Chiron in Gemini with those whose capacity for verbal communication was wounded. One man, with Chiron in Sagittarius, was brought up in an ardently Catholic household. He was on the point of entering divinity school when he admitted to himself that he neither believed what he had been taught, nor had he enough faith to continue on the path that had been set for him. He sacrificed the traditional religion in which he had been raised, and was thus forced to find his own way to reconnection with God.

Sometimes life itself arranges the sacrifice; sometimes people take it into their own hands, to the consternation of their friends and family, and perhaps also themselves. Kerenyi notes that human sacrifices were offered to Peleus, who lived on Mount Pelion, and dismisses a suggestion that this was also done in honour of Chiron.[8] It was, however, the custom to offer human sacrifices to dangerous chthonic gods, and Kerenyi gives no reason for assuming Chiron to be an exception, other than emphasizing his noble qualities. I believe that careful consideration of events occurring during Chiron transits gives us cause to include this metaphor as an image of a misplaced or literalized sacrifice, an externalization, or acting out, of an impulse which in the story of Chiron himself results in the surrender of his immortality and thus his healing.

Many traditions have a history of human and/or animal sacrifice, a practice which continues secretly today in many countries. Although we may recoil in horror at the idea, the Christian sacrament of the Eucharist is a symbolic version of the same thing, featuring the *omophagia* (eating of the body of the god) that was part of the famous rites of Dionysus. The metaphor of blood sacrifice lies closer to the surface of our consciousness than we might like to think.

Sacrifice can be performed for many reasons, but there are several principles which occur frequently throughout diverse cultures and have importance for us in psychological terms. A sacrifice may be performed to ingratiate the suppliant with the gods, to incur their favour, or propitiate them in anticipation of their wrath; sacrifice may induce or reduce sanctity. In other words, when something becomes too numinous it is dangerous and must be sacrificed to restore life's balance. On the other hand, when the 'spirit has gone out of something', a sacrifice may be performed in order to bring it back. Thus sacrifice 'consists in establishing a means of communication between the sacred and the profane worlds through the mediation of a victim, that is, of a thing that in the course of the ceremony is destroyed.'[9] It is a focus of energy designed to achieve a purpose far greater than the ceremony itself.

In psychological terms, the metaphor of sacrifice is activated when we become imbalanced, when part of us is developed at the expense of the whole. The psyche may arrange the killing of the fatted calf, so to speak: for the sake of wholeness, our most cherished projects, self-images and aspirations must be allowed to die so that something else can live. We may take upon ourselves the act of sacrificing something dear to us, hoping to give life to something else; alternatively, we may make an act of self-sacrifice in order to support another person. A woman with Chiron in Aries had become very ill at her Chiron return, and eventually admitted that she wanted to leave her husband. The fear of sacrificing the marriage, with all the repercussions she imagined, including worrying about how he would cope without her, had contributed to making her ill. She eventually decided literally to sacrifice her marriage. At other times, the symbolic meaning of the urge may be more relevant. For example, one woman with Chiron in Virgo worked part-time as a secretary and was also building up a practice in massage and healing, both of which are Virgoan activities. When transiting Chiron made the waning square to her natal Chiron, she felt intense pressure to 'kill off' her secretarial job, and yet knew she could not afford to, as she also had two children to support. When she examined the situation more closely, she realized that what needed to happen was for her to integrate into her massage practice some of the organizational skills and groundedness that she exhibited in her secretarial job.

The desire to 'kill off' her secretarial job served to separate her from it emotionally, and enabled her to begin rechannelling the energy that she was putting into it. Had she acted out this impulse and simply left the job, it might have taken much longer to retrieve the qualities which were invested in it, and which she urgently needed to develop her massage practice into an economically viable occupation.

I have sometimes heard people express suicidal feelings during strong transits affecting the Chiron configuration, when a transformation of some kind is trying to occur. If we are very attached to something, or unconsciously identify with it, when it needs to die, we may literalize it into our feeling suicidal. One woman with Chiron in Scorpio felt suicidal when transiting Pluto was conjunct her Chiron. When she examined more deeply what it was that needed to be sacrificed, she realized that it was in fact her old attitude to herself, which was in essence: 'I am no good', and 'Life isn't worth living.' Although, or perhaps because, recent experiences had been proving the contrary, it was very frightening for her to let go of this old pain and invite something new to take root in her life. Another person felt suicidal when transiting Chiron was square his 10th house Saturn in Virgo, and opposite his natal Chiron in Sagittarius. He was a mature student finishing a full-time university degree for which he had worked very hard. He eventually realized that he was afraid of losing the security of the world of the campus; he was being challenged to find his way in the world again, but in a new way. Having finally achieved his dearest wish, a void seemed to be opening up ahead.

In Tarkovsky's brilliant film *The Sacrifice* we are shown the inner journey of a man who apparently 'goes mad': he refuses to speak, burns down the family home and is carted off to an asylum. In the light of his inner experiences, however, these actions make perfect sense to us the audience. He was trying to prevent a nuclear holocaust, and struck a bargain with God, pleading that if He would avert the holocaust, he would in return give up everything that was precious to him: his family, his possessions and even his speech.

It may be useful to consider this metaphor if catastrophic illnesses or crises occur during strong transits of Chiron. An illness may be an attempt to 'bargain with God' in one of the ways described above. We may unconsciously choose to sacrifice our health rather than give up something else: this may be equally unconscious and often comprise a one-sided or inflated attitude of some kind to which we have become accustomed, but which needs to change for the sake of our wholeness. In the words of Kahlil Gibran, 'Your pain is the breaking of the shell that encloses your understanding.'[10] Chiron in the horoscope often indicates where and how we are called upon to give up our inflations, positive or negative, and sacrifice our false sense of immortality. Behind our symptoms may lie thoughts such as: 'If I will say my prayers every day . . . or give all my money to charity . . . or be nice to everybody . . .' then 'please will you let me off the hook.' Thus we perpetuate our own suffering.

6 · The Question of Rulership

It has been suggested that, owing to its 'maverick' nature, Chiron cannot be pinned down to rulership of one specific sign.[1] Other opinions favour either Virgo, Libra, Scorpio and/or Sagittarius.[2] In discussing this, Richard Nolle even calls into question the whole notion of planetary rulership, which dates from the time of Ptolemy, possibly earlier.[3] In this chapter, the concept of 'rulership' is used in the traditional way when referring to the individual horoscope, but it is also expanded to include Chiron's relevance to the larger context of the incoming Age of Aquarius.

From the Age of Pisces . . .

Chiron seems to be a planet of transition. At an individual level, this quality can easily be appreciated through observing what occurs during its transits; at a cosmic level, its discovery at the present time accompanies the shift from the Age of Pisces to the Age of Aquarius.[4] Since the famous musical *Hair*, even people who know nothing about astrology are aware that 'this is the dawning of the Age of Aquarius'. What does this actually mean, astronomically and symbolically?

Students of astrology will know that a *precessional age* is defined by the vernal point (0° Aries) moving backwards relative to the constellations of the sidereal zodiac. This motion is called the precession of the equinoxes, and is caused by the wobble of the Earth's polar axis about the pole of the ecliptic. It takes about 25,800 years for the vernal point to precess once around the entire sidereal zodiac, and thus a precessional age is approximately

2150 years; its moment of beginning cannot be exact, as the size of each constellation varies.

Each precessional age corresponds in a striking way with the dominant civilizations of the period, especially as regards their religious orientation. For example, during the Age of Taurus (beginning *c.* 4000 BC) various cults of bull worship flourished; great temples and pyramids were built as earthly representations of cosmic principles. The Age of Aries (*c.* 2000 BC) was characterized by conquest and exploration; in the Jewish traditions of the Old Testament lambs were sacrificed. Some gods formerly worshipped in the Taurean Age metamorphosed, their attributes changing in a manner congruent with the new Age of Aries. Thus the Persian god Mithras, previously the 'Sacred Bull', became the 'Slayer of the Bull', while the Assyrian Ashur formerly known as the 'Great Bull' became a Martian god of war.[5] As discussed in Chapter 3, the disintegration and transformation of religious forms are currently affecting our civilization, as we move from the Age of Pisces to the Age of Aquarius. Let us further explore what this might mean, for:

History and anthropology teach us that a human society cannot long survive unless its members are psychologically contained within a central living myth. Such a myth provides the individual with a reason for being . . .[6] It is the loss of our containing myth that is the root cause of our current individual and social distress, and nothing less than the discovery of a new central myth will solve the problem for the individual and for society.[7]

Taking a panoramic view of the last 2000 years of the Piscean Age, we can see reflected in Christianity not only the qualities of the sign of Pisces, but also those of the other three signs belonging to the mutable cross. Early Christians identified themselves by the symbol of the fish, and many of the original disciples were fishermen whom Jesus chose to be 'fishers of men'. The compassionate God who sent his only Son into incarnation in order to redeem the suffering of humanity is a truly Piscean figure. The doctrine of *imitatio Christi*, as well as promoting altruism and charity, however, can become literalized as self-sacrifice, martyrdom and guilt, also familiar Piscean motifs. Longing for the

Kingdom of Heaven, separate from and superior to human life, led to the mortification, indeed to the *demonization* of the world and the flesh. Sagittarius looms large in the wealth and grandeur of the Vatican, and also the fanaticism of the Inquisition and the Crusades, when mass conversions were forced by military conquest as devotional fervour joined hands with imperial ambitions. The sign of Gemini depicts the dualism which permeates Christianity, and is also reflected in speculations that the historical Jesus in fact had a brother, who may have even been Judas, his betrayer.

Virgo is represented in Christianity by the figure of the Virgin Mary. Materialism can be seen as the worship of matter (Virgo), and in capitalism there is a curious earthly parallel to the Christian emphasis on the afterlife: accumulating wealth and possessions is also supposed to ensure a better life in the future. The Virgoan qualities of austerity, pragmatism and simplicity can also be seen in the Protestant sects which reacted against the characteristically Piscean abuses rife in the Roman Catholic Church, where 'indulgences' were sold to sinners seeking pardon, and trafficking in bogus relics of saints had become big business. Interestingly, the significance of the Virgin Mary was minimized in Protestantism, but devotion to the Virgin Mary is currently increasing. In 1950, the Doctrine of the Assumption was officially ratified by the Vatican: the Virgin Mary was decreed to have ascended bodily into Heaven at her death, thus being sanctified at the same level as Christ himself. In 1983, Pope John Paul II expressed the doctrine of Mary as Co-Redemptrix; many suspect this will eventually become an official Catholic doctrine which will in effect give Mary equal spiritual status with Christ, thus extending her role as *Theotokos*, or Mother of God.

Since 1900 there have been an extraordinary number of apparitions of the Virgin Mary: over thirty have been recorded, some of which have been endorsed by the Vatican.[8] At Fatima in 1917 a secret was revealed to one of the visionaries and sealed until 1960, as instructed; rumour has it that Pope Pius XII fainted when he read it. In May 1981 it was purported that the document contained a prophesy that the Devil would gain power in the Vatican.[9] On 13 May 1981 Pope John Paul II was nearly assassinated. On that day, the Moon was in Virgo, sign of the Virgin Mary, and trine a triple conjunction of Sun, Chiron and Mars in Taurus. In addition, the Sun and Chiron were opposite Uranus in late Scorpio. Given the revelation of the Fatima documents, one cannot but wonder whether the shock of this experience may have prompted Pope John Paul II to propose the Doctrine of Mary as Co-Redemptrix.

About a month later, on 23 June 1981, there began at Medjugorje in Yugoslavia the longest recorded series of daily apparitions of the Virgin Mary, still continuing at the time of writing, although due to end soon with the promised appearance of a visible sign, an event eagerly awaited by the faithful and the sceptical alike. At the closing of the Piscean Age, Virgo is seeking to manifest at both a literal and a transpersonal level, and the current interest in older pagan cults associated with goddess-worship has resulted in an explosion of interest and literature concerning images of the goddess as whole-in-herself, or Virgin.

Chiron and the Mutable Cross

Using the traditional concept of rulership, from what I have observed Chiron co-rules Sagittarius with Jupiter and is in detriment in Gemini; it is exalted in Virgo and has its fall in Pisces. This links Chiron with all the mutable signs and the houses which they naturally rule, namely the 3rd, 6th, 9th and 12th houses. The traditional images are evocative here: a planet in domicile (the sign it rules) is like a person in his own home, functioning easily and without hindrance. In detriment, it is a visitor in someone else's home, where its own nature may be at a disadvantage, and is repressed or expressed with effort and restraint. In exaltation, a planet is compared to an honoured guest in someone else's home, able to express its best qualities with dignity and control, but as it is on show, not as spontaneous and natural as when in domicile. Finally, when in fall a planet is like an exile: its qualities have no home; they are under stress and unhappy, and consequently may express themselves in a weakened, distorted or negative way.[10]

Chiron as Co-ruler of Sagittarius and the Ninth House

Sagittarius is currently ruled by Jupiter and, as we have seen from the mythology, it was Zeus (Jupiter) who imprisoned Prometheus, with whom Chiron's fate is so intertwined. The traditional symbol for Sagittarius is a Centaur, but note that in esoteric astrology the Centaur's arrow points downwards, a fitting symbol for Chiron's emphasis on the embodiment of gifts and individuality, the reconnection with the instinctual realm and the commitment of human life. The esoteric ruler of Sagittarius is the Earth, to which Chiron eventually had to surrender in order to be released from his pain. [11]

Zeus Akraios of the sky and mountain peaks is Chiron's half-brother and shares a sanctuary with him on Mount Pelion, the traditional home of the Centaurs. The temple of Zeus is on the south side, facing the Sun; the Chironian, or cave of Chiron, is on the shady side, facing north. This symbolizes Chiron's complementarity with Zeus, who rules over all the gods and goddesses on Olympus, the place of eternal light. Below Chiron's cave is the valley of Pelethronion, where healing plants grow in fertile abundance. At the foot of Mount Pelion lies a deep lake named Boibeis, sacred to the moon-goddess Phoebe, ancestress of the Apollonian line, whose descendant Apollo fostered Chiron when he was abandoned. On the shores of this lake, at the dawn of time, a union was said to have taken place between the primeval goddess, the first woman and a phallic god representing virility. The goddess of Lake Boibeis was also called Brimo, the Northern Greek name for the goddess Persephone who gives birth to the Divine Child (sometimes called Brimos) during the Eleusinian Mysteries, a connection which we shall pursue in Chapter 11.

Chiron's half of the mountain thus depicts chthonic, feminine and lunar qualities symbolized by the cave, the lake and the valley with its healing plants. Chiron retains his animal self and his earthiness; he complements, grounds and balances the inflationary tendencies of the 9th house and Sagittarius as ruled by Jupiter. Chiron safeguards our humanity, prompting us to look down as well as up, to humble ourselves before our pain, and to value the dark recesses of our imagination as well the bright light of our Olympian visions of possibility. The Sagittarian Centaur holds a bow and arrow: ironically, in his own hand he carries the instrument of his wounding. Those with Chiron in Sagittarius or the 9th house may need to discover this potential self-wounder within themselves to avoid constantly shooting themselves in the foot. Indeed, the Inner Wounder lives in the same place as the Inner Healer, whether its energy is directed towards ourselves or others.

It should be noted that although Chiron and Zeus share the same father (Saturn) and grandfather (Uranus), Chiron is an outsider to the glory of Olympus. The planet Chiron, however, is an 'orbit-crosser', and thus represents the possibility of 'cosmic fecundation', to use a term Dane Rudhyar applies to Pluto, whose orbit crosses that of Neptune. Although the centre of our solar system is the Sun, the entire system revolves in turn around the Galactic Centre, which is currently located at 26°42' Sagittarius (1988) in zodiacal terms, moving about 8' forward every decade. This late-Sagittarius/Gemini axis is said to have a specifically religious connotation,[12] and as the Galactic Centre is considered to be the source of most of the gravitational energy permeating our galaxy (the Milky Way), it symbolizes the Sun of our Sun, so to speak, an organizing principle or centre of a higher order than the individual centre represented by our Sun. Chiron's discovery chart has the Ascendant conjunct the Galactic Centre, at 26°3' Sagittarius, congruent with Chiron's role as herald of a New Age and the influx of cosmic energy which this implies.

Detriment in Gemini

Chiron seems uncomfortable with the extreme dualism with which Gemini struggles. The Twins are an image of irreconcilables, mortal and immortal following each other in alternating cycles, never meeting. In mythology, twins are often numinous beings with a special destiny; the appearance of twins in dreams and imagery may herald something coming into consciousness, emerging from unity into a pair of opposites which can be distinguished from each other by contrast and comparison. The warfare which often ensues is reminiscent of the battles between the Lapiths and the Centaurs, mentioned before. The Gemini mind is often dominated by either/or thinking: it may work against the instincts in order to differentiate itself, struggling for rationality and objectivity; it may split mind from body, and thus make it difficult for the instinctual and intuitive side of Chiron's nature to find a place. Surrender to mortality may be difficult, because in the sign of Gemini this often means separation from the splendour of the realm of the immortal twin, bringing an acute sense of loss and depression.

Exalted in Virgo

Chiron functions in a more integrated way in the sign of Virgo. Being a feminine Earth sign ruled by Mercury, Virgo has both the gift of intellectual discrimination and also connection with the wisdom of the Earth. In addition, Virgo is traditionally associated with the healing arts, the medicinal use of plants and other substances, and with apprenticeship; all of these themes are apparent in the myth of Chiron. Barbara Hand Clow suggests that Chiron rules Virgo, pointing out that 'the virgin or Virgo is the Great Mother who births the Christos or Pisces'.[13] In this context, Chiron's discovery signals the possibility for individuals to find the Christ principle *within*. As mentioned in Chapter 3, the shamanic paradigm which Chiron represents is the means by which this process of internalization occurs. Through the process of crucifixion on the cross of the opposites within us and in our life, we may eventually give birth to a new self which is fruitful in terms of our human life. Like Chiron, who surrendered his immortality, Christ submitted to the cross; both died and were subsequently immortalized.

Fall in Pisces

On a personal level, the Piscean fluidity and lack of boundaries may make it difficult for those with this placement not to be swept away by the connection with the numinous realm that is natural to them: inflation, confusion and sacrificial distortions may be the result. Chiron's need for both individuality and connection with the transpersonal is not easily met in Pisces. Often the balance is weighted towards dissolution, and emotional chaos erupts. Those with Chiron in Pisces often suffer through lack of a suitable vehicle through which to express their depth of compassion for others. During this century, we have witnessed on a global scale many of the more negative characteristics of this sign: mass chaos, wars, gurumania and the abuse of drugs. These themes will be explored in detail in later chapters. However, in the context of the current transition, we can perhaps see in all this the last gasps of a dying age.

. . . to the Age of Aquarius

Just as echoes of the entire Mutable Cross can be seen through the Age of Pisces, so we can discern traces of the Fixed Cross in the myth of Chiron and also in current collective preoccupations. As the sign of Aquarius describes something of the emerging religious context within which civilization will unfold in the future, these traces perhaps offer some hint of what lies beyond the threshold on which we are collectively poised. What would an Aquarian religion look and feel like, we might wonder? What kind of God-image will develop to dominate the next 2000 years?

A major theme of the Age of Aquarius is likely to be conflict between the individual (Leo) and the tyranny (Saturn) which can be exerted by collective ideas (Uranus); these may be political, scientific or religious, or even the apparently benign aspirations towards brotherhood which already abound within New Age circles. The steps from brotherhood to conformism to tyranny can be alarmingly small. A group, a group leader (Leo) or an ideal of revolution in society or change in consciousness (Aquarius) may become the god for many and, like anything invested with powerful transpersonal energy, it may become dangerous, as others are trampled underfoot in its name. For example, Chiron was conjunct Pluto in Leo when the Third Reich reached the apex of its power.

On the positive side, Leo as the opposite sign to Aquarius suggests the importance of discovering our own individual creative centres (Leo), since only on this basis can we participate in the ferment of our times without getting swept away in 'groupthink' (Aquarius). The motif of personal revelation and religious experience (Leo) again suggests Chiron as representing the archetypal pattern of the shaman, and emphasizes the essentially religious nature of the quest of individuation. The sign of Leo prompts each of us to find our own sense of specialness and individual worth, lest we become subsumed and dehumanized by the identity of whatever group or system of ideas we might subscribe to (Aquarius).

The watery and emotional Piscean qualities of Christianity are well expressed in the great classical oratorios, where the suffering experienced by biblical characters is often dramatized with great pathos. In contrast, Aquarius is a fixed air sign, notorious for its quality of detachment from personal feelings, although emotionally involved with *ideas*, usually dedicated to perfecting something, or bringing intuitions of a cosmic plan or divine order far removed from the stuff of human life. In Greek mythology, where many of the gods were anthropomorphic, Uranus represents a principle so remote that he was not worshipped at an altar. The current interest in UFOs and science fiction symbolizes the search for a connection with this strange, distant, alien being, usually considered to be of vastly superior intelligence. The fantasy of humanoid creatures, or sometimes angelic beings from outer space, who contact us earthlings is now widespread, as illustrated by movies such as *E.T.*, *Close Encounters of the Third Kind* and *Wings of Desire*. Rather than 'Jesus Loves You' (Pisces), the message is now 'You Are Not Alone' (Aquarius)! The theme of personal revelation (Leo) is also present in the phenomenon of 'channelling', which often involves information described as having been received from extraterrestrial beings.[14]

The twentieth century has seen a surge of interest in Eastern religions and, furthermore, the New Physics has described a view of reality that supports these ancient traditions. Apart from isolated esoteric mystery traditions, in the West there was until recently an unbridgeable schism between the materialistic view of reality and personal inner experiences of a mystical or unitive nature, which are elaborately conceptualized and articulated in shamanism and the major Eastern religions. In the words of Laurens van der Post, 'We have become the greatest collection of human know-alls that life has ever seen. But the feeling that our knowing is contained in a greater form of being known has gone.'[15] The idea of a divine plan (including our own discipline, astrology), or a super-intelligent extraterrestrial being certainly addresses this need, as the *individual mind* cannot know itself through rigorous self-scrutiny, psychoanalysis, astrology or spiritual disciplines.

Western psychology knows the mind as the mental functioning of a psyche. It is the 'mentality' of an individual . . . we have already become so accustomed to this point of view that 'mind' has lost its universal character altogether. It has become a more or less individualized affair, with no trace of its former cosmic aspect as the *anima rationalis*.[16]

Wisdom, or 'knowing the mind', comes rather through awareness of *being known* by the One Mind beyond, as a raindrop might suddenly recognize its origins in the cloud from which it has fallen.

From an astrological perspective this universal mind is represented by Uranus, while wisdom is the quality of Jupiter, the inner planet through which we may experience *being known*, unless prevented by our hubris or intellectual pride. Jupiter is also the esoteric ruler of the sign of Aquarius. In the myth, Chiron is half-brother to Zeus, while the planet Chiron links together the orbits of Jupiter, Saturn and Uranus, all three of which relate to the sign of Aquarius. On the Mutable Cross, Jupiter co-rules both Pisces and Sagittarius; on the Fixed Cross it is the esoteric ruler of Aquarius. Together Jupiter and Chiron co-rule Sagittarius, through which energy from the Galactic Centre reaches us, and thus both are intimately concerned with the transition from the Age of Pisces to the Age of Aquarius.

With regard to the Taurus/Scorpio axis, Chiron was discovered at 3°8' of Taurus, and it was also in Taurus when Uranus and Pluto were discovered, or 'given substance' (Taurus). During the last few transits of Chiron, several people were born who bridged different levels of consciousness in true Chironian fashion; many have profoundly affected our view of reality. Several made extensive excursions into Eastern philosophy, and made it more accessible to Westerners. The list includes Franz Anton Mesmer (pioneer of hypnotism and teacher of Freud), Lewis Carroll (of *Alice in Wonderland* fame), Alice Bailey, Madame Blavatsky, Pablo Picasso, Paul Klee, James Joyce and Igor Stravinsky; more recently, Colin Wilson (author of *The Outsider*), Jane Roberts (medium of the discarnate 'Seth'), Bhagwan Rajneesh, Stanislav Grof and Baba Ram Dass (Richard Alpert), and Einstein himself, whose theory of relativity revolutionized physics so that matter (Taurus) will never be the same again!

There are several typically Scorpionic motifs in the story of Chiron: he was poisoned by the blood of the Hydra, often associated with Scorpio, and he endured death, dismemberment, suffering and rebirth. Although an apocalyptic ending of the world has been prophesied many times, mankind now has the capacity literally (Taurus) to annihilate itself (Scorpio). Chiron's recent discovery in Taurus has coincided with an increase in ecological awareness (discussed further in Chapter 11). In the 'Gaia' theory, James Lovelock describes the earth as a living system which is self-regulating and thus can survive even severe ecological crises. *Homo sapiens*, however, will need to discover the 'right use of resources', or he may become extinct as a species.[17] Indeed, according to one current prophecy, biological life as we know it will depart from the planet Earth at around the beginning of the fourth millennium.[18] Use of resources is a Taurean theme, while the life–and–death nature of the issue is clearly Scorpionic.

In summary, at present, Chiron's themes in the lives of individuals can clearly be observed to operate most strongly through the Mutable Cross, especially Sagittarius and Virgo. However, in a few hundred years' time, when the Age of Aquarius is more established, perhaps it will be seen to work through the Fixed Cross, possibly ruling Scorpio and being exalted in Leo. Working with the personal issues that Chiron represents in our horoscope provides a means of grounding ourselves in our humanity and also defining our unique contribution to this transition, in which we are all participating just by being alive at this time.

7 · Chiron by Sign and House

Some individuals will be more sensitive to Chiron's energies than others, as they may be to any other planet. If there are one or more of the conditions listed below, Chiron may be considered focal in a particular horoscope: in this person's life Chironian themes may be dominant, and will be strongly activated when any outer planet transits part of the Chiron configuration.

i)   Chiron conjunct any of the angles.
ii) Chiron conjunct or square the Moon's Nodes.
iii) Chiron aspecting many planets, especially if the Sun, Moon, and/or Ascendant ruler are among them.
iv) Chiron focal according to the shape of the chart. Examples would be Chiron as the handle of a 'bucket-shaped' chart, or as the leading planet of a 'bowl-shaped' chart, or in the middle of a stellium, or in hard aspect to the midpoint of an empty hemisphere or quadrant.
v)   Sagittarius or Virgo on the Midheaven or Ascendant.
vi) Chiron in either Sagittarius or Virgo.
vii) A stellium of planets in Sagittarius or Virgo.

In the following descriptions, houses and signs are grouped together, so you will need to refer to two sections to explore the house and sign placement. In addition, if Chiron is strong in the horoscope you are working with, you may want to explore the associated network of factors in the Chiron configuration. For example, if you have Chiron in the first house in Libra, then Venus, being the ruler of Libra, may be touched by typically Chironian themes. Equally, Mars, as the natural ruler of this house, may express these themes. Venus and Mars will form part of the Chiron configuration, as described above.

Richard Nolle has suggested the image of Chiron's cave, the Chironian, for the house in which Chiron is found. This evocative image certainly seems applicable, in that by house Chiron focuses on those areas where we may feel pain and encounter difficulties, as well as where we seek to express our unique individuality. We may avoid 'coming out into the light' of this area of life-experience, hiding ourselves away in pain like Chiron with his incurable wound; we may only be able to enter this domain of life in a supercharged or heroic manner, like Chiron emerging as the healer and mentor of heroes. However, we can also regard Chiron's house position as a *temenos* – a sacred enclosure where we may encounter the numinous side of life. Another image for Chiron's house position is taken from Buddhism: when we consider Chiron to be the Inner Teacher, as described in the previous chapter, its house and sign often describe important lessons which we are here to learn. These lessons represent the inner goal of the journey, rather than anything external, and involve the Middle Path, or 'right' way. This is not 'right' as opposed to 'wrong', but rather that which is *appropriate* in order for us to fulfil our individual *dharma* – our realization of universal law and our part in the totality of existence. Before the Middle Path is found and appreciated, Chiron tends to manifest in a wounded, all-or-nothing way, as amply described in the following chapters. With maturity and surrender, however, a feeling of 'rightness' may come, often having overtones of religious meaning and/or connection with the *dharma*, with some context larger than ourselves: this is Chiron's gift. In addition, planets aspecting Chiron here represent inner and outer forces with which we must contend, lest they pull us away from the *dharma*. Here are some typical examples, listed by house, taken from 'lessons' which various people have reported learning through a period of sickness or crisis involving their Chiron.

1st house: Appropriate initiative, or action
2nd house: Appropriate values, or use of resources
3rd house: Appropriate communication, thought and speech
4th house: Appropriate emotional bonds and attitude to family
5th house: Appropriate self-expression and creativity

6th house: Appropriate form of services to others, and respect for the body

7th house: Appropriate relationships

8th house: Appropriate attitude to death and sexuality

9th house: Appropriate attitude to possibilities

10th house: Appropriate vocation and participation in society

11th house: Appropriate ideals and friendships

12th house: Appropriate renunciation

When we add the quality of the sign in which Chiron is placed, it fills out this description and suggests a *way of being* which supports us in the area of life represented by Chiron's house. For example, a person with Chiron in Virgo in the 5th house suffered for many years what she felt was a complete blockage in her creativity; she had wanted to be a dancer, but an early marriage and children had interrupted her career. She eventually redis-covered her creativity by learning eurhythmics, which is more about the process of inner development and its outer expression than performing set pieces before an audience. Chiron's sign position may also show how we seek to protect ourselves from our inner pain, what we draw on to try to deal with an area of our life which may be blocked. For example, someone with Chiron in the 1st house in Sagittarius may have difficulties with self-assertion, and may develop a philosophy (Sagittarius) of optimis-tic passivity, believing that everything comes right in the end. A woman with Chiron in Scorpio in the 7th house felt very vulner-able towards others, and hid her need behind an intense, pseudo-independent and emotionally abrasive way of relating to others. Thus the sign may provide a kind of bandage over our wound as expressed by Chiron's house position; this bandage is often removed during a strong Chiron transit, as we shall see in the chapter on transits.

Needless to say, what follows does not describe how Chiron will or 'should' manifest, as its varying expressions are as unique as the life of the person whose horoscope you are examining. Nevertheless, if a client should bring a specific problem to discuss, you may recognize obviously Chironian themes within what he or she is saying. By examining the Chiron configuration, as well as looking into the psychological process and events coinciding with the Chiron cycle through that person's life, you may be able to assist the process of healing by helping the client to get a clearer idea of what is trying to happen, and of the purpose behind the suffering or crisis.

Chiron in Aries and the First House

> First and last, man is alone.
> He is born alone, and alone he dies
> and alone he is while he lives, in his deepest self.
>
> D. H. Lawrence, 'Deeper than Love'

The first house and Aries bring the basic feeling 'I exist', the desire to emerge into life with conquest, self-assertion and initiative; the 'I am', the inner sense of beingness and primary identity also belong to this house. The physical appearance is said to be described by the Ascendant, and is often used to help rectify unknown birth-times.

With Chiron in Aries or the 1st house we find a wound in this area, often a deeply buried one. After all, if you feel you have no right to exist, then self-assertion and initiative may be accompanied by the fear of non-being. Therefore, with this placement we may unconsciously feel that we only exist as a mirror to someone else (echo of the 7th house); we only feel motivated to champion a cause on someone else's behalf, like a knight in shining armour, but with no will of our own. Grandiose displays of bravado and fighting spirit compensate for the pain, self-doubt and fear underneath, which could drive us into a repeating cycle of futile and self-destructive endeavours; we tend to take action prematurely, translating emotional tension immediately into action. With this Chiron placement, we may wound ourselves with a militant self-sufficiency, becoming unable to ask for help and support in our conviction that we must 'go it alone'. Underneath, however, there may be despair and an identification with non-being, a 'death-wish', and a deep fear of doing anything that truly expresses what we want. Either we do not know what this is, or we conceal it for fear it will be taken away, spoiled or destroyed. One person with Chiron in the first house said, 'Where there ought to be a sense of *me*, there is an enormous hole and a pain beyond my ability to endure it.'

With Chiron in the 1st house or Aries, our spontaneous expressions of passion, being or will may have been crushed in childhood, either subtly or overtly with stock phrases such as: 'I want never gets', or 'Children should be seen and not heard'. Repressive child-rearing methods such as schedule-feeding, lack of physical holding and mirroring and premature systematic toilet-training often accompany the early wounds of this placement. If the interference with, and rejection of, our natural rhythms are serious enough, they result in deep confusion and the belief that what we want – indeed *who we are* – is not acceptable, and that we must not reach out to satisfy our desires. A paralysis of the will follows and, understandably, a deep, often misplaced rage lies underneath. Later on in life, we may feel that we must conceal what we truly want, or it will be destroyed by outside forces. Hence, we find ourselves instead getting exactly what we do *not* want. Owning up to what we *do* want might initially create panic because it touches our wounded area.

Sometimes the early environment of those with Chiron in the 1st house or Aries is hostile and full of suppressed or overt aggression, which compounds feelings of timidity and lack of self-worth and personal rights. Then survival becomes equated with learning how to please and placate others (7th house-echo). One woman expressed this as a capacity to 'fill the holes' in other people or situations, and stay anonymous herself; 'being seen' was too dangerous. Conversely, we find individuals with this placement who struggle until their will is so inflated that they appear as virtual personifications of will, drive, energy and enthusiasm. A rugged, pioneering quality sometimes characterizes this Chiron placement. Albert Schweitzer, doctor, pioneer and missionary had this placement, and so did Jan Smuts, who led the Boer guerrillas against the British and rose to being Prime Minister of South Africa. Margaret Thatcher, present Prime Minister of Britain, has Chiron in Aries in the 6th house (of work and service!), and it is not for nothing that she is nicknamed the 'Iron Lady' (iron is the metal associated with Mars). However, sometimes this powerful energy is fragile like a bubble. When it bursts, the person may deflate into a sorry mess of pain and insecurity, and even wish for death. Relationships where dependence/

independence issues arise, as an echo of the 7th house, frequently cause this, as do situations which create a feeling of impotence.

With Chiron in Aries or the 1st house, we may be prone to suicidal fantasies or feelings. Sometimes these are a response to anger, frustration or not being in control of a situation; they may be a wish to regain some sense of power, or a reaction to not being able to get our own way. With this placement, a wilful adolescent, who brooks no interference with his or her omnipotence, often lives side by side with an uncomfortable timidity, vulnerability and awareness of the ephemeral nature of physical life. One person with this placement described herself as living with an acute awareness that when she died there would be nothing left, no trace – she would depart like a will-o'-the-wisp.

If Chiron is conjunct the Ascendant, beginnings may be difficult. We either rush into starting something, or we hesitate – even get ill – rather than make decisions; we may collapse at the threshold of what seems to be an exciting new phase of life. Behind this, we find the experience of physical birth is often particularly significant or traumatic; from then on, every 'birth', every beginning of a new life-cycle, may be fraught with fear, resistance and tumult. The nature of this struggle is frequently described by the sign in which Chiron and/or the Ascendant are placed and the aspects to them, which in turn usually express characteristics of the physical birth.

Some examples will make the point clear. A man with Chiron in the 1st house in Pisces would retreat into confusion, 'space out', and sometimes drink too much whenever he approached a new phase of life and had decisions or initiatives to take. His mother was anaesthetized during his birth; he described himself as likewise feeling 'anaesthetized' – numb, confused, unable either to think clearly or know what he was feeling. A woman with Chiron conjunct the Ascendant in Aquarius always consulted an astrologer or medium before making decisions, as she was terrified of 'getting it wrong' (see the section on Chiron in Aquarius). She concealed this fear by never consulting the same person twice, contemptuously dismissing the various readings as useless. When I innocently asked her if she had ever seen an astrologer before, she 'confessed' the issue. She was ready to talk about it and did so at length. This enabled her to begin to face and contain the real feelings which were underneath: she had been 'making *them* wrong' as a defence against the terrifying feeling of not having a right to exist and being fundamentally 'wrong' herself. These were the emotional conclusions she reached shortly after her birth; her mother initially rejected her and did not want to feed her, as she had wanted a son. With Chiron in Aquarius we are quite capable of rejecting people who do not fit the bill, and this is reminiscent of Chiron's rejection by his mother. A person with Chiron in the 1st house, with a Scorpio Ascendant, squared by a 10th-house Pluto, provides a second example. This person nearly died in birth, and was pulled out by forceps. She later connected her lack of will-power with having been 'twice defeated' during birth: first, when she was struggling to get out and couldn't; second, when she had given up, was dying, and was then pulled out against her will. Her basic attitude to life was one of defiance and determination to defeat it by refusing to co-operate; underneath was a profound death-wish which, once faced, began a remarkable transformation.

Any 1st-house planet, especially if near the Ascendant, represents a strong archetypal energy encountered early in life, which often develops into a pseudo-identity that must be shed in the search for our true inner nature. In extreme cases, planets conjunct the Ascendant seem to 'possess' the person, if his or her ego is weak. With Chiron present, there may then be an identification with the Wounded Healer. Eve Jackson's research found that indeed this is a common placement for healers and therapists.[1] Very early in life, even in the womb or during birth, a person can take on the role of the healer as regards his family and friends, and this continues throughout life, perhaps even becoming a career. It is frequently a way of concealing a deep feeling of woundedness, similar to the well-known pattern of 'identifying with the aggressor'.[2]

With this Chiron placement, we may take our sense of identity from others, pouring ourselves into their mould, taking on their allegiances, ideals, thoughts and even feelings – another echo of the 7th house. As one person put it: 'I'm just becoming aware of the horror of the fact that I always take my cue from the outside, from other people, and underneath I feel utterly unreal.' Previously in his life, he had suffered from an apparent lack of motivation. However, when transiting Chiron squared his Sun he began to realize what was underneath: a feeling that it was not worth doing anything because the person who was doing it was unreal, so anything he did would therefore also be unreal.

Sometimes, people with Chiron in the 1st house or in Aries struggle hard to find something they can *do* which will bring them the sense of being they lack. They may set themselves wellnigh impossible tasks, loaded with all the intensity of a search for confirmation that they exist. Often, this is the futile struggle which has to be given up, but this placement is also frequently found in the horoscopes of people who are in fact originators, unique one-off individuals, perhaps precisely because the inner being has had such a struggle. Jung has Chiron in Aries; his conflict with Freud (a typical 7th-house echo) led him to originate a new model of the psyche based on his pioneering exploration of his own inner world. Isadora Duncan has Chiron in Taurus conjunct the Ascendant in Aries, and through her unique sensual style of dance pioneered the development of dance-forms characterized by flowing, sensual and earthy movements (Taurus). Samuel Hahnemann has Chiron in Capricorn in the 1st house; he rediscovered and formulated the principles (Capricorn) of homoeopathic medicine. Mick Jagger and Muhammad Ali ('I am the greatest!') both have Chiron in the 1st house in Leo and Leo rising! Although Muhammad Ali has recently fallen from grandeur, both he and Mick Jagger *embody* the qualities of animal instinctuality in their performances. Even lesser mortals with this placement have an urge to be the first, the best and the only!

With Chiron in the 1st house or Aries, we may project on to our bodies our inner sense of shame and embarrassment at existing; we may feel mortified by features which others do not even notice, but which to us seem monstrously ugly or misshapen. We might cringe inwardly at our ears, which stick out too much, or our legs which are too fat. We feel too tall, too short. We feel uncoordinated or awkward, and situations of physical exposure, like sport or sex, turn into potential nightmares. Cecil Rhodes, who had Chiron in the 1st house in Capricorn, had a foreshortened finger on one hand, which acutely embarrassed him; even his aggrandizement of the British Empire could not compensate for this deformity, which he always carefully concealed when being photographed. See the section on Chiron in aspect to Mars for further details of his horoscope.

Lon Chaney, perhaps the most famous 'Hunchback of Notre Dame' has Chiron in the 1st house in Taurus; both his parents were deaf and dumb, and Chaney's familiarity with the pains, vulnerabilities and frustrations of the handicapped contributed to his moving portrayal of this figure, an archetypal victim indeed. The theme of physical disability or life-changing initiatory illness is a frequent one with Chiron in the 1st house or Aries. It seems that we are asked to include in our sense of being our sickness, woundedness or disability, and our struggle might be not to identify with it completely, and become 'the wounded one'. Just as some with this placement will identify themselves as healers, others will identify themselves as victims, without realizing that they are caught in an archetypal pattern which is blurring the truth of their feelings and their situation.

Those with Chiron in the 1st house or Aries have the capacity to enable and empower others, being so aware of their own deep powerlessness in the face of the immensity of the universe. Living close to the edges of existence, they often give the impression of being rather wild and untameable; they are often loners, even if married or in a committed relationship. They may also *personify* qualities for others: see the horoscopes of Martin Luther King (pp. 246–7) and Dr Ian Player (pp. 327–33) for examples of this. I have met several people with this placement who have spent long intense years searching for a missing and elusive sense of identity, only to discover that when they gave up the search and accepted their nothingness, an enormous vitality and sense of being followed: the spark of being finally ignited.

With this Chiron placement often comes a knack for timing actions intuitively to 'grasp the moment'. Yours may be a unique combination of compassion and appropriate action, an ability to be highly innovative and to take initiative, especially where the welfare of others is at stake. You gain strength through conquest and fighting difficulties, but you must also learn the lesson of how to be a 'noble rival' to those with whom you compete. If you succeed in treading the narrow path of neither succumbing to passive aggression nor obliquely acting out destructiveness, you may come to feel the 'will of life' flowing through you. You are not omnipotent, and you don't have to do it all! Whether or not you work in the healing field, you probably have the capacity to act as a catalyst in situations, and to touch the inner being of others; although your wound is your doubt of your own existence, you are probably quite magnetic as a personality, so don't be surprised if others react strongly to you.

Chiron in Taurus and the Second House

> No man unless he has died, and learned to be
> alone, will ever come into the mystery of touch.
>
> D. H. Lawrence, 'Initiation Degrees'

The 2nd house describes what gives us a sense of safety and solidity; it is also about our values, what we cultivate and make our own, the nature of our inner and outer resources in life and how we relate to them, including money, property and possessions. Developmentally, we begin here to separate from mother, and to derive our sense of substance from our own body and from objects other than her. Our sense of self is still rooted primarily in our instincts and bodily experiences and, if there is wounding during this transition, we may later project our instincts and body-sense on to other people or material objects.

Although we have already explored some of the more metaphysical implications of Chiron in Taurus, let us look at its meaning in the individual horoscope. With Chiron in Taurus or the 2nd house, we may lack a sense of self-worth, being unable to value ourselves, feeling insecure and insubstantial. We never quite feel solid and safe, and may therefore attach great importance to material possessions. 'I own, therefore I am' could be an underlying feeling, although we come to discover that even acquiring possessions does not help. People with this placement may be deeply possessive and materialistic, clinging to people and possessions in the hopes that they will provide the missing sense of substantiality.

The body itself may be felt to be unreliable, faulty or wounded; as with Chiron in the 1st house, when it is in the 2nd house there may be some actual disability, injury or physical trauma to cope with. The body may also be feared and controlled rigorously, since from it emanate powerful and unacceptable sexual and territorial instincts. Many people with Chiron in Taurus have great sexual magnetism: Isadora Duncan and Marilyn Monroe, both already mentioned, are examples of women with Chiron in Taurus. Marilyn Monroe, with Chiron in Taurus conjunct the MC and Venus in the 9th house, tried to get a sense of substance from her public image (10th house), and also from her relationships (Chiron/Venus). With Chiron in Taurus or the 2nd house, we may also unconsciously identify with the wounded instincts; the collective legacy of rejection of the instincts may be felt personally, unless we are able to come into a healthy relationship with our own powerfully sensual and instinctual nature. If we do not learn to recognize and consciously experience these feelings and drives, we may become possessed by them, or use up a great deal of energy trying to repress them. The body may then speak through symptoms that are embarrassingly graphic. One man with Chiron in Taurus, for example, had left a great many things unsaid in his life, especially to those he loved; later on in life he was plagued by a sore throat. One woman with Chiron in the 2nd house in Cancer was unable to 'stomach' her own feelings of possessiveness and territoriality; she would often be unable to eat, unable to 'take in substance'.

If you have this placement, healing often comes through learning to trust the instinctual wisdom of your body. As far as possible, learn to listen to it: eat what your body tells you, and sleep when you need to. If you have a legacy of having your instincts ignored or programmed according to others' standards, some gentle undoing may be necessary. Initially, you may feel that physicality, the body and the material world are your enemies, and you therefore may spend your energy trying to ward off, control and dominate them. The lesson of this placement may be one of learning to befriend these realms; massage, pleasurable exercise with awareness (not military regimes of fitness!) and taking pleasure in personal grooming can be very healing activities.

Conversely, some individuals with this placement have a horror of being tied down by possessions, and a reluctance to own things. A woman with Chiron in Scorpio in the 2nd house felt wounded in her childhood by the values of her parents, who attached more importance to their material possessions and wealth than to feelings; her unconscious anger about this continued to manifest as a sabotaging of her painstaking efforts to build up material security. A man with Chiron in the 2nd house in Sagittarius suffered from a poignant feeling of the transitoriness of material life; he felt a contempt for it which actually compensated for his fear of it. Eventually, he embraced an Eastern philosophy of life which encouraged the renouncing of worldly goods; instead of facing his fear, this belief system (Sagittarius) actually supported and concealed it.

Chiron in Taurus or the 2nd house often signifies issues concerning wealth and money. Some individuals who must come to terms with great wealth feel unable to accept the responsibility that goes with it; others may have a genuine desire to share their resources with others. Either way, the control of resources is a theme of this placement. Negatively, such people may obsessively control their instinctual and sexual needs, or be very controlling towards others (8th-house echo); positively, they may make excellent managers for others' resources. Fortunes may be won and lost, and those with this placement may have an uncannily good financial sense, perhaps accompanied by difficulty in managing their own finances. One woman with Chiron in Virgo in the 2nd house found it difficult to prevent her own affairs from sliding into debt and chaos, but successfully ran the office of a debt-collecting agency! Here again is the theme of Chiron able to do for others what he cannot do for himself. Alternatively, Chiron in the 2nd house or Taurus sometimes signifies material poverty, which is felt as wounding and humiliating; frequently it creates an exaggerated sense of the importance of material possessions. One woman with Chiron in Taurus who spent several of her formative years as a refugee said she had to learn to recognize that 'man is fed not by bread alone'.

Another frequent manifestation of Chiron in Taurus or the 2nd house is the inability to see things symbolically and the tendency to make everything too literal. At times, practical reality may seem to grind to a halt in a welter of problems or decisions which need to be made; the person feels stuck in the mud, unable to turn right or left; situations and dilemmas become over-concretized and paralysing. When this occurs, the route to resolution often lies within the body; instead of trying to solve a problem or work out practical details, it may be more creative to step back – go and dig the garden or do the dishes – to allow the energy time to disperse. Letting go is not easy for those with Chiron in Taurus, who frequently show the bull-like obstinacy and stubbornness for which Taurus is anyway well known! Insecurity within the material realm is often the underlying reason for why people inappropriately or prematurely make things solid and literal; their ability to think symbolically seems wounded simply because they find this way of thinking too frightening.

People with Chiron in the 2nd house or Taurus might have felt wounded by values that are foreign to their true nature; they are frequently unable to accept the value system which they inherited from their parents or the society in which they live, and must struggle to find out what is really important to them. They sometimes have to accept financial hardship in order to uphold their own values; although this is very threatening for some with this Chiron placement, it may also bring a sense of inner strength.

The horoscope of Stanislav Grof has Chiron in Taurus in the 5th house, sextile Pluto in the 8th house; both are quincunx the Ascendant, which is the focus of a yod, or 'finger of God' pattern. He is a psychiatrist and researcher into altered states of consciousness, who began using LSD in his therapy work and later developed non-drug techniques with similar effects. His conceptual and experiential work bridges all levels from the instinctual through to the archetypal, and encourages the expression (5th house) of deep woundedness. The title of one of his books encapsulates his Chiron configuration: *Beyond the Brain – Birth, Death and Transcendence in Therapy*. In it he expresses (5th house) a conceptual framework (Sagittarius Ascendant) that encompasses and synthesizes most major therapeutic models (Chiron) to date. The context is birth (Ascendant), death (8th house) and transcendence (Sagittarius).

As mentioned in Chapter 6, there is a parallel between the figures of Chiron and Vulcan – the Roman smith-god and also the name of an undiscovered planet said to be located between the Sun and Mercury, which in Alice Bailey's system rules Taurus. In the world of myth there is often a connection between shamans and blacksmiths; in some early-European cultures one person often performed both roles. Hephaestus is the Greek name for Vulcan, who made the paraphernalia of the gods and goddesses. It was he who forged the chains that kept Prometheus bound to his rock; he also made the thunderbolts of Zeus and the arrows of Artemis and Apollo.

Like Chiron, Hephaestus was wounded: he was rejected by his mother Hera, who found him so ugly that she threw him out of Mount Olympus shortly after he was born, and thus one of his legs was lamed. Unlike Chiron, however, Hephaestus took revenge on his mother by trapping her in a golden throne which he made for her, and refusing to release her, even though the Olympian gods implored him to hand over the key. He eventually agreed, on condition that he would be granted any wish. He asked for Aphrodite as his wife, and she was powerless to refuse in the circumstances. His fate of being rejected continued, as Aphrodite was notoriously unfaithful and unkind to him. Undaunted, however, he continued to create beautiful things.

Hephaestus represents a creative energy which does not turn in upon itself and destroy its own potential in response to the pain of having been rejected. Although ridiculed by the high and mighty Olympians, being lame, sooty-faced and awkward, Hephaestus was a fine craftsman and metal-smith, and played a key role as catalyst, helping the gods and goddesses to perform their functions. He was not servile; he made spirited retaliation by setting various traps and thus humiliating them in return. Hephaestus enables others to express their individuality and their selfhood, or inner divinity, and this gift is part of his own individuality. He is dedicated to his craft in spite of being wounded. He refuses to be crushed by rejection and humiliation, but instead honours and expresses his own creativity, often with materials drawn from the earth itself, such as metal.

The figure of Hephaestus represents the potential, through self-respect and perseverance, to turn one's area of woundedness into a place from which fine creativity can issue. Although those with Chiron in the 2nd house or in Taurus may suffer through feeling unable to give substance to their own creativity, they are often gifted midwives to the creative endeavours of others. They may initially admire and envy others' creative gifts, but undervalue their own. If they can encompass this pain without inflicting it upon their own sense of self-worth, those with this placement can develop a reverence for the creative process itself; once their own creativity is transpersonalized in this way, it often begins to flow. With the territoriality of Chiron in Taurus or the 2nd house, creativity may need to be experienced as something we participate in, as a process which we serve, rather than something we own. One woman with this placement said that she found the process of creating very laborious, and would dream of figures like Hephaestus in his forge.

Another woman with Chiron conjunct Mercury in Libra in the 2nd house, remembers being asked by a friend in class to write a story, as he had not done his homework. She quickly dashed off a story for him, which to her horror got higher marks than the one she had written for herself. (The friend's surname was Terranova, and his father owned the local nursery!) Later in life, she longed to write, but felt blocked; however, in her work as an editor, her creativity, spontaneity and generosity flowed easily, and she was able to understand and support the writers with whom she worked. She said, with true Chiron/Mercury wit, 'What I need is someone like me in my life.'

Chiron in Gemini and the Third House

Two souls, alas! within my bosom throne;
One from the other wildly longs to sever.
One, with a passionate love that never tires,
Cleaves as with clamps of steel to things of earth,
The other upwards through earth's mists aspires
To kindred regions of a loftier worth.

Goethe, *Faust*

In the 3rd house we begin to communicate verbally, to explore the environment, relate to it, take it apart and attempt to understand it. Our ability to reflect and think begins here; we look at details and associate them with our own reactions in a personal and subjective way; we begin to differentiate outer from inner. This house is also associated with siblings (the twins of Gemini), short journeys (like a child going a short distance from its mother and needing to return), with reading and writing, learning, speaking and problem-solving.

With Chiron in Gemini or the 3rd house, we might feel our mind to be wounded, unreliable, in danger of disintegrating, or subject to storms of incomprehensible activity. We may indiscriminately absorb ideas from anywhere in the scramble to understand what is happening. We often have difficulty believing in our own ideas; perhaps we worry about whether or not we are right, and so resort to parroting the ideas of others, which we even take as our own, or which we use like a safety net to hold together the scattered fragments of our thought. The drive to understand everything often reaches obsessive proportions with this placement: we become 'mentally identified', nervous and stressed, as confusion or dissociation develops.

However, if there is enough basic personal security and maturity, the minds of those with Chiron in Gemini or the 3rd house may be very open to transpersonal sources in a creative and healing way, being prophetic and mediumistic in a positive sense.

Ruth White, the well-known medium of the discarnate 'Gildas', has Chiron in Gemini in the 7th house. Her book *Seven Inner Journeys* tells the story of her inner relationship (Chiron in the 7th) with Gildas. Through communication (Gemini) with him, she has an extraordinary ability to provide healing and clarification on a soul-level for people seeking reassurance and guidance.

Individuals with this placement often have great originality and brilliance, their ceaseless probing and questioning taking them into areas where others prefer not to look. Ken Kesey has Chiron in the 3rd house; he introduced many people to LSD, either by giving it to them, or by writing of his experiences (3rd house). Sigmund Freud, originator of the 'talking cure' also has Chiron in the 3rd house, in Aquarius; he developed a painful cancer which ate away his jaw and interfered with his speech (3rd house), a poignant image of the link between the wound and the capacity to heal. Freud rediscovered, and began to explore, the inner world we now call the unconscious, and thus radically altered the collective perceptions of reality, an expression of his Chiron in Aquarius in the 3rd house. We will be referring again to Freud's chart in the section on Chiron in aspect to Pluto (pp. 254–5).

Werner Heisenberg, founder of quantum mechanics, has Chiron in the 3rd house, in Capricorn. His famous 'principle (Capricorn) of uncertainty' was formulated in 1926–7, during a series of exact transits of Chiron, quincunx his 1st house Mercury in Scorpio. In June 1926, as discussions with colleagues reached a critical stage, he suffered a severe attack of hay fever (a Mercurial ailment, affecting the breathing and upper bronchial membranes). He sought refuge on a rocky island (a suitably Capricornian place!), began to recover his health, and one night during the week the quincunx was exact, he awoke to a 'peak experience' which deeply confirmed the direction of his research. He writes: 'I had the feeling that through the surface of atomic phenomena, I was looking at a strangely beautiful interior, and felt almost giddy that I now had to probe this wealth of mathematical structures nature had so generously spread out before me.'[3] The theoretical formulation of this vision took place during the next two exact quincunxes of Chiron to his natal Mercury, through written correspondence with colleagues, a 3rd house/Gemini activity.

During the last exact quincunx, he coined the term now bearing his name: 'Heisenberg's Principle of Uncertainty'. This is a typical Chironian experience: the 'breakthrough in plane', as mentioned in Chapter 1, the unexpected finding of a key or solution from a higher dimension of consciousness, the clarification of one's purpose in life, and, most obviously, an illness being the catalyst for the entire experience. Note also his humble attitude and typically Capricornian sense of responsibility towards his experience: he regarded it as his duty to follow up and ground his vision. During the war, Heisenberg remained in Germany under Hitler; although he disagreed with the political regime, he felt obliged to stay and preserve the German scientific tradition. He later re-established many scientific research

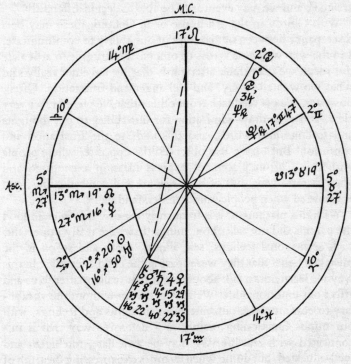

Werner Heisenberg

institutes (Capricorn again). Louis de Broglie, who won a Nobel Prize for the discovery of the wave nature of the electron, also has Chiron in the 3rd house.

With Chiron in Gemini or the 3rd house, we may need to become conscious of self-defeating and destructive thought-patterns which have their origin in childhood hurts, or which constitute the unspoken attitudes and beliefs inherited from our childhood environment. Very early in life we may have made unconscious decisions based on painful emotional reactions. For example, one woman who had Chiron in Virgo in the 3rd house vowed she would never be a dry intellectual like her mother: she grew up denying her own intellect, but habitually fell in love with intellectual men. The process of unearthing these destructive thought-patterns acts like the 'sword which heals the wound it created', and we may eventually be able to decide differently.

With Chiron in the 3rd house or in Gemini, there may be a discrepancy between our concept of our ability to communicate, and the way we come across to others. We struggle to articulate our ideas; we may think afterwards that we have not really said what we wanted to say, and feel anger and frustration. Often, however, we get feedback from others that we were in fact very clear, and even draw admiration for our ability to put thoughts and feelings into words, and this adds to the frustration and confusion! But I have also observed the opposite, where people with this Chiron placement express ideas in a confused and idiosyncratic way, full of *non sequiturs* and contradictions, and are amazed when people cannot understand them.

With this placement, it is frequently the case that in childhood the parents did not talk about things that were really important, such as personal feelings, sex, illness, death and so on in the mistaken belief that they were sparing the child's feelings. In this way we learn not to talk about things that really matter to us and affect our emotional life. We may grow up without the vocabulary to communicate our innermost thoughts and feelings, with our minds functioning mainly in a defensive way that is unconnected with real life. We may be articulate, intelligent and well-educated, but dumb when it comes to expressing the truth of our own inner feelings.

The mind of a person with Chiron in the 3rd house or Gemini can function in an intuitive or associative way – the so-called 'primitive' mind which tends to focus on the whole picture rather than the parts. In education where logic is the god, such a person may have 'learning difficulties' in childhood. However, this is often due to a mismatch between the child's natural mode of thinking and the method of teaching. I have met several such people who later learned to value their own original thoughts and perceptions by expressing them through images and other non-verbal means. It may be useful for those with Chiron in Gemini or the 3rd house to discover a synthesizing framework (echoes of Sagittarius) within which their fears of being crazy can subside, and which can serve to conceptualize and validate their intuitions; it might be helpful to read the current literature linking the findings of the new physics with various states of consciousness.[4] When the associative or transpersonal mind has not been acknowledged, people with Chiron in Gemini can become paranoid or overwhelmed by strange subjective perceptions; they may feel themselves at the centre of an inexplicable and hostile maze of impressions, unable either to let it go or to separate inside from outside. When the Logos function of clarifying, separating, dividing and discriminating is wounded, this can be quite terrifying. Here again a suitable framework of meaning (echoes of Sagittarius and the 9th house again) may spell the difference between disaster and a true healing process.

Sometimes people with this placement are intellectually arrogant, deifying the mind and not valuing the irrational, regarding those who are not intellectually cultivated as inferior beings. They seem to benefit from some kind of religious attitude, with which they can recognize that as human beings they cannot know it all, that only God is all-seeing and omniscient (the 9th-house polarity again). This is especially true in our culture where we have not only lost our humility in the face of Creation, but have also enshrined the Logos as the one true God: this results in the distortion that to become godlike means to know more, understand more and thereby to control the universe. This is expressed in *Faust*:

> In vain I have amass'd,
> Within me all the treasures of man's mind,
> And when I pause, and sit me down at last,
> No new power welling inwardly I find;
> A hairbreadth is not added to my height,
> I am no nearer to the Infinite.[5]

On the other hand, people with this placement can be so aware of the puniness of the human mind that they give up on it, and do not respect or develop it; they may emphasize their feelings or intuitions instead. But if the horoscope shows an emphasis on air signs, this tactic may result in a feeling of emptiness, dissatisfaction, and a subtle feeling of cheating oneself.

Sometimes, with this placement (especially with Chiron in Gemini), the issue of duality is critical. We may feel almost paralysed by acute awareness of our inner opposites, knowing that whatever we do or choose, the other polarity will complain and interfere, or create moods and depressions. We may have to resign ourselves to never reaching the synthesis we long for (9th house); our inner resources may seem to dry up, or our wound may be too deep, or time may run out. We might have to accept the pain of being lop-sided, and mourn the aspects of ourselves that will remain unexpressed or unfulfilled; conscious acceptance of this brings healing compassion for ourselves and others.

The 'other twin' or 'soul mate' may be a preoccupation for those with Chiron in Gemini; he or she may be sought (and sometimes found) in obsessive relationships characterized by intense mirroring and feelings of *déjà vu*. For example, one woman with Chiron in Gemini as her only air planet, trining a Libran Ascendant met and married a man who was her total opposite in every way (and very intellectual); he represented everything she did not want in a man. She said she felt an 'intervention from another level' (a typically Chironian statement) when they met. The relationship proved to be the focal point of her life, and survived much conflict; both she and her husband eventually made successful careers as healers.

Sometimes with this placement, a brother or sister is literally wounded: he or she is physically ill, deformed, or mentally retarded, or very important in our lives for some other reason. These relationships may be especially wounding or healing. There may be rivalry and hostility; we might feel that our brother or sister was somehow favoured. On the other hand, we might have to deal with the discomfort and guilt of knowing that we ourselves were the favourite child in the family. Relationships between brother and sister may have intense sexual overtones: sometimes they are enacted literally; sometimes we later seek a partner similar to the beloved sibling. The brother or sister could also be like a mentor and wise person, with a positive influence in our lives.

A gift of this placement is the ability to express feelings and emotions in words, to speak out about contentious issues, and to articulate experiences of other dimensions of reality. D. H. Lawrence has Chiron in Gemini in the 8th house; he was a spokesman for the wounded instincts, especially sexuality (8th house). He died of a lung condition (Gemini/8th house); when it was acute he would bleed from the mouth, a poignant image of the quality of his poetry: his words are like blood flowing from his wounds (Chiron in Gemini). His major biography (written by Harry T. Moore) was originally entitled *The Intelligent Heart*, a symbol of the gift of Chiron in Gemini or the 3rd house.

Chiron in Cancer and the Fourth House[6]

> Even as you have homecomings in your twilight, so has
> the wanderer in you, the ever-distant and alone . . . For
> that which is boundless in you abides in the mansion of
> the sky, whose door is the morning mist, and whose
> windows are the songs and the silences of night.
>
> Kahlil Gibran, *The Prophet*

The 4th and 10th houses have long been the subject of controversy: which relates to the mother and which to the father? For
our purposes, I will regard both houses as indicating our *image*,
and therefore experience, of our parents. The 4th house describes
the 'hidden' parent,[7] the one less present physically or emotionally, and therefore more unknown and mysterious. Considering
that many men 'marry their mothers', and that in our culture
fathers are often absent all day from the home, it is perhaps not
surprising that many astrologers find in practice that the IC
usually refers to the father.

Chiron in the 4th house highlights the relationship with the
father. He may have been experienced as wounding and hurtful,
or inadequate in some important respect; the relationship may
have been fraught with conflict. He might be totally unknown,
having died or left before the child was born. He could have been a
priest or doctor, a Chironian healer or saviour-figure, with which
neither mortal son nor suitor can compete. The variations are
endless, but the nature of the wound is usually described by
Chiron's sign, and the aspects to it. For example, one man with
Chiron in Sagittarius in the 4th house was always in conflict with
his father, overtly about religious issues (Sagittarius). The father
was a staunch Catholic, but his own Chiron in the 4th house in
Sagittarius was restlessly searching beyond this inherited religion.
After one argument which threatened to erupt into physical
violence, the young man left home. At the time, Neptune was
exactly conjunct his 4th-house Chiron, also activating a 12th-

house Sun/Pluto conjunction which trines Chiron natally and describes the emotional volcano which accompanied his departure; his leaving home was experienced by the whole family as a wounding event (Chiron in the 4th house). During this Neptune/ Chiron transit, he contracted polio (Neptune signifies wasting and paralysis), which left him partly crippled. His bitterness was later healed when he fathered a son, and thus became the wounded father himself.

Chiron in the 4th house in the chart of a woman may accompany the theme of an incestuous desire for her father. Whether or not there is explicit sexual contact, the 'family romance' may have been between father and daughter, not father and mother, and such a woman may continue this pattern by always falling in love with men who are unattainable. If the father was the only parent, or showed more empathy than the mother, the woman may later try to fulfil unmet mothering needs through men: women also can 'marry their mothers'. Whether the conscious attitude to her father is one of idealization or contempt, a woman with this placement is often fixated on him – or indeed, he is fixated on her: he is God, and he must be obeyed. Sometimes women must struggle to avoid identifying with strong images or 'anima figures' that their fathers may have projected in the form of expectations about how they should or should not be. It can be difficult, however, to risk the fear of rejection and disapproval that might follow should one step outside the image and 'disobey'. For example, one woman with Chiron in the 4th house in Gemini was encouraged from an early age by her father to value intellectual pursuits; she went to university flying high on the energy of her father's approval. However, as her horoscope showed an emphasis on water and fire signs, she eventually felt as though she were firing on her weak cylinder; her studies became a torment, and she became very unhappy. She left after her first year, although quitting felt a frightening thing to do, because it meant 'leaving father'.

If separation does not occur, a woman with Chiron in the 4th house can become 'Daddy's little princess', getting her own way either by flattery and seduction or by more high-handed means. For example, a woman with Chiron in the 4th house in Libra judged her father for lacking cultural sophistication, and felt contempt for him. Later she became very snobbish, which alienated many people who could have been her friends (Chiron in Libra, wounding her relationships). Eventually, she realized that she was 'doing it for father': the strident quality of her cultural pretensions came from her father's unfulfilled longing to be sophisticated and artistically educated. She had sensed his pain and wanted to alleviate it, yet also felt contempt for him.

The 4th house is also our 'point of deepest sustainment and most secure foundation for the building of anything that is to rise above the ground',[8] in the words of Dane Rudhyar. It refers to our personal history, our ancestry, the psychic and emotional inheritance that we received from our family. It is our roots, ultimately our rootedness in the inner core of ourselves. A plant absorbs nutrients from the earth through its roots; they anchor it so that it does not blow away. Likewise the 4th house is about needs, receiving nourishment, standing our ground, being anchored and rooted in the soil of our inner being.

With Chiron in the 4th house or in Cancer, our wound is inevitably connected with early mothering and basic security needs. Many a person with this placement feels a longing to reunite with mother, outrage at being cast out in birth, the search for a home, for belonging and security. With this placement we may be forced on a long inner journey to find our roots within our own psyche, a journey prompted by a feeling of being exiled from human life. Eventually, strength comes from an inner sense that all life belongs to us and we do not need to possess it because we already have it. One woman, after a strong transpersonal experience, said she had realized that 'we are all babies in the womb of the universe'.

The issue of belonging is frequently externalized and idealized, however, and we then sacrifice our own feelings and potentials in order to belong to another person or group. Feeling homeless, we search for a womb where we can stay forever safely contained by mother: 'Take care of me and I'll be anything you want me to be', is the unspoken attitude to others. We may belong to a Capricornian structure, such as a business corporation, a school or society where principles are important, but we still feel like exiles.

However, the womb that we choose usually has strong boundaries which eventually curtail our development, like a shell that has become too small for the growing crab, and we must then fight to get out. Life begins to feel like a series of prisons or 'bad wombs', until, like Jonah in the belly of the whale, we are forced to retreat for sustenance into our inner depths, where within ourselves we may find our spiritual origins.

With Chiron in Cancer, mother may have been experienced as wounding on account of specific traumas or sudden separations that have left us feeling stunned and unable to figure out what on earth happened; we may then conclude that we did something wrong, and later on tend to be over-sensitive to disapproval. Peter Fonda has Chiron in Cancer in the 2nd house; when he was ten years old he shot himself in the stomach (ruled by Cancer) in response to his mother's suicide. A woman with Chiron in Cancer in the 2nd house has a vivid memory of her mother saying to her: 'You don't exist!' Later she was unable to be independent emotionally and financially (2nd house). Because all that existed was mother, she broke down when her own daughter left home: if she was not being mother, as instructed, she did not exist.

The Chiron-in-Cancer wound is one which all humanity shares: that of the original ejection from the womb and separation from the mother. If you have Chiron in Cancer, you are very sensitive to the emotional suffering of others, and able to empathize with them; people find it easy to express their feelings, especially their pain, in your presence. You have an ability to nourish others emotionally, to accept them when at their most vulnerable without feeling threatened. However, your difficulty may be with relationships not modelled on the mother/child dyad, in which you are supremely comfortable, and which you may never leave. You find separation difficult; you need to be needed and can even resort to subtle emotional deals in order to recreate 'umbilical unity' with people. You do not find it easy to let others be independent, and might become very crabby if your role as nurturer and good breast is threatened. If you feel your good intentions abused, you can be quite vitriolic and hold grudges.

If you have Chiron in Cancer you might have difficulty

receiving emotional and/or physical nourishment, always feeling hungry and full of longing, starving in the midst of plenty. You then hide away: you feel too vulnerable to open yourself to receiving nourishment from others, but shrivel inside your protective shell. Your stomach could be a vulnerable area of your body, and express the strong emotions that you feel; you might translate into physical hunger your other emotional needs, eating when what you really need is emotional sustenance. The naturally cyclic life-rhythm typical of Cancerians may be disturbed or unconscious when Chiron is in Cancer; it could be useful to become aware of the ebb and flow of the tides of your energy so that you do not unwittingly go against this, when you may become over-emotional and clingy, or morose and withdrawn.

Men with Chiron in Cancer often spend at least the first half of their lives 'in the womb': they choose partners who are 'good mothers', and perhaps envy the attention given to their children. Divorce or separation hits them very hard, as the original wound of separation from the mother is opened up again. Once they have come to terms with this, however, such men turn out to have strong nurturing abilities and a well-developed connection with their inner world; they are often psychically intuitive and know what is happening to those they love even at a distance.

Those with Chiron in Cancer or the 4th house may have come from a family that has been hurtful through overt bullying or sadistic emotional manipulations in the name of 'fun' or 'good-intentioned teasing'. If we are mocked or accused of melodrama when we express our emotions, we learn that they are not welcome or acceptable, that we must try and hide them from others, or worse, from ourselves. Then we become manipulative or emotionally explosive, and spend much energy trying to control and suppress our feelings (shades of Capricorn here). It may take some time for us to learn how to defend ourselves against further emotional wounding, especially in close relationships where issues of dependence come into focus.

Walt Disney has Chiron in Capricorn in the 4th house. His chart provides an interesting comparison with that of Werner Heisenberg, mentioned in the section on Chiron in Gemini and the 3rd house (p. 115): Their birth-times are only a few hours apart, but their respective house positions of Chiron clearly illustrate their unique contributions to the world. Heisenberg, with Chiron in Capricorn in the 3rd house, gave form (Capricorn) to inspired new ideas (3rd house) in the field of science. Walt Disney, through his films, gave form (Capricorn) and expression to simple and childlike sentiments and feelings (4th house), using cartoon characters which became household names. His work has universal appeal not only because it expresses archetypal themes and stories in contemporary form, but also because it retrieves and portrays their feeling tone and content (4th house). Although some condemn him as sentimental, he has touched the hearts of millions of children and adults alike with his films. We see mirrored the rawness and directness of our own feeling child. The path for many people with Chiron in Cancer is discovering, and caring for, the vulnerable, needy child *within*; when we become the healing mother to ourselves, this ends the search for the accepting womb.

Chiron in Leo and the Fifth House

> The lion sits within his cage,
> Weeping tears of ruby rage . . .
>
> Stevie Smith, 'The Zoo'

The 5th house concerns the time in childhood when we begin to separate from mother and encounter the world of father, a change in focus which symbolizes the birth of a separate sense of individuality. The child, both human and divine, is also an image of the self, whose hallmarks are joy in life, spontaneous self-expression, innocence and simplicity, and love that radiates from the heart. This house describes how we enjoy ourselves: here we have romantic encounters which may be brief but touch us deeply and make us feel special; here we also experience our inner nature and are rejuvenated through the process of creative expression.

With Chiron in Leo or the 5th house, our ability to be spontaneous can be wounded; we feel unable to let go and enjoy the moment in a carefree way, or, when we do, we perhaps go to potentially destructive extremes. Often those with this placement have had their spontaneity severely crushed during childhood and are hypersensitive to ridicule. Some deal with this by playing the clown, pre-empting ridicule by *making* people laugh at them. Others develop a noble, almost regal persona, always seeming cool and in control; they make *others* feel scruffy and ridiculous.

Our creativity and capacity for self-expression may be wounded with this Chiron placement. In childhood perhaps we had to forgo a cherished creative outlet, or were forced to be showpieces for our creative parents – the 'watch little Johnny play his violin' syndrome! A physical injury or inexplicable failure may have aborted a promising career in the performing arts. I have met several people with this placement who 'failed' in their own careers in the performing arts but who became very gifted at fostering, promoting and facilitating creativity and self-expression in others, often through techniques that address the whole person rather than merely teaching skills. For example, one woman became an art-therapist; another, rather than taking it up as a career, used writing as a means of connecting with her inner experience. One woman with Chiron in the 5th house loved to play the piano as a child, but had to give it up when her family came by hard times financially and sold the piano. At her Chiron opposition, she remembered this love which was in painful contrast to the nature of her life then, with no creative outlets. She tried taking lessons again, but did not enjoy them; struggling to play the piano opened up a great deal of pain that dated from the time she had to stop. This prompted her to seek help, and thus began her inner journey of self-discovery – another important theme of this Chiron placement. Eventually she was able to mourn the loss of this creative potential and trust that something else would grow in its place.

If Chiron is in the 5th house or Leo, we might have learned early on that what we express is not welcome. Urine and faeces are our first creations and, depending on our parents' attitude to our excretions, we may come to believe that what we produce is dirty, unacceptable, and a nuisance. Later on, if we struggle to express anything genuinely our own, we may encounter inexplicable terror, creative blocks, resistance and inner conflict. We may long more than anything to release ourselves into some form of creativity, but be quite unable to. Often behind this apparent inability lie painful feelings and experiences from the past and, if we are able to embrace these wounds, the flow may unblock. Some people with Chiron in Leo or the 5th house become ill when faced with the possibility of doing something creative, especially if it involves a performance in front of an audience. The opportunity to put themselves on show plunges them into a sense of woundedness which in turn expresses itself in physical sickness. On the one hand we may feel a lack of confidence; on the other hand, however, we may also harbour an unconscious desire to be superstars shining brighter than anything else in the environment, heroes or heroines of enormous proportions. Usually people are more aware of the former, and may have great difficulty with their need for admiration. A little boasting in front of the mirror goes a long way for those with Chiron in Leo or the 5th house, as they may be using a lot of energy trying to keep their fantasy superstars under wraps!

The generation born between late 1940 and mid 1943 has produced several megastars with a characteristically Leonine flavour; all of them also have Pluto in Leo, which increases the intensity of their drive to express themselves no matter what the cost. Janis Joplin and Jimi Hendrix are two people with Chiron in Leo who expressed themselves with almost superhuman intensity; they bared their souls on-stage, expressing pain and joy that were both personal and collective. The self-expression of those with Chiron in Leo or the 5th house can be raw, visceral and uninfluenced by concern for what others might think, even revelling in being offensive or iconoclastic.

With this Chiron placement, although we may wish for beauty, fame and adulation, these may be denied us. We perhaps put others on a pedestal; then the curse of envy may get to work, like the queen in *Snow White* raging at not being 'the fairest of them all'. If these uncomfortable feelings of wanting to spoil the success, good fortune and artistic achievements of others are not acknowledged, we may gradually sour and destroy the things we have created in our own life. We merely perpetuate our sense of woundedness by hiding our creative aspirations, by pretending they are not important, or by denigrating things that really do matter to us. We often fear others' envy, and may attract envious and vindictive people into our lives when we risk being creative.

With Chiron in the 5th house or Leo, it may be useful for us to distinguish between creating to impress others and to gain power and prestige, and creating for the sheer joy of it. One woman with Chiron in Leo had such high standards of what she was supposed to achieve (shades of Aquarian perfectionism) that she was eventually unable to enjoy any creative endeavour, having failed in her career as an actress. On her second Chiron square, she went into therapy and began drawing and painting images from her dreams. Rather than trying to achieve an external standard of excellence, she began to participate in the creative process itself and to feel healed by it. This in turn enabled a deep insecurity to surface, which she had staved off in the 'futile struggle' to become a famous actress. Eventually she began to view the whole of life as a creative process, in which we are both creators and also continually being created and recreated. This perspective is indeed a gift of this placement: living creatively does not necessarily mean painting pictures or writing poems.

With Chiron in Leo or the 5th house, we may be incurably naive, believing that, if we behave nobly, then life will treat us accordingly. If it repeatedly does not, however, we may become perplexed or depressed. Although we have faith in people's basic goodness, we may also long to be saved from the meanness of the world and its ways. In situations that call for self-assertion, or for appropriate self-defence and creative retaliation, we perhaps pull back and, considering ourselves above such petty dealings, hide our fears with contempt and such attitudes as: 'I'm above that.' It is difficult for us to come to terms with the base and ignoble side of life. We prefer to see things in terms of grand gestures, theatrical sweeps, archetypal dramas of the heart and its passions. We might view with disgust the mediocrity, pettiness and self-betrayal which are part of life, yet also feel ashamed of our own meanness of heart.

Suffering may come through children if we have Chiron in Leo or the 5th house. We may be unable to have children, although greatly desiring them; they may be born ill or handicapped, or die young; we may feel wounded by them, through lack of appreciation, mutual envy, and so on. But equally, with this Chiron placement, children can bring us joy and healing through their open-heartedness, spontaneity and natural wisdom. Either way, relationships with children, whether or not they are our own, are likely to be characterized by the Chironian themes of learning experiences, wounding and healing. For example, one woman with Chiron in Leo in the 5th house felt anguish over not having had a child, and became severely depressed as she passed child-bearing age. In the course of her therapy, she rediscovered her inner child, with all its spontaneous life energy. She was a successful artist and, during this period, the style of her work and her attitude to it changed; she began to find healing for herself through full emotional participation in the process of her painting, allowing the raw Leonine passions to pour through into her work.

With Chiron in Leo or the 5th house the journey may involve finding the creative centre of our own inner being, rather than putting on a show or perfecting a creative technique. If our sense of being special is wounded, this could drive us towards ever more grandiose and perhaps futile attempts to win the appreciation from others that we lack within ourselves. However, it can also initiate an inner quest for our lost sense of self. We feel as if we are missing something; we mourn for some lost or dimly remembered spontaneity. Our journey to find this might include taking some risks in the area of self-expression; drama classes, singing lessons, or free drawing may help us to reconnect with our lost sense of self. If we can enjoy these activities for themselves, or for the healing they bring, rather than needing to impress others, a great deal of vitality can be awakened.

Having Chiron in Leo or the 5th house often makes a woman blind to the destructive side of the masculine principle. She may repeatedly experience being let down, hurt and betrayed by the men in her life, and this will probably echo her relationship with her father. She may from an early age take on masculine values, striving after excessive intellect, ambition and control at the expense of her feelings and her body. Alternatively, her masculine side could be wounded or negative (perhaps also echoing her relationship with her father), and result in difficulties with creativity. She may encounter persistent feelings of lack of self-worth or guilt should she try anything creative; she may even give up the struggle to honour her own creativity and experience it vicariously through her husband and children. Here again envy could be an issue: she may only encourage her children in directions which she would have taken herself, but did not. Equally, many people with Chiron in the 5th house or Leo have had to contend with this from a parent: in order to discover their own creativity, they have had either to conform or risk envy.

A well-known theme from the world of story, myth and legend is relevant here. An old king suffers from sickness, and his kingdom becomes increasingly sterile. The king awaits the arrival of a successor who can redeem the kingdom and allow him to die in peace. He has several sons who must prove their worth, including one who (depending upon the story) may be lame, ugly or stupid. Perhaps he is mocked by his brothers, but certainly nobody considers him a suitable heir to the throne of his father. In the end, however, it is he who redeems the kingdom and succeeds his father. The image of the innocent fool (like Parsifal) who through suffering eventually becomes wise and thus redeems the kingdom, is often meaningful for people with Chiron in Leo or the 5th house.

Healing comes through accepting this apparently 'worthless son' within us, for he represents the part of us that is awkward, ill-adapted and unsophisticated, the part that feels inferior and infantile. The sterile kingdom of our lives may indeed be redeemed through coming to terms with past experiences of failure, rejection and suffering, a coming to terms that brings compassion for our own pain and that of others. On the other hand, people with this placement often play the tragic hero or heroine, preoccupied with their pain, their inner dramas and their tragedy, and in this way lose both the momentum of their journey and also any sense that there could be a purpose to it. The 'sick old king' often represents repressive and negative experiences that we suffered in the childhood home, and can be connected with the father. If these patterns are internalized they become a restrictive and punishing super-ego, a wounding internal critic who tears down our creative efforts and whose negative attitude spoils our joy in life. With Chiron in Leo or the 5th house, any change in this pattern seems to require that we embrace our own suffering: then our Parsifal nature may come to the fore. This means the desire to take responsibility for the health and expression of our inner being, and the commitment to build the kingdom of our life in accordance with it. We then receive the gift of deep respect for our own inner self and that of others, as well as the ability to see and honour the spark of divinity within everyone.

Chiron in Virgo and the Sixth House

> If you have love, you will do all things well.
>
> Thomas Merton

In the 6th house we develop discrimination, and begin defining ourselves by what we are not (in Leo and the 5th house we still think of everything as an extension of ourselves); we begin thinking reflectively and desire self-improvement; we develop skills and the perseverance to apply them. Virgo is the sign of the harvest, where we acknowledge and receive the fruits of our labour, and then work to perfect and improve them.

With Chiron in Virgo or the 6th house, control is often an issue – either too much or too little! Life in general and the body in particular may be controlled rigidly, or subjected to disciplines of exercises and special diets. Purity and order is important to us, and we may feel the need to be constantly organizing our thoughts, our life and others in an attempt to ward off the chaos that always seems to be just around the corner. We might have to learn through trial and error what can be controlled and what cannot. We eventually find relief through learning to accept chaotic emotions and/or practical situations. By risking the delegation of responsibilities to others we see that the universe does not fall apart if we don't organize it all.

Virgo rules the intestines, and with Chiron here we may have difficulty with processing information, thoughts, emotions and life-experience in general. We might collect scraps of material, photographs, ideas or information without being able to digest them and create something of our own; we find it hard to let go of an experience before it has been ordered, so that it can be filed away in our memory; we can chew on a hurtful experience for years, replaying every nuance; when under stress, we can become obsessively pragmatic, analytical and preoccupied with apparently meaningless details. However, as an example of the healing side of these qualities, note that Fritz Perls, founder of *Gestalt* therapy, had Chiron in Virgo. His techniques are characteristically Virgoan in their attention to the here-and-now details of voice, movement and posture; through this, people recognize, discriminate and separate (all Virgoan activities) conflicting parts of themselves that are usually engaged in internal dialogue or even warfare, and to enact outwardly this exchange, often releasing deep feelings in the process.

When Chiron is in Virgo or the 6th house, our emotional issues are often mirrored in a particularly direct way through physical symptoms. We may have phobias about getting serious illnesses, loathe or feel embarrassed about parts of our body, or have eating disorders. Piscean/12th-house feelings with their oceanic quality are uncomfortably close, and we may eat to give ourselves a sense of substance, to conceal our fear of dissolution, or to intercept deep feelings or instinctual drives which threaten to overwhelm our Virgoan control. Alternatively, we may starve ourselves to keep matter and substance at bay, taking some comfort in controlling our own bodies. With this placement, however, our bodies not only serve to connect us with the emotional pains of our past, but also are sources of healing, vitality and powerful sexuality.

Some people with Chiron in Virgo or the 6th house seem to bypass the analytical mind altogether, being instead rather Piscean/12th house in nature, hiding from others their obsessive Virgoan qualities. Those with this placement are often able to organize for others, but not for themselves. They can be rather 'spaced out', disorganized and chaotic, but are sometimes also very mediumistic. Bernadette of Lourdes, whose horoscope is explored in Chapter 9, had Chiron in Virgo, as does the woman whose visionary dream features in the Epilogue.

With this placement, there is often an experience of sterility on some level. We may be unable to have children, or to give substance to our thoughts; even if we should do both, however, we may subjectively feel sterile, a source of great pain. If we learn to bear this wound gracefully without lapsing into bitterness, we may be able to rediscover motherhood or fatherhood in another way, by working in the caring professions, by teaching, or by providing assistance and positive guidance to those who ask. We may have to be beware of a periodic sense of martyrdom and the accompanying feelings of guilt and blame; these are the less pleasant aspects of the 6th/12th axis, and result from dedicating ourselves to serving others without taking enough care of ourselves. This placement of Chiron gives us the gift of instinctively understanding how to foster and cultivate the best in others and ourselves.

If you have this placement, typically 12th-house/Piscean activities or experiences can facilitate healing for you, and you are probably instinctively drawn to these. Periods of solitude in which to let things dissolve quietly, being near the sea, or getting drunk and chaotic are some typical ways of releasing the tension of this placement. Taking care of your body, learning its dietary needs and its particular signals, will also be helpful, for emotional issues, life-stresses and activities which are leading you off-balance will immediately take their toll physically. Instead of regarding this as a nuisance, try opening an on-going dialogue with what your body is experiencing, and you may be surprised at how it can guide and support you. Learning how to allow the wisdom of the body to speak and how to listen to it is often a feature of the journey of those with Chiron in Virgo or the 6th house.

Healing the split between spirit and body, between corporeal and non-corporeal is an important theme here, as, in my opinion, Chiron is exalted in Virgo. Archetypally, the image of the Black Madonna has associations with this sign and symbolizes this union. Statues and shrines of the Black Madonna are relatively rare, but are renowned for producing miracles and healing.[9] They are sometimes located on sites where pagan goddesses, such as Diana of Ephesus, were once worshipped. The Black Madonna represents a bridge between the older fertility cults and the more recent images of the Virgin Mary, which, in contrast, are somewhat asexual. Sometimes – for example, Our Lady of Guadalupe in Mexico – the Black Madonna represents a mixture of Christian and pagan ingredients from indigenous religions that still flourish and are closer to what D. H. Lawrence called 'the religion of the blood' (he has a Sun/Jupiter conjunction in Virgo, both square Chiron in Gemini).

However, in the individual psyche this image is usually split in half, and the two figures resulting may be at odds with each other: the Virgin and the Whore.[10] With Chiron in the 6th house or in Virgo, one of these figures may be apparently absent, wounded or indeed inflated, and profound healing usually accompanies the recognition and acceptance of both. One figure may be prominent, while the other is unconscious and erupts from time to time, as illustrated in the case study in Chapter 10. Relationships with men may be difficult for women with Chiron in Virgo or the 6th house. The Whore may seek power over men through her sexuality, exploiting them rather than relating to them, or she may abuse herself by giving herself indiscriminately to anyone. The Virgin, on the other hand, dreads physical or psychological penetration, and often defends herself against it through becoming a diffuse and compassionate mother-figure (shades of Pisces/12th house) and therefore impossible to penetrate. She may also freeze up emotionally or physically, perhaps withdrawing from sexual relationships altogether. She may have pseudo-Platonic relationships with men, where the sexual undertones are never openly acknowledged and often sour into a mutually critical and destructive liaison which seems to give each partner a curious sense of sado-masochistic satisfaction. Positively, however, this placement of Chiron represents the opportunity for a woman to travel on a journey of spiritual unfoldment firmly rooted in the body, a journey which is not a mortification of the flesh, but an exaltation of it. The ancient image of the temple priestess, discussed in Chapter 4, is perhaps another guiding image for this placement.

Men with this placement sometimes fear and seek to control women, or display the 'split anima' pattern, alternating between these two figures in the women they fall in love with or choose to marry. One man with Chiron in Virgo was a devout Roman Catholic who regularly prayed to the Virgin Mary; he eventually sought help because his compulsion to visit prostitutes was driving him into debt. Another was emotionally shattered by the discovery that his docile wife was earning pocket-money through prostitution while he worked night-shifts. In each case, it was the appearance of both opposites together that precipitated a crisis which was ultimately one of healing.

Virgo is traditionally associated with crafts and skills, including those of medicine (especially herbalism and homoeopathy); these enhance the quality of our earthly life, and involve the working of actual materials. To make and perfect a skill with patience and care can almost enslave a person to the process. People with this placement will often be heard to say, for example, 'But I cannot imagine life without being a violinist (or a teacher, etc.).' If our chosen craft or vocation is a suitable vehicle of expression for our true nature, we will find fulfilment and meaning through work and service. But if it is not, this will be a potential crisis area, and the 6th-house area of life will be painful. It will then be difficult to apply ourselves to the task at hand; practical details will elude us and domestic life have no order.

To be apprenticed to a service or craft requires surrender to the process of creativity, a willingness to reap the harvest of what we have sown, to follow through and guide our children or perfect our creations. However, if we are too obsessed with 'getting it right', this urge to improve, craft and perfect things may invert into a drive for perfection which withers everything it touches. It is sometimes this that lies behind the sterility that plagues some people with this placement. For Chiron in Virgo or the 6th house is rather about learning to work *with* the imperfections inherent in life incarnate, accepting them and including them. To quote Marion Woodman: 'Somewhere in us there is a perfect image, a perfect work of art, a well-wrought mask that is cutting us off from our own flesh and blood.'[11] If this is our wound, we might become slave-drivers, intolerant of our own and others' 'imperfections' and weaknesses, and feel compelled to present ourselves through a perfect mask. However, learning to accept that which is imperfect, wounded, ugly or messy is both the trial and the gift of this placement.

People with Chiron in Virgo or the 6th house are often keen on self-development, and if they work in the healing field they can unwittingly be seduced by this drive towards perfection. Where there is glib talk of curing depressions or 'becoming who you truly are', we may need to determine whether this is merely a subtle kind of exorcism of anything not perfect and ideal, or a genuinely organic growth process seeking a wholeness which can include our imperfections. People with this placement can eventually develop a deep acceptance and compassion for others, although their own self-acceptance is often a long time coming. Equally, their drive to perfect themselves or their craft may leave them no peace, unless they are working for wholeness rather than perfection, as described above. To quote Jung on the subject, 'The individual may strive after perfection . . . but must suffer from the opposite of his intentions for the sake of completeness.'[12]

Virgo also traditionally has links with the employer/employee, slave/master, guru/disciple relationship. People with Chiron in Virgo or the 6th house often find that work colleagues open up their deepest wounds. One woman with this placement worked as a technical assistant to an art-teacher and fell in love with him; after a tempestuous affair, he returned to his wife and their relationship could go no further. Through this painful situation, she became aware of the hitherto unconscious side of her relationship with her father, and this in turn began a process of healing. Sometimes people with this placement have difficulty with issues of equality in a relationship, and assume a teaching role or believe that they know what is best for someone. Superiority and aloofness can result; although they are often unaware of this, and genuinely astonished at people's reactions to their well-meant gestures, which come across as gross interference. Some people with Chiron in Virgo or the 6th house habitually take on the role of the inferior or the servant. A gift of this placement, however, is the ability to serve life as a whole by serving one's true self and that of others. Beyond the wound of too much control and separateness may lie a profound sense of connection with all of life, and an experience of being totally interpenetrated by it.

Chiron in Libra and the Seventh House

> I searched, but I could not find Thee; I called
> Thee aloud, standing on the minaret; I rang the
> temple bell with the rising and setting of the sun . . .
> I looked for Thee on the earth; I searched for Thee
> in the heavens, my Beloved, but at last I have found Thee
> hidden as a pearl in the shell of my heart.
>
> Hazrat Inayat Khan, *Gayan, Vadan, Nirtan*

With this placement, relationships are of prime importance, and Chiron will be met here in all his varying facets; we may walk into the fire and be hurt many times. This situation is often a repetition of our early relationship with the parent of the opposite sex, and can make us believe that relationships are dangerous and should be avoided, or at least approached in full battle-gear. This may lead us into sorrow, isolation and defensiveness until we have recognized the source of the repetition. Our early environment may have been characterized by destructive relating, or perhaps non-relating, a mask of politeness being kept up to conceal hostility, vengeance, and competitiveness (shades of the first house and Aries).

We may, therefore, have learned more how to defend ourselves than how to form relationships, and matters are complicated by the enemy being essentially unseen: feelings that are not expressed can wound us more than feelings which are openly acknowledged, even if they are unpleasant. We may have learned how to please everyone, how to be all things to all people, how to smooth over potential conflicts. We may have an overdose of Libran diplomacy and tact, leaving us fearful, brittle and defensive, for, with Chiron in Libra or the 7th house, we are more than usually disturbed by interpersonal conflict, perhaps because of this overt or subterranean conflict in the early environment. Paradoxically, here may be another example of the wound being healed by the sword that inflicted it: with Chiron in Libra or the 7th house, we are empowered by learning how to stay creatively in situations fraught with conflict, how to fight cleanly and trust the relationship through the process.

In Libra and the 7th house we also first meet the 'other': both 'other' people different from us, and also our own internal 'other', the shadow or unconscious side of our nature. Qualities represented by planets in the 7th house are often first met 'out there', projected on to others towards whom we experience strong emotions. With Chiron in Libra or the 7th house, many learning experiences come through recognizing ourselves through the mirror of others, and also by learning to respect others' differences and separateness. 'Where there is other, there is fear', is a saying in the Upanishads. This Chiron placement increases our tendency to react to people as if they are extensions of ourselves; our emotional reactions to others may be more to do with ourselves than with them. We could experience difficulties in relationships where others seem to fight us: in reality they are fighting not to be the image we project upon them. Situations of emotional bondage may develop in this way; relationships may eventually become wounding for both people concerned and probably will self-destruct.

As Chiron's image already involves an uneasy yoking of irreconcilables, when it is in the 7th house, it increases the tendency to enact our Chiron issues vicariously. For example, we might unconsciously cast ourselves into one of the roles associated with Chiron: the wounded one, the healer or teacher, the apprentice, the outcast, the saviour, the hero and the one who wounds. We then attract to us people who represent the opposite; indeed, with this Chiron placement, we learn a lot about ourselves by looking at the kind of people we are drawn to, and who are drawn to us, as they symbolize our own potentials or weaknesses. For example, if we always attract 'lame ducks', it might mean that we are not acknowledging a painful failure of our own, or that we need these people in order to feel powerful; if we always relate to dominating people, it may mean we are not owning up to our own power. If we frequently end up feeling victimized in relationships, we will need slowly to discover the mechanisms with which we unwittingly cause this to happen. For if we persist in seeing the 'one who wounds' as outside ourselves, we may blame others and ignore our own part, thus leaving ourselves open to it happening again and again. The attitude of being an innocent bystander does not work very well when Chiron is in the 7th house or Libra.

With this placement, there is often one major relationship which we experienced as very wounding, from which we cannot escape, or from which we take a long time to recover. For we meet the archetypal world through other people, and the accompanying emotional voltage and pain may be a feature of our lives. Although our relationships on one level echo a relationship with a parent, with this Chiron placement healing often seems to come through recognizing the archetypal level. For example, one woman, whom I shall call Veronica, had Chiron in Scorpio in the 7th house; her mother had Sun conjunct Pluto in Gemini, and had several mental breakdowns during which she would lash out verbally in storms of abuse over trivial things. Later, Veronica lived in fear of this happening with others, and was always on tenterhooks; she did indeed have several relationships which included similar episodes of sudden critical outbursts. During the course of her therapy, she allowed her feelings of fear and outrage to be elaborated through drawing and painting. An archetypal figure, whom she called the Death Woman, emerged: 'the enemy of life, who could strike you down without warning, when you least expect it.' Working with this, Veronica realized that she had not yet come to terms with the fact of death: it was always 'out there', personified as her mother, and later others, waiting to cut her down. Working with this figure over time while transiting Pluto was conjunct this 7th-house, Chiron she began a process of slowly reclaiming her own sense of power.

With Chiron in Libra or the 7th house, we could have unwanted periods of separation and isolation forced upon us. We might continue in hurtful relationships until one day we feel: 'That's it! I've had enough', and we close the shutters of our hearts and cut ourselves off from people. However, this withdrawal can also be a creative time, if we are able to use the space behind the barrier to do some soul-searching and discover what is really happening. With this placement, we have a strong need to be separate, and an equally strong resistance to it. We periodically need space and distance from others to reclaim what we may have projected on to them. We might also tend to displace our feelings and emotions. For example, someone with Chiron in the 7th house was in a relationship in which he felt constricted, hurt and unappreciated; as he had difficulty confronting the situation directly, he tended to vent his feelings elsewhere – the 'kick the dog' syndrome! His feelings of anger spread into several other relationships, which all suffered and became increasingly strained and unreal; he longed to escape them all and be totally alone.

With Chiron in Libra or the 7th house, we learn a great deal through encountering the less pleasant aspects of relationships: the Martian qualities of Aries and the 1st house are echoed here. We could become involved in subterranean power struggles, wanting only to relate on our terms and surreptitiously asserting our own will. We are very competitive, but perhaps blissfully unaware of it; we could unconsciously provoke others and stir up conflict in order to divert ourselves from our own inner tension. Conversely, we might also be very afraid of these qualities and fall foul of them in others. However, with Chiron in Libra or the 7th house, we might need to accept the fact that not everyone is going to like us if we are being true to ourselves, and that having enemies does not make us bad people. Your sense of individuality need not stand or fall on whether others like it.

If we are in a relationship with someone who has Chiron in Libra or the 7th house, we need to learn to stand our own ground and not get drawn into being their opposite number. Although those with this placement long to grow through being challenged in relationships, they often make it difficult for this to happen, as their own wound or blind spot is in this very area; we are likely to receive venomous reprisals or stony silences if we tread near it. On the other hand, if we do not, the relationship may grind to a halt. People with this placement are very sensitive to being judged or scrutinized; they may experience the feeling of separateness as an attack, or judge us as cold and detached. They have a horror of being irrational and unfair, and may therefore be over-diplomatic and cautious in expressing their feelings. They are often afraid of their own negative feelings, which can build up and erupt in scenes of mutual accusation. It seems that with Chiron in Libra or the 7th house, if we cannot honour the need to be alone, separate and unrelated, we will act it out literally: we (or our partner) may pack our bags and go, when a little more emotional honesty might have sufficed.

People with Chiron in Libra or the 7th house seem often to marry or have close relationships with people who work in the healing field. They might even assume the role of the wounded one, and, in this case, a very destructive situation results. People who have one or both parents who are doctors, priests, healers or teachers are especially vulnerable to this. A woman with Chiron conjunct Neptune and Jupiter on the MC in Libra was the daughter of a lay minister, and she later married a man who was a doctor. She was crisis-prone, with frequent emotional collapses and serious physical symptoms; the relationship continued for many years, in spite of the palpably destructive quality of it. Predictably, the career of her husband, the 'healer' half, flourished while she took on the role of the Sick One! During the marriage, she had several intense affairs, in which she was usually the 'healer', or served as a catalyst for the other man; at these times her husband was plunged into his own woundedness.

People with Chiron in Libra or the 7th house have a great deal to offer in areas of healing where the quality of the relationship is a central factor. Although relationships are important in any therapeutic situation, these people excel when the dynamics of relating are worked with directly and consciously – for example, in situations of transference as encountered in psychoanalytic therapy. This is yet another example of the wound being healed by the spear that caused it. There is a version of Chiron's story in which he took a wounded Centaur into his cave. Because the wound was poisoned with the blood of the Hydra, it infected Chiron, who thus received his incurable wound. People with Chiron in Libra or the 7th house who work in the field of healing may find themselves always confronted with their own pain through their clients. This placement gives the gift of being in touch with both the human and the archetypal levels within relationships. The experience of being truly seen in this way can be very healing, and those with Chiron in Libra or the 7th house have much to offer those to whom they relate, both in terms of insight and also in terms of the ability to 'let them have their space'. Ira Progoff has Chiron in Aries in the 7th house. He was the originator (Chiron in Aries) of a system of journal-keeping for personal psychological growth. He was initially trained as a Jungian analyst, and worked within the traditional dyadic analytic relationship (7th house). Later he came to question the validity of this method: true to Chiron in Aries, he had to go his own way. His Chiron in the 7th is expressed in his belief that true spiritual growth could only occur through relating privately and deeply to one's inner world (Chiron in the 7th), without dependence on another person (Chiron in Aries).

Finally, in the *Oresteia* the goddess Athene appears as a figure of reconciliation, justice and respect for potentially negative forces; she provides us with an evocative image of Chiron in the 7th house or Libra. Athene was as famous for her prowess in battle as for her benevolence in peace and her civilizing influence: she never actively provoked a battle, but nor did she ever lose one. In the *Oresteia* Orestes slays his mother to avenge the murder of his father, and thus invokes the wrath of the Furies who pursue him relentlessly into exile and madness. He finally seeks refuge in the temple of Athene, and she appoints a court to decide his fate, a suitably Libran scenario. However, the votes are equally divided, and Athene herself has the casting vote: she sets Orestes free, purging him of blood-guilt, but thus invoking the rage of the Furies upon herself. She gradually wins them over with respect: 'I will bear with your anger. You are older.' She assures them that: 'No house can thrive without you.' She guarantees them a place in the new order 'where pain and anguish end', and actually begs them to stay.[13] Eventually, their wrath is appeased by her compassionate persuasiveness, her frank admission of the similarities between herself and the Furies, and her willingness to include and respect them. Likewise, with Chiron in Libra, we might continually be 'confronted by the Furies' in relationships, until we learn to include and respect their world without being dragged back into it. For just as the 7th house and Libra represent another important threshold of separation, here the Furies of our own regressive desires may confront us, and Athene's treatment of them perhaps provides a metaphor of how to proceed.

Chiron in Scorpio and the Eighth House

All men are so shining-bright
as if they were going to the great sacrificial feast . . .
Only I am reluctant, I have not yet been given a sign:
like an infant, yet unable to laugh;
unquiet, roving as if I had no home.
All men have abundance,
Only I am as if forgotten.
I have the heart of a fool: so confused, so dark . . .
as if locked into myself . . .
All men have their purpose,
only I am futile like a beggar . . .
But I consider it worthy
to seek nourishment from the Mother.

Lao Tzu, *Tao Te Ching*

In Scorpio and the 8th house we seek personal transformation, to overcome our separateness and become more than ourselves; we grow through our deep encounters with others and our desire to be at one with them. Here we find the powerful themes of sexuality, birth, death, loss and abandonment, emotional destructiveness, rebirth and regeneration. Through this house and sign we may be reborn through experiencing deep feelings from pre-verbal times that were hitherto buried, but which surface within our intimate and sexual relationships; these may resemble emotional mine-fields. With Chiron in Scorpio or the 8th house, our deepest wounds are present, and our emotional lives may be fixated at an infantile stage. Thus it is important to become familiar with the emotional life of our early instinctual self, with its extremes of rage, greed, destructive envy, love and guilty depression, as well as its deep vitality and capacity to thrive, important also to experience deeply the positive side of our emotional life and connection with others.

With this placement, we may encounter death very early in our life, for example in severe birth trauma as illustrated in Chapter

10; we may have had a life-threatening illness, lost a parent very early, or had near-death experiences. Freud believed that there were two powerful but contrary drives within us, one towards life (*Eros*) and the other towards death (*Thanatos*). Although this is a controversial idea, it will probably make sense to us if we have Chiron in Scorpio or the 8th house, for we are often uncomfortably aware of our own destructiveness or fascination with death. *Thanatos* may sometimes feel like the stronger of the two, making us very aware of the frailty of life. We may then become very controlling of others to try and protect ourselves against loss and abandonment. We may also meet this in the area of money, struggling hard and perhaps failing to gain financial independence. Like any Scorpionic type, however, we are adept at hiding our vulnerability and dependency behind moodiness, or a façade of being powerful and inscrutable.

Many people with this placement have suicidal feelings at some point in their lives, and fantasies about suicide and death frequently accompany major changes and transitions. This can be seen as an expression of the desire to return to the source. This source, with Chiron in Scorpio or the 8th house, is not a rarefied and transcendent spiritual source; the desire is rather to return to the deep womb of the primordial Mother, to a rich darkness and a kind of cellular consciousness from which to be reborn. A useful question to reflect on might be: 'What *within me* needs to die in order that I can be reborn?' Personal growth is often rather tumultuous with this placement, and sometimes everything feels like a matter of life and death.

In some primitive societies, it is believed that there is only a certain quota of good in the world, and so if someone starts to outshine his peers he is taking something away from others. Similar feelings are present in those with Chiron in Scorpio or the 8th house, who often feel inexplicably nervous and guilty at every success they achieve, and expect that disaster will follow any minute. Needless to say, it often does, and a little black humour goes a long way with this placement! We might have low self-esteem, easily feeling bad, worthless and somehow wrong; underneath, we perhaps fear our own potential destructiveness, and develop a rigorous emotional control designed to protect others from it. With this placement our unconscious emotional destructiveness can be projected on to others; we then become rather paranoid or preoccupied with warding off the imagined or actual persecutor, trying to outwit or placate him. We might read a potential threat into situations where, in reality, although it might be there, it is not necessarily directed against us personally. We may also tend inwardly to assume blame for misunderstandings or things that go wrong with others. We can be superstitious over small things; for example, we may feel doomed to a bad day if our bus is late! All this can be described as a negative inflation, where we identify with our imagined badness, and may indicate deep wounds from our pre-verbal life which have not yet been allowed into consciousness.

The roots of these uncomfortable feelings lie in our early relationship with mother: we want her, need her for survival, yet we fear her awesome power to fulfil or deprive us. We wish to devour her totally, to eat her up so that she can never leave us again; all our emotions are experienced in an all-consuming manner, whether positive or negative. These strong feelings are normally mitigated by enough good mothering, but with Chiron in Scorpio or the 8th house, they often resurface in our adult life when we strongly desire something, be it power, fame, sex, money, food, status or whatever. We long to fuse completely with another person, become them, and be someone other than what we are, somewhat like Chiron's mother Philyra in the myth. If someone evokes strong feelings of love and/or hate in us, we may feel ourselves to be at their mercy, and, by 'becoming them', we seek to regain some sense of power. Thus we become intensely devouring, consuming and passionate in our relationship; we want to incorporate physically and psychically the object of our desire. One person with Chiron in Scorpio had several dreams of eating people she loved. Although we are all wounded by having to separate from our mothers, with Chiron in the 8th house and Scorpio, we may take a long time to forgive those who have wounded us, and we cannot fake feelings of forgiveness. We might have an uncomfortable taste for punishment and vengeance, which we can only grow out of by acknowledging.

The uncovering of this terrain was the speciality of the

psychoanalyst Melanie Klein, whose pioneering but controversial work recently made its way into 'pop psychology' through the book *Jealousy* by Nancy Friday (well worth reading if you have this placement). Klein has Chiron conjunct Neptune, Pluto, Saturn and Jupiter all in Taurus, and trine Uranus in Virgo, a placement describing her ability to analyse (Chiron trine Uranus in Virgo) and work with powerful fantasies (Chiron conjunct Neptune) coming from areas of the psyche still intimately linked with physical and instinctual experience (Chiron in Taurus conjunct both Saturn and Pluto). Our earliest fantasies of sexuality, destruction, love and death are all typically 8th-house/Scorpio themes.

People with this placement often benefit from rebirthing therapy, as sometimes the actual birth trauma is an important focus of woundedness and therefore also of healing. The patterns established at birth may repeat at the beginning of every new cycle of life, as illustrated in Chapter 10, and healing may begin by their becoming conscious of what they are and releasing the emotions holding them. With Chiron in Scorpio or the 8th house, we know, or imagine, that we were not wanted; our birth might have severely injured our mother or created financial hardship; our mother may have unwillingly sacrificed a career in order to bear children, repressing her resentment but making us painfully aware of it. Later, 'leaving mother' in a deeper sense means leaving behind these negative self-concepts and reactions to life. With Chiron in Scorpio or the 8th house we eventually need to find the good mother within ourselves, drawing on the resources of the deep psyche to find acceptance and love for ourselves and others.

People with this placement often feel wounded in the area of their sexuality: incest, child abuse and frightening episodes of sadism, rape and violence frequently occur in their real or fantasy life. They may both give and receive tremendous wounding and/or healing through their sexual experiences – always an area of confrontation with their deepest feelings. One woman with this placement felt her partner's penis like a spear, causing not physical but psychological pain; another bled profusely from some untraceable vaginal wound when making love with a man with Chiron in Scorpio. A man with Chiron in Scorpio managed to keep sexual relationships with four or five women who all knew they were not the only one; he said he was 'determined not be possessed by any woman'. Wilhelm Reich has Chiron conjunct both Uranus in Scorpio and Saturn at the beginning of Sagittarius, and this placement suitably describes his work. He was one of the first to work directly to break down (Uranus) rigid armouring (Saturn) within the musculature of the body, releasing pent-up emotion held locked within it (Chiron and Uranus in Scorpio), and thus reawakening sexual energy and orgasmic potency (Chiron in Scorpio).

Men with this Chiron placement often experience their masculinity as having been wounded in their relationship with their mother, and may constantly seek out women more powerful than themselves; they may try to bring them down, compete with them sexually or professionally, or look up to them from a distance. However, if they can come to terms with their early feelings of powerlessness, they are very nurturing, and make loving partners, fathers, therapists or teachers, as they understand what emotional suffering feels like. Men with this placement are often very charismatic, with the typical Scorpionic aura of sexual promise and intense pent-up feelings; they are usually very attractive to women, and not above exploiting this.

With this placement, at some point we may be confronted by our power drives, our hidden motives and attempts to control and dominate others. Alternatively, we could find ourselves in situations of powerlessness containing typically Scorpionic ingredients: love-triangles, jealousy, and unconscious power-struggles. Learning about power, its use and abuse, is often a feature of the life-journey of those with Chiron in Scorpio or the 8th house. More than we realize, we could have charisma, sexual magnetism and the ability to influence people deeply through both our words and our powerful emotions. This can be abused where there are unconscious infantile patterns at work, or indeed if we pretend it is not there. For example, a woman with Chiron in Scorpio felt wounded when she inherited a considerable amount of money (an 8th-house issue), and suffered agonies when it gradually changed her life-style. She was afraid people would no longer love her just for herself; she felt despair at the power she imagined it gave her over men, whom she feared would feel castrated by her wealth, and either be envious and sponge off her, or feel too inferior to approach her sexually. Another woman, with Chiron in the 8th house, felt bitter and angry at the powerlessness that was her dominant pattern, but equally afraid of the feeling of power that rushed through her when she sought to take the reins of her life in her own hands. Eventually, by acknowledging the destructive fantasies that made her fear her own power, she was able gradually to feel more comfortable with it. Uri Geller has this placement; he can bend spoons by tele-kinesis, thus acting as an agent for a power that can affect the structure of matter. He has also earned a fortune through this gift; Pluto, ruler of the 8th house and Scorpio, is also the god of wealth! Prince Charles has Chiron conjunct his Sun, both in Scorpio in the 4th house, quincunx both Moon in Taurus in the 10th and Uranus in Gemini in the 11th. He belongs to the most powerful family in England (Chiron in Scorpio in the 4th house, of family and ancestry). He is also a controversial figure in his own right; he has become a spokesman (Moon in the 10th sextile Uranus in Gemini) on behalf of alternative medicine and other contentious issues – a suitably Chironian role (Moon in the 10th/Chiron); true to Chiron in Scorpio, he has the ability to raise or lower the temperature of public emotion and to elicit both strong criticism and passionate support. He is preparing for his future role during a time when there has been an unprecedented series of media attacks on the public image of the royal family (which is perhaps a collective expression of some of the patterns of destructive envy mentioned above). Separating personal feelings from emotionally charged political issues is often an important theme for those with Chiron in the 8th house or in Scorpio, who are sometimes prone to politicizing their feelings.

The paths of those with Chiron in Scorpio or the 8th house may take them into the 'heart of darkness', for they experience things deeply, and to outsiders might seem to dwell unnecessarily on the negative and morbid aspects of life. However, we must respect this, as we may lose their friendship if we interfere; well-meant attempts to cheer them up may provoke outbursts of rage or rejection. With Chiron in Scorpio or the 8th house, our journey usually includes a confrontation with death or the experience of emotional and mental dismemberment. However, if we can also recognize the transpersonal elements in our experience, they can lead us to inner security and regeneration; we may be reborn with trust in life, compassion and depth of personality. With this Chiron placement, we perhaps also must let go of our preoccupation with our suffering and our dark moods; our difficulty may be in allowing joy, hope and other positive experiences to touch us. This pain may be less bearable for us than the familiar pain of our suffering.

With Chiron in Scorpio or the 8th house, we see beneath the surface of life into the darkness which most people try to ignore. If we are also by nature full of sweetness and light, this is a burden, but we cannot avoid it. We may even feel our dark vision to be a punishment or a sickness, but it is really neither: Chiron in Scorpio or the 8th house brings the possibility of a deep acceptance of the dark side of life, without identifying with it or trying to change it. We are asked to encompass our own emotional depths and a wide range of positive and negative feelings; we may begin to feel more at home in life after confronting death consciously in some way. We perhaps need also to learn not to discredit or scorn the vision of others who may be more light-hearted than ourselves. People with Chiron in Scorpio or the 8th house often have a powerful presence, and others often instinctively trust them, sensing their emotional depth and familiarity with inner suffering. As healers, they may be able to reach people who are trapped in pain and darkness, for knowledge and experience of this area are their gifts.

Chiron in Sagittarius and the Ninth House

> Oh seekers, when you leave off seeking
> You will realise that there was never anything to seek
> for.
>
> D. H. Lawrence, 'Seekers'

In the 9th house we begin to expand our mental and philosophical horizons; we pursue our special interests, and search for the patterns of meaning in our personal life-experience. We broaden our understanding of life through travelling, experiencing or studying other cultures, their religions and their mythology. With Chiron as co-ruler of this house and sign, its themes are strongly expressed here.

With Chiron in Sagittarius or the 9th house, the driving force of our life is of a religious nature, although it might not appear so at first sight. Often, our inherited religious framework does not suit our inner needs, and we must travel a long and sometimes lonely path in search of our own individual meaning and purpose in life. Sometimes this search is literalized, and we become great travellers: we feel healed and nourished by making pilgrimages to shrines or holy places, and we also enjoy the food, music and customs of other cultures. Mankind has always undertaken ritual journeys of healing, whether to grand churches and famous sacred sites or simply to commune with a favourite tree. We may have recurring dreams or inner images of sacred places to which we can return in our imagination; we also feel replenished by communion with nature, particularly in wild areas. With this Chiron placement, we might have been raised in a foreign culture, or in one where our religion is not recognized; we perhaps feel persecuted by our peers for our beliefs; we could live in a country where a cultural transition is taking place; our parents might be foreigners, exiles, or hold religious beliefs that set us apart from others.

One woman with Chiron in Sagittarius in the first house and conjunct the Ascendant had several hair-raising experiences while travelling alone. Reflecting on this later, she felt she had almost deliberately exposed herself to danger to see whether God would come to her aid. She was testing whether he was there and on her side; although she had an indefinable faith in 'something', she was brought up by parents who were both atheists, and had therefore to make this inner connection without their help. With Chiron in Sagittarius or the 9th house, we may feel 'wounded by God' for some reason; perhaps our parents fought over religious issues. We will be very sensitive to ideas such as original sin and may believe that when things go wrong it means that God is angry with us; we might have a heritage of religious conflict or confusion to come to terms with.

Unlike Freud, Jung believed that the religious instinct and the search for meaning and right connection with the gods was a natural human drive, and could not be merely reduced to its biological counterparts or explained away as pathological. With Chiron in the 9th house or Sagittarius, this religious instinct often awakens very young; from childhood onwards we ponder deeper questions concerning the meaning of life, and may never receive satisfactory answers. I have met several people with this placement who in childhood came to the conclusion that 'grown-ups are stupid'!

With Chiron in the 9th house or Sagittarius, we will usually have a deeply devotional sense, a passionate zeal which longs to devote itself to something; literally anything can become our god if this religious instinct is misplaced. We may unwittingly deify food, education or even the latest cult movie, and pursue the object of our devotion with fervent enthusiasm. However, the divine discontent which is our wound cannot be satisfied in this way. A useful question might be: 'Where (or who) is the god (or goddess) in my life?' Our devotional drive could take us into perilous waters if we embrace causes or follow spiritual paths where our questions and personal beliefs (Gemini/3rd house) are swept aside in a wave of fervour. Worse, if our god (or goddess) image is projected on to a guru or leader, we may then be vulnerable to exploitation and psychological rape. As Chiron often indicates where we meet our early wounds, unless we have done some homework resolving our early parental issues, we might fall foul of them when our devotional energy is mobilized. A little Geminian rationality and light-heartedness may usefully balance our tendency to make zealous commitment to an erstwhile mentor or spiritual teacher: he or she may turn out to be merely a glorified father- or mother-figure. With Chiron in Sagittarius or the 9th house, we could become inflated with a feeling that we have found the Truth, and the desire to tell everyone else about it may wreak havoc in our personal lives. We may even limit our friendships to those who hold the same beliefs as ourselves. One can see shades of Gemini here, in the either/or stance: if I have the Truth, then I am right and you are wrong. I am doing you a favour by trying to convince or convert you, because then you too can join the elect who *know*. You cannot be right because that means I am wrong.

The importance of the religious question for this placement is illustrated in the life of a woman (I shall call her Diane) who has Chiron in Scorpio in the 9th house, square Saturn and Pluto in the 7th house (her story also clearly illustrates the themes of Chiron in aspect to Saturn and Pluto). Diane's conception and birth were preceded and surrounded by 9th-house elements. Her parents were missionaries (a 9th-house activity); three generations of her family had been actively involved in the church and mission societies. During World War II, her father was in Burma (foreign travel is a 9th-house experience). He made a bargain with God (very 9th house!) that if he got out alive, he would go to Africa and serve him by being a missionary. Eventually, he returned to England and started a theology degree (9th house) to fulfil the bargain. Diane was born during this time, her first home being the typically 9th-house environment of a university. Once her father had qualified, however, the family's departure for Africa was delayed by Diane developing primary tuberculosis. At the time, Chiron was conjunct her MC by solar arc, and exactly square her Ascendant, and we might perhaps wonder whether she was instinctively rebelling at being part of a bargain with God. Having sought a second opinion about whether it was safe to go, the family eventually went to Africa, and Diane's mother later dedicated her to Africa, in thanksgiving; her mother's Sun is conjunct Diane's Chiron in Scorpio.

Diane believes her path has been to internalize the religious drive within her family heritage. When Chiron was conjuncting her Sun by transit, her quest took her through several different religious frameworks, from Billy Graham and evangelical Christianity to Sufism; she eventually settled into another esoteric tradition. She married a man from the Caribbean, which caused a crisis in the family, forcing her parents to re-examine some of their racial attitudes, and hence their religious convictions. Chiron squares her Saturn and Pluto in the 7th house, here an image for the transformative potential of this relationship. Diane's 9th-house Chiron also addresses these themes: she married a man from a foreign country and a different race, which caused a family crisis that led to a re-evaluation of her parents' religious beliefs and a deepening of contact between all of them. In a curious way, she also fulfilled her mother's dedication of her to Africa.

With Chiron in Sagittarius or the 9th house, we might suffer because of our sense of vision and possibility, as we often have difficulty with commitment and finding a suitable direction in life. The arrows of our intuition fly everywhere, but we may be dismayed to discover that things do not happen by themselves, and feel reluctant to take active steps to make things happen. Like Chiron, we might be 'shot down' by others; the balloon of our enthusiasm and over-extension of ourselves may be pricked many times before we accept the gap between what can be made to happen and what cannot. It may cost us great pain to let go of a vision or hope, and, if our whole sense of individuality and identity is bound up with it, we could then feel as though we are dying. However, with this placement, life often brings exactly such a crisis. If we can let go, we discover that not only does our vision remain alive, but we are in fact in a healthier relationship with it, not driven by it or identified with it.

The image of the Chironian, Chiron's cave on the dark side of Mount Pelion, is an evocative one, as it points to an important aspect of the journey of those with this placement. With Chiron in Sagittarius or the 9th house, we cannot get away with a sense of vision or meaning that excludes our suffering, the painful and limiting aspects of existence, and our mortality. We need a personal philosophy of life which can embrace contradictions and different points of view without splitting them apart and setting them against each other. Finding this may be a difficult task if we were raised within a traditional Judaeo-Christian framework, where the Devil is the enemy of God and the true faith, but not really supposed to be part of it. The feminine image of deity is likewise split: on the side of the Good is motherhood, virgin or otherwise, while other feminine aspects are ignored or condemned. Women with Chiron in Sagittarius or the 9th house often have to struggle to shrug off negative attitudes resulting from the inherited Judaeo-Christian stereotype that presents women as evil and dangerous creatures who bring the temptations of the flesh and lure men away from their quest for enlightenment. They often have a natural wisdom way beyond their age and life experience, and it may initially be difficult for them to recognize or value it. In Western cultures, for many centuries most women have had no transpersonal image of a wise woman who has not rejected her sensual self. Apart from the Virgin Mary, women have had no divine image to worship, no holy name to call upon. If you are a woman with Chiron in Sagittarius or the 9th house, you might find it enriching to study the stories and images of goddesses in the great religions of the world. Both men and women with this placement are especially sensitive to images of the divine, and need an appropriate, natural expression for their urge to worship and pay homage.

With Chiron in Sagittarius or the 9th house, we may develop a tendency to see personal meaning in everything. Although we may be inspired and energized, we may get into difficulty when the meanings we find do not tally with what others find meaningful. We need to learn that meaning is not an absolute, but a subjective quality. Our facility for finding meaning can also be a defence against suffering. We may compensate for underlying feelings of despair, hopelessness and depression by strained attempts to appear positive and outgoing. Alternatively, with this placement we sometimes have difficulty finding meaning in anything at all. Underneath, however, we could be harbouring an unconscious and unfulfillable vision or hope, perhaps from childhood, like Chiron's unhealable wound. Allowing this into consciousness can bring a great sense of relief. For example, a man who had Chiron in the 9th house in Cancer became obsessed with his family's past history; he scrutinized the lives of his ancestors, suffered over their tragedies and felt a burdensome sense that he was supposed to be 'doing something about it'. He eventually realized that he was trying to take on the burden of the family's unconscious pain and heal it. He felt that he had already disappointed his parents' high hopes for him (9th house), and before he had come to terms with that, he embarked on a self-appointed but unconscious mission (Chiron in the 9th house) to feel the pain of his family's past on their behalf.

Many people with this placement receive a powerful vision of other dimensions at some time in their lives: they are infused with a strong sense of purpose and meaning, sometimes through the use of drugs and often during a strong transit of Chiron. Later they may suffer terribly, unable to continue believing what they once believed. They feel intense frustration, knowing there is something inside them which they want to give, but they cannot find a way to do it, and nor do they know what it is. Often, however, with Chiron in Sagittarius or the 9th house, the natural sense of expansiveness and optimism is blocked in order to facilitate an expansion of consciousness and inner understanding. Chiron in this house or sign may introvert the Jupiterian qualities; if we can accept this process, we develop earthy wisdom, humour and an open-hearted attitude to life. Vision may be more a quality of consciousness than a possibility that we must do something about, and the compulsion to externalize and go upwards and outwards must perhaps be resisted in order to allow this to happen. Ultimately, the gift of this placement is the capacity to devote ourselves to life as an expression of the divine, here and now: once we trust its presence we no longer need to pursue it (see the writing of D. H. Lawrence in the Chiron/Jupiter section – pp. 223, 226–88. This trust may be hard-won with this placement; we periodically fall into a dualistic view where some things are sacred and some are not, like the twins of Gemini. The frenzy of our search may resume only to have to be relinquished time and time again.

Chiron in Capricorn and the Tenth House

> But you who are strong and swift, see that you do not
> limp before the lame, deeming it kindness.
>
> Kahlil Gibran, *The Prophet*

The 10th house describes parental issues. Our attitude to the world 'out there' and to authority figures is strongly coloured by our experience of our mother, and her qualities are usually symbolized here. Saturn is the natural ruler of this house, and our first sense of boundaries is provided by mother. Also, until recently, in our culture many women lived the Saturnian principle through their husbands, taking their roles from them, interfacing with the world through them, and even using their surnames. Thus the 10th house may describe the mother's *unconscious* ambitions, her drive for success, independence and power in the world; if this is so, then her unlived life and unfulfilled ambitions will deeply affect us.

The 10th house describes our natural place in the world, our heritage and the way we seek to express it. It also concerns the laws, institutions and structures of society and the material world and, on a deeper level, how we aspire to give form to our potentials, manifest ourselves and participate in the world. With Chiron in Capricorn or the 10th house we often experience difficulty in setting and achieving goals, and finding our place in society. We may have to be patient in our longing for a vocation through which to contribute to the world, as it may only come later in life, preceded by many false starts. On the other hand, we perhaps find it difficult to enjoy the prestige which others perceive us as having, and are plagued with feelings of failure no matter how successful we appear. It is usually helpful to examine some of the deeper reasons behind this: we may be setting ourselves impossible standards, or hoping that each new mountain we climb will be the last. We could be struggling under a burden of parental expectations that can never be fulfilled; we are perhaps trying to succeed where they fa~~iled~~, or ~~ra~~ not dare to aim for. We could even~~tually be~~ to disappoint our parents, and thi~~ might~~ success. However, if this is uncons~~cious~~ ourselves short and fail in order to pun~~ish~~ lack the ability and drive to succeed. With ~~Chiron in~~ the 10th house, we could eventually find ~~joy in struggling to~~ climb the mountain of our own ambitions. ~~We perhaps cling to~~ external façades and role-playing to conceal our ~~vulnerability~~ and feeling of being somehow out of place. We ~~may either~~ place undue emphasis on material success, prestige and status, or shun worldly power and position, only to find ourselves falling foul of the system, always getting parking-tickets, having our tax affairs investigated, or clashing with authority figures!

With this placement we might seem to lack a sense of responsibility. On closer examination, however, a different picture emerges: we may be assuming responsibility for things over which in reality we have no control. This hinders our ability to be independent in the world, and we then look for someone to take care of us (shades of the 4th house). We may need to relinquish a futile struggle with difficulties and burdens that really are none of our business. If we carry others' burdens, hoping for some reward or recognition in return, we may be disappointed and become bitter, resentful and refuse to participate in life. We sometimes misjudge our own capacities, take on too much, fail and then feel guilty for not living up to our responsibilities.

Although we may fear being conspicuous or in a position of control and authority, we perhaps also harbour fantasies of inflated and despotic power, usually suppressed through shame and fear. If these uncomfortable feelings remain unconscious we could sabotage ourselves on the threshold of success. For example, one woman with Chiron in the 10th house was convinced that in a past life she had been a member of a royal family in ancient Egypt. She was depressed and preoccupied with trying to discover what awful thing she must have done to cause such a fall from grace that, in this life, she was struggling for money and living in a humble flat in London, along with millions of others who did not recognize her noble origins. Through working

...y over time, she realized that she could only ... self-worth in terms of power and status in the world. ...image of the princess she felt she had been represented her goal, and was preventing her from achieving things that were well within her means to achieve. Eventually she began to see this figure as symbolizing the inner qualities of dignity, presence and self-containment. Once her sense of self-worth began to improve, the issue of success or failure in worldly terms lost some of its intensity and she gradually set about setting and achieving more realistic goals. One of the gifts of this placement is success flowing from a healthy sense of self-respect and self-worth, rather than success as a compensation for a lack of it. Many people with Chiron in Capricorn or the 10th house have a natural sense of authority and dignity that invites respect from others.

With Chiron in Capricorn the wounded area may be the relationship with the personal father, and thus the father principle in general. The father may have been unknown; he may have been seen as weak and incapable, or rigid and authoritarian, or both: 'Don't do what I do, do what I say', is a familiar message to many with this placement. Men and women alike may grow up determined that they will never be like their fathers; they then struggle hard against his model, only to discover later in life that this wounded or authoritarian father looms large within their own psyche, and threatens the positive outcome of conscious goals they may be striving for. Many men become fathers with the intention of 'doing it different', only to discover later on, to their horror, that they have repeated exactly, but in another form, the characteristics of their own fathers which were so distasteful to them.

In the following example, however, the pattern was redeemed by the person having had the courage and the opportunity to face his own wounds first. This young man, whom I will call Roger, had Chiron in Capricorn in the 5th house, and part of a T-square: Chiron opposite Uranus conjunct Jupiter in Cancer in the 11th house, all squaring Neptune in Libra in the 2nd house. Roger's father was a self-made man who rose considerably in status through his own efforts and provided a suitably Capricornian model for his son. His business activities and urge to succeed (in fact, to outdo his own father) meant spending long periods of time away from home, and Roger was thus brought up mainly by mother, hardly knowing his father. When his father took to drink (Roger's Chiron in Capricorn squares Neptune in Libra) and became vicious and unpredictable (Chiron opposite Uranus) Roger protected his vulnerability by refusing to react (Chiron in Capricorn); he also rejected his father's values of success and material achievement. Later in life, however, Roger found himself imprisoned in this emotional non-reactiveness; he felt inwardly paralysed, and was often at the mercy of a ruthless and critical inner judge. When transiting Saturn and Pluto were conjunct his Neptune and therefore square his Chiron, Roger entered therapy. He had a series of dreams about being attacked and raped by a gang of violent frenzied men. Through working with these dreams a vulnerable and hitherto unseen child part of himself emerged (Chiron in the 5th house). Initially, Roger felt only contempt and fear for this child; he had learned from his father that to show any sensitivity was a sign of weakness. Shortly after this, his wife became pregnant; he wanted her to have an abortion, but changed his mind at the last minute, in spite of his fears of 'not having enough substance' to be a father. Eventually, through his relationship with his new son, he was able to put into further practice his hard-won respect for his own feeling of vulnerability.

One woman's father was in the Territorial Army and often away from home. Her Chiron configuration shows Pluto in the 12th house, Mars in the 1st house, both in Cancer conjunct the Ascendant and all quintile Chiron in the 10th house; Saturn, natural ruler of the 10th house, is in Sagittarius, sesquiquadrate Mars. Her father joined the Army the year she was born, and she became convinced over time that he had gone away because of her. Her mother was often angry and found it difficult to cope alone and this reinforced the message of it all being her fault: this is symbolized by Chiron in the 10th (here both the wounding mother and the absent father) quintile Mars (being hurt by anger). This feeling of being responsible for her father's absence went underground until he died when she was fifty-three. The unconscious conclusion that she was somehow bad had meanwhile taken a tremendous toll on her feeling of self-worth.

Another woman had Chiron in Capricorn in the 4th house; it was in close aspect to almost every planet in the chart. She came from a well-to-do family of distinctly patriarchal quality; her rejection of her father and everything he stood for was so all-consuming that she eventually became a lesbian and radical feminist. She overtly hated men and sought to cut them out of her life as fully as possible; she belonged to a group which campaigned for the reform of laws dealing with rapists. Underneath her anger, however, lay painful feelings of vulnerability and dependence (Chiron in the 4th house), as well as intense love for her father.

Sometimes the wound of Chiron in the 10th house reflects issues concerning the mother. She may have been the wounder; and women with this placement may struggle not to repeat the patterns inherited from their mothers. This is a common placement for people who work in the healing field, and sometimes their choice of profession is a direct attempt to counteract the wounding effects of an early relationship with their mother, by becoming a 'good mother' themselves. They may also be making reparation for unconscious rage against their mother. If the mother was wounded or incapable in some way, they may when still very young have become capable in dealing with the world and looking after others. Later on in life, people with this placement often have jobs with a great deal of responsibility, and are good at holding situations together; they may not, however, be able to take in nourishment from life (echoes of the 4th house here). For example, a woman who ran a healing centre was told she was like a dealer in healing, not taking it in herself. Initially, she found it impossible deeply to avail herself of what was there on offer, like Chiron giving to others the healing he could not find for himself. On the other hand, a gift of this placement is the ability to foster the growth of others, by 're-parenting' them, showing love and giving guidance which may have been pre-viously lacking. Those with this placement also can take seriously their duties towards themselves and others, and are not afraid to struggle with difficulties and burdens which others might shy away from.

Chiron in Aquarius and the Eleventh House

> Human salvation lies in the hands of the creatively
> maladjusted . . . honesty impels me to admit that
> transformed nonconformity, which is always costly
> and never altogether comfortable, may mean walking
> through the valley of the shadow of suffering.
>
> Martin Luther King, *Strength to Love*

In the 11th house, we seek groups of like-minded people in order to widen our social sphere. We stand back from society to reflect on and perhaps to criticize the wider collective context of politics and history. We may want to reform the world we see and become involved in social or political causes dedicated to improving the human lot. Individuals with Chiron in the last two houses and signs, as well as those with Chiron in the 8th and Scorpio, are often intensely connected to the deeper psyche and the collective unconscious, but also vigorously defended against it. It takes considerable strength to be able to give expression to collective ideas (11th house) or feelings (12th house) without being carried away by them and losing our individuality in the process. However, Chiron in these houses and signs offers the possibility of our being able to do just this, although we usually pay a price in terms of feeling somewhat isolated in our journey.

Saturn and Uranus are the dual rulers of the sign of Aquarius; with Chiron here or in the 11th house, we see the themes of these two planets interwoven. Some individuals with this placement will appear more Saturnian, others more Uranian, but, as explored in Chapter 5, Chiron's place between them suggests a both/and perspective. Those with Chiron in Aquarius experience Chiron opposite its natal place just before their Saturn return. This creates problems with the Saturn return, as the Chiron/Chiron opposition may make us impatient with limitation and reluctant to face issues from the past which tend to surface around the Saturn return: we perhaps try and skirt responsibilities in a bid for freedom, with the result that a crisis erupts at the next Saturn/Saturn square, at about the age of thirty-five. However, some people experience this Chiron/Chiron opposition as an influx of creative energy and may take strides forward in self-expression and social participation.

With Chiron in Aquarius or the 11th house, we are vulnerable to the collective unconscious in the sphere of ideas and ideals. Although we have the potential to be original and iconoclastic thinkers, we are also prone to taking on stereotyped attitudes. Rather than risk expressing our own opinions, we may adopt a party line of some kind, following the political or spiritual aspirations of the group to which we belong. We could become enslaved by the ideas of another person, not realizing that these hinder our own development; we may take on and subsequently reject many different systems of ideas on our quest. With this Chiron placement, we benefit by learning to use our own individual minds creatively, concretely, and with rational discrimination. If we can build a suitably Saturnian vehicle for the Uranian energy of our thoughts, we may find ourselves able to make an important contribution to others through our truly independent thinking. In this process, we will perhaps discover many useless 'shoulds' and 'oughts' which we are slavishly believing or obeying. With Chiron in the 11th house or Aquarius, we can usefully direct our iconoclastic tendencies towards our own belief systems – allowing the quality of our own thinking to be revolutionized first – rather than participating unthinkingly in collective movements dedicated to social or political change.

Some people with Chiron in Aquarius or the 11th house become the vehicle for controversial collective ideas, and often suffer from the response they receive, as they may be way ahead of their time. They could be writers, poets, teachers, or philosophers, all of whom influence people's thinking by formulating what is ready to become conscious within the collective mind. Amongst those with this Chiron placement, we find many people whose names have become almost synonymous with a system of ideas. For example, the French playwright and philosopher Jean-Paul Sartre has Chiron in Aquarius: he was the existentialist *par*

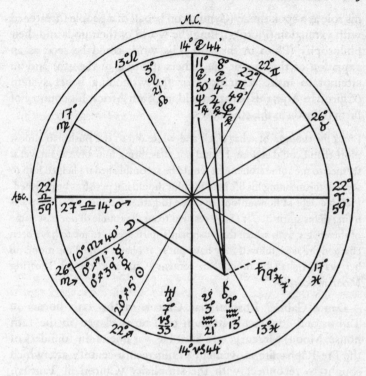

Laurens van der Post

$$\text{⚷} = \text{♄}/\text{♅}$$

excellence. The English playwright George Bernard Shaw was notorious for his vehement support of Socialist philosophy.

The author Laurens van der Post has Chiron in Aquarius in the 4th house. Through him many people have become aware of the beauty of the inner world of the Khoikhoi and other tribes that are vanishing from Africa. His Chiron squares Moon in Scorpio in the 1st house, a suitable image both for the wilderness, and also the inner pioneering symbolized by his work. Africa is sometimes called the cradle of mankind, here echoed by Chiron in the 4th house, aspecting the Moon. Chiron is sesquiquadrate Pluto in Gemini in the 9th house, symbolizing the power of his words, and his role as a spokesman (Gemini) on behalf of a people threatened with extinction (Pluto), telling the world of their gods and their philosophy (Pluto in the 9th). His work could be seen as an expiation of the sins of the fathers (Chiron in the 4th) and an attempt to make reparation for the wounding belief system (Chiron in Aquarius) of apartheid in South Africa, his country of birth (Chiron in the 4th house).

I find the thought of what black and white did to the Bushman almost more than I could endure. I could not, alas, bring him alive again: yet it seemed to me some atonement would be accomplished if I helped him to see that the meaning his life held for him should not perish as he perished. I felt it a debt of honour long overdue to gather into our own what was living in his spirit . . . If I have rescued from the rubble of our past some of this magic with which the Bushman's spirit seems to me to have been charged or, as he himself may have put it, if I have 'helped the moon on her way', I shall be more than content [Chiron in the 4th squaring Moon in Scorpio].[14]

Dante Gabriel Rossetti has Chiron in the 11th house, in Taurus and conjunct a stellium of Taurus planets in the 12th house: Moon, Mercury, and Sun. He was one of the founders of the Pre-Ràphaelite movement in nineteenth-century art, which sought to reconnect with the simplicity (Chiron in Taurus), purity and idealism (11th house) of earlier art (12th house), and to convey spiritual realities through skilled representational painting (Chiron in Taurus, conjunct 12th house stellium). He usually chose mythological or pastoral subjects, both of which are symbolized by his Chiron configuration. His principles and ideas (11th house) addressed the longings of the collective of his time (12th house) for the re-spiritualization of matter (Chiron in Taurus). Like Hephaestus (Chiron in Taurus), who fashioned the attributes of the gods, Rossetti depicted them with luminous reality.

With Chiron in Aquarius or the 11th house, we may be intensely critical of society, or reject it as far as possible; underneath, however, we may have a strong desire to make a positive contribution. We might become depressed and angry if we cannot find a way to do this; the urge then sours into acts of rebellion, destructiveness and anarchy. We find it difficult to accept how things are now, and to work for change on that basis. If we embrace spiritual or Utopian ideals and study revolutionary political frameworks, we will probably become progressively disillusioned as we realize that there is no perfect system or person on earth. Although we perhaps fervently believe that we know how things ought to be, we also need to learn humility lest we espouse 'new' ideas, ideals, or ways of life with as much rigidity as the old system we have rejected, and thus fall into our own shadow.

With Chiron in Aquarius or the 11th house, however, we potentially have the gift for balancing the opposites represented by Saturn and Uranus. We then truly bridge the old and the new: we are able to embrace innovation without wholesale rejection of the past, incorporating it as a firm foundation to our individual life and connection with society. We positively influence others by our example of creative non-conformism, rather than by trying to convince them that our ideas are 'right'; we uphold our own individuality (Leo/5th-house echo) and make a positive contribution to the collective in which we live, although we are unlikely to belong to the 'status quo'. Through acceptance of limitation and imperfection, we can allow others to find their own way, rather than imposing our ideas upon them.

Some individuals with Chiron in Aquarius find it almost impossible to relate in a feeling way to people whose mental constructs are different from their own. You may begin to feel somewhat unreal yourself around such a person, as you do not exist for them unless you subscribe to the same ideals and political or spiritual beliefs! Astrologers, psychotherapists and those involved in various metaphysical arts or spiritual disciplines are not exempt from this. The whole of life can be seen through the binoculars of our own system of beliefs and anything that does not fit is ignored, dismissed or pruned to fit. Our clients may be subtly manipulated to conform with our own reality system or pet beliefs. In these fields, once something becomes a 'should' we are treading near the perilous area of mind control, and perhaps need to remember that 'the map is not the territory'. It is sobering to realize that the media brainwashes us every day, influencing us to think in certain ways, to hold certain attitudes, and so on. Even this book is doing it! With Chiron in Aquarius or the 11th house, useful questions might be: 'Whose ideas am I actually receiving?' or 'Whose truth am I believing?' Collective images and ideas, from news reportage to advertisements, create our world-view and influence our attitudes, aspirations and ideals; without an exercise of Aquarian detachment, we succumb to subtle forms of thought-control, reminiscent of George Orwell's *1984* (he has Chiron in Capricorn and Saturn in Aquarius).

With Chiron in Aquarius or the 11th house, we could be over-sensitive to 'getting it right' and tie ourselves in knots trying to live up to spiritual ideals. We have perhaps transferred on to our belief system an attempt to win love from a cold and distant parent. This attachment to perfection is destructive, for if we can only allow the perfect to live, many creative projects, relationships, and careers could go down the drain as a result. Until we have found a measure of inner freedom, we might fear commitment. However, Chiron brings the possibility of individual freedom *within* commitment to life, and, when it is in Aquarius, this theme is particularly strong. The story of Prometheus illustrates this: a condition of his release from bondage and suffering was the wearing of a ring to remind him of his period of enchainment.

With this Chiron placement, we might have a horror of groups and the collective, partly because we are sensitive to being influenced and taken over by collective ideas. Perhaps we only feel comfortable when we are in charge ourselves or playing the role of the outsider or dissenter. We could project the figure of the Wounder on to the group, and become paranoid and seek to protect ourselves by withdrawal or aggressive behaviour. Martin Luther King said: 'There is nothing as powerful as an idea whose time has come.' Some people with this placement have consciously opposed the collective; they have been creatively iconoclastic and facilitated social change. Emmeline Pankhurst, who won voting-rights for women in Britain has Chiron in Aquarius in the 12th house; it is square Mars in the 8th house in Scorpio, trine Jupiter in Gemini in the 3rd house, and quincunx Moon in Virgo in the 7th house. When transiting Uranus was exactly conjunct this Chiron, the suffragette movement was staging increasingly vehement protests. One of her followers threw herself under the King's horse (!) at the Derby and was killed, in a curious reversal of the Chiron myth. However, some biographers believe this event made Parliament realize the depth of the movement's determination for change, and thus shortened the struggle. Emmeline Pankhurst is also an example of a woman expressing the archetypal pattern of the Amazon, as discussed in Chapter 4.

Women with this placement frequently have trouble in their relationships with their fathers, who perhaps personify the more difficult Aquarian qualities – they may have been cold, critical, distant, unfeeling or authoritarian. Conversely, one woman with Chiron in Aquarius said she felt that her mind was wounded through recognizing at an early age that she was the most intelligent person in the family. Her father was a particularly earthy person; she learned to deny her superior mental development and her own abilities in order to feel her father bigger and stronger than herself. Clarity, detachment, a highly developed sense of political or social potential and an ability to articulate current trends within the collective are some of the gifts of this placement, but these too are double-edged swords which need tempering by the humility of having felt our own suffering and accepted the imperfections inherent in life.

Chiron in Pisces and the Twelfth House

> Can you educate your soul so that it encompasses the
> One without dispersing itself?
>
> Lao Tzu, *Tao Te Ching*

In the sign of Pisces and the 12th house – the last of the cycle –
forms disintegrate; the past is dissolved and our separateness is
relinquished so that a new and more inclusive cycle of life can
begin, hopefully accompanied by the wisdom of the previous
cycle. This sign and house link us to the feeling life of the
transpersonal and the collective – especially the longing for the
return to unity. This may be experienced in many ways, from
the chaos of a football match to the rarefied atmosphere of a
meditation on universal love – for collective and transpersonal
feeling can be savage as well as uplifting. Jung has written at
length about the dualism inherent in the sign of the fishes that are
yoked together but eternally swim in opposite directions.[15] Here,
things may not be what they seem: deception, emotional manipulativeness and genuine transcendental experiences can weave together in a confusing blend which defies rational understanding.

In this sign and house the urge to be reborn as an individual
with a more inclusive consciousness is eternally at odds with the
urge to destroy individuality and regress into a preconscious state
of womb-like bliss. With this Chiron placement, we often have
difficulty gaining a sense of personal individuality and separateness; steps in this direction may initially be fraught with guilt or
even illness. On the other hand if we are too defended against the
oceanic experience of Pisces and the 12th house, and too enclosed
in a shell of brittle defensiveness (echoes of Virgo/6th house), we
might regress, drown our sorrows in drink, seek refuge in drugs,
pursue a life of crime or exile ourselves from society. If you have
Chiron in Pisces or the 12th house, loss of personal identity
through the experience of ecstasy and the feeling of unity with the
entire cosmos is probably a strong psychological need for you,

and your dilemma will be how to honour this without getting swept away and regressing to an enwombed state and ignoring the tides of material or emotional chaos which then surge through your life.

Poseidon (the Greek name for Neptune), was Chiron's half-brother and also fathered by Saturn, and thus helps us glimpse the meaning behind some of the themes that appear in the lives of those with Chiron in Pisces or the 12th house (Dionysus too is often associated with the sign of Pisces[16]). Horses were sacred to Poseidon: he assumed horse form in his conquest of the goddess Demeter, and the Centaurs are sometimes said to have been born from their union. At any rate, Poseidon's connection with horses points to his originally lunar character: horses were sacred to the moon-goddess, their hoofprints being shaped like a crescent moon. Poseidon's trident is said to have been the labyris, or double-headed axe of the moon-goddess. This line of associations goes deep into pre-Hellenic mythology, into the realm of goddess-worship, and connects us with mare-headed Demeter, whose ancient cult precedes the story of Chiron.

Poseidon's name is derived from Ida, a water-goddess, and thus alludes to the primal waters of Pisces and the meaning of the 12th house: our individuality is called home to the sea of our origins, our future and our return – to *mare, mater*, mother – and is dissolved in chaos in order to be reborn. Chaos is a name for the *prima materia*, the substance on which the alchemical work of inner transformation is performed. An engraving by Marolles depicts the unfettered opposites in chaos: dark clouds surround images of the various beasts of the zodiac, all warring in their respective pairs. The Water-carrier is trying to put out the fire of the Lion, the Archer is about to shoot the Heavenly Twins, and so on. It is well worth studying if you have Chiron in Pisces or the 12th house – for its humour as well as any deeper implications![17] The impossibility of sorting out the inner world, Virgo-style, is made abundantly clear. With Chiron in Pisces or the 12th house, we may struggle to establish inner order and neglect the practical aspects of life (Virgo/6th house), or become preoccupied with this only to have it threatened time and again by our inner chaos.

After Poseidon assisted his brothers Zeus and Hades to overthrow their father Cronos, Poseidon was allotted rulership of the sea, while Zeus and Hades were given dominion over Mount Olympus and the Underworld respectively. Poseidon resented this and coveted the earthly kingdoms. He was notorious for his truculent character and periodic rages; he occasionally made territorial conquests, sending storms and huge waves to wash over cities and destroy their walls. If forbidden to do this, he could inflict a crippling drought instead. Usually, some form of treaty or bargain was necessary in order to deter him, and often a sacrifice was required in exchange for his protection – a theme which we have already noted as relevant to the meaning of Chiron.

In order to prevent the sea from flooding and destroying his city, King Minos made a bargain with Poseidon: he would sacrifice his best bull if Poseidon would restrain the seas. However, when King Minos had to honour his side of the bargain, he substituted an ordinary bull, saving his magnificent white bull for himself. When Poseidon discovered the deception, he was enraged; he took revenge on Minos with the help of Aphrodite, who struck his wife Pasiphaë with a consuming passion for this bull. Eventually Pasiphaë contrived to mate with it, and from this union was born the Minotaur. This monster was shut up in a maze, the labyrinth, and required regular human sacrifice. Eventually he was vanquished by Theseus with the help of Ariadne and her famous thread.

When we pause to reflect on the meaning of these mythic patterns as regards Chiron in the 12th house and Pisces, we can see the theme of sacrifice here showing two distinct forms – perhaps like the two fish. Whether or not we are ready and willing, this placement requires that we sacrifice our separatist notions of individuality and take a wider perspective into account. However, as we cannot sacrifice something which we do not have in the first place, we may have to struggle hard to gain any sense of separate individuality. Those who have Chiron in Pisces have transiting Chiron square its own place later than any other sign, at about the age of twenty-three. By this time most of the first Saturn cycle has passed, providing the opportunity to be grounded in the world of form before the first Chiron/Chiron square, when the Piscean themes of the natal placement often erupt.

With Chiron in Pisces or the 12th house, we may experience this grounding process itself as a sacrifice, for our natural dwelling is in the realm of oneness and the process of differentiating is felt as exceptionally painful. If this first sacrifice is not made, however, we may instead destroy the outer structures of life, and this creates difficulties in the world of solid objects, material reality and Saturnian requirements. Relationships, jobs, projects or homes may be swept away if we cling to an undifferentiated state of unity and refuse the world of form: we then sacrifice the 'ordinary bull' of our ordinary life instead of the 'special bull' of our inflated sense of specialness. We may have a horror of ordinariness; for all the suffering it entails, we perhaps feel a certain comfort in hanging back where all is possible but nothing actually happens, thus sacrificing form before it has even had a chance to manifest.

The bull is an ancient symbol of phallic power, instinctual fertility and procreation; its sacrifice is also a relevant image here. He who performs a sacrifice often wishes to incorporate into himself the qualities and attributes of his victim, human or animal. Here again is the *omophagia*, the eating of the body of the god, mentioned in Chapter 5. Indeed, the Minotaur is sometimes said to represent such ceremonies, which were held annually in Crete: amidst orgiastic rituals a bull was torn to pieces and eaten raw in honour of bull-gods such as Zagreus, Dionysus Omadius 'the Raw One', or even Zeus, whose Idaean shrine was cemented with bull's blood.[18] Note the mention of Ida, incorporated into the name Poseidon, and that Jupiter (Zeus) was the traditional ruler of Pisces. Behind this looms the spectre of human sacrifice, mythologized by later cultures in order to avoid the peril of blood-guilt by relegating responsibility for sacrificial acts to mythic gods and monsters.

When a people has outgrown in culture the stage of its own primitive rites, when they are ashamed or at least a little anxious and self-conscious about doing what yet they dare not leave undone, they instinctively resort to mythology, to what is their theology, and say the men of old did it, or the gods suffered it.[19]

With Chiron in Pisces or the 12th house, then, the first sacrifice is like the *omophagia*, where in order to claim some sense of separate individuality and power to enter into life we may need to 'eat the bull' – to re-embrace and honour the primal phallic potency that lies within us. This may mean encountering for perhaps the first time our selfishness, powerful will and the destruction we can wreak with great subtlety if we are crossed. Chiron connects us with the primitive underside of any house or sign in which it is found, and here the territory at first looks very foreign indeed, being so different to the Piscean stereotype to which we have become accustomed. With Chiron in Pisces or the 12th house we perhaps feel deep envy for people who seem to possess a solid sense of personal identity, like Poseidon coveting the solid land his brothers inherited. We may then react by sending 'floods' of emotional moods and deviousness calculated to wear away the 'city walls' of the victim we envy, and on whom we have projected our latent sense of individuality. We then develop complex relationships with people, trying to absorb by osmosis their individuality, for with this placement our struggle for personal territory is rarely overt.

A sense of guilt may accompany the development of our sense of individuality. With Chiron in Pisces or the 12th house, we could have difficulty with angry feelings that accompany the process of growing beyond the role of a child dependent upon parent figures. In ancient-Greek rites, he who murdered someone of near kin was stoned by the community and ritually put to death, cast out of the city as the *pharmakos* – the remedy, the purifier of evils. The pervasive feelings of worthlessness and self-blame that may plague us often have their roots in suppressed anger; in extreme circumstances we may identify with the lonely outsider, scapegoat or exile, the guilty *pharmakos*.

The second sacrifice, to pursue this analogy, takes the form of the *consecration* of the bull of our active potency and creative power. Instead of the love of power which unconscious instinctual energy can demonstrate, we become imbued with the power of love, offering our individual talents, fertility and self-expression for the good of all. This surrender as a conscious choice fulfils our individuality rather than dismembers it, and provides an opportunity to be of service to others. However, if we should cheat or defy Poseidon, another theme of this Chiron placement comes into being: unfulfillable longing. We may be consumed with passionate longing for someone unattainable: it could be a film-star or a character in a book over whom we secretly weep; it could be someone else's husband or wife. Like the special bull of King Minos, it might be someone who embodies a powerful, proud and instinctual sense of individuality. Whoever is the object of this passion, however, it has the effect of dismembering us; thus the sacrifice comes to pass with the help of Aphrodite, the goddess of love (note Venus is exalted in Pisces). But these painful longings, lying like the Minotaur in his labyrinth, can also be the means by which our heart is opened to the suffering of others.

With Chiron in Pisces or the 12th house, the life of our imagination can be experienced as totally real, especially when we are young. We initially lack sufficient Virgoan discrimination of the different levels of reality, and might become confused or alienated. However, Poseidon can also send the affliction of drought, and some people with this placement retreat into an uncomfortable Virgoan cynicism, pragmatism and hyper-rationality, with a corresponding tendency to be over-literal and rigid. With this Chiron placement, we may deeply fear the experience of surrender and dissolution, and hence increase our Virgoan boundaries, mental divisiveness and emotional control. This also leads to suffering, as our need to experience oneness with humanity will remain unfulfilled. We may then seek this at one remove, through friends involved with the occult, drugs, or other Piscean pursuits.

With Chiron in Pisces or the 12th house, we may need to sacrifice our urge to redeem others. Poseidon's kingdom is under the sea, and our personal wounds will remain unseen if we are preoccupied with the suffering of the world at large. With such a preoccupation we tend to sacrifice our own health and well-being for others, doing voluntary work, or entering professions such as nursing. Feeling that we must help others may be our downfall if our concern with humanity at large means that we unwittingly do violence to our own needs for separation, isolation and individual enterprise. Chiron in Pisces or the 12th house may ask us first to accept suffering as part of the fabric of life, without being tempted to take it upon ourselves and perhaps to identify with a Christ-like figure who redeems others by taking away their suffering or by feeling it for them. If we are so tempted, we then identify with the victim, and the burden of unjustified suffering may seem to be our lot; we believe in the redemptive power of innocent suffering without considering whether there is an alternative; we may be repeatedly drawn into situations guaranteed to result in more pain. Although the meaning of our life will be intimately bound up with our experience of suffering, with this Chiron placement we might eventually be asked to sacrifice our suffering. What will we do without the familiar pain we know so well, the constant friend and companion who never leaves us?

If you have Chiron in Pisces or the 12th house, you may enter the profession of healing in one form or another in self-defence! You will probably attract people who need comfort, compassion, support and make unceasing demands on your time and energy. I know several people with this placement who coped with this by deciding to drift with the inevitable: through their professional work they accommodated this fate in a very Virgoan/6th-house way, with strong boundaries and specific skills. As they could not stem the tide, they decided to organize it so that they could benefit from it too! If you have this Chiron placement, a healthy dose of practicality and self-interest can be useful, although the pragmatism and Mercurial opportunism of Virgo might at first seem rather alien. Commitment to form and structure, for both the benefit of yourself and others, is sometimes a creative solution to the dilemma of this placement. On the other hand, with Chiron in Pisces or the 12th house, you also need periods of creative isolation, although you may at first resist and fear this. Your sensitivity may leave you at times feeling drained and overwhelmed, and you may periodically need to retreat.

With this placement, we often have difficulty tolerating separation. We may erode our spouse's or children's sense of personal initiative, or demand sacrifices from them with our unspoken demand for unity, which can escalate into emotional blackmail. We may become ill or even threaten suicide if those we love become too separate from us; we can be adept at stirring up emotional chaos, making tempers rise around us and retaining an air of vague innocence throughout. One man whose parents both had Chiron in Pisces encountered this every time he chose to do something outside his parents' wishes. Words such as: 'You've no idea how much this will hurt your father [or mother, depending on who was talking]', accompanied his struggle to assert himself.

With this placement, there is often a deep wound connected with grief. Perhaps we feel a chronic 'existential grief', often crying for no apparent reason; we grieve for the pain we imagine others to be feeling, even if they are not aware of it themselves. Our feelings may be archetypal rather than personal: we may mourn the loss of original unity and bliss which inevitably accompanies the initial stages of psychological maturation. In addition, with this placement specific traumas of blocked grief and incomplete mourning frequently occur, for to grieve means to acknowledge death, duality and separation – and we may find this impossible unless we already have some sense of the overall continuity of life. We may deny the feelings that accompany the mourning process and maintain a spaced-out and precarious happiness instead. Later, this may wreak havoc with our health and well-being. However, our first experience of deep mourning may also unlock our inner world and send us on our journey of self-discovery, where the illusion of duality may finally be dissolved: we may discover we are already where we long to be, no more an exile or a stranger to life.

With Chiron in Pisces or the 12th house, we may feel deep compassion for others, and the central struggle of our life may be to create a suitable vehicle (Virgo/6th house) to offer this compassion. Astrologer Eve Jackson found Chiron in the 12th house prominent in the charts of healers. Illness often expresses disconnection from the sense of unity with life, and those who remain in touch with this 12th-house experience are natural healers. With this placement we may eventually feel the 'wisdom realizing emptiness' spoken of in Buddhism: just as the process of minutely analysing something reveals ever more void and less form, so we may eventually relinquish our search for a personal sense of identity and instead base our security in the mysterious process of life as a whole.

Several famous composers and musicians have this placement; music speaks to the feelings and directly addresses our longings for unity, love and redemption. Yehudi Menuhin has Chiron in Pisces in the 2nd house; during his Chiron return he made extensive personal and musical excursions into Eastern philosophy. Singers Ella Fitzgerald, Billie Holiday, Mahalia Jackson and Muddy Waters all have Chiron in Pisces; blues music expresses many subtle nuances of sorrow, longing and unrequited love. Richard Wagner has Chiron in Pisces in the 11th house, square Sun and possibly Ascendant both in Gemini, and quincunx a focal Jupiter in Leo in the 4th house. The search for redemptive love is a central theme in his operas; he was preoccupied in his personal and artistic life with the idea of the woman who would sacrifice everything for love. Indeed, he managed to make his wife, mistress, colleagues and friends sacrifice a great deal for himself and his aspirations, unashamedly drawing upon their support, emotionally and financially – an interesting expression of Chiron in the 11th house! Chiron quincunx Jupiter in Leo in the 4th house describes the dramatization of emotional extremes within his music; Chiron in Pisces indicates its hypnotic and evocative effect on the deep unconscious. The theme of tragic or unrequited love is also common in Wagner's work, and is often seen in the lives of those with Chiron in Pisces or the 12th house, whose attunement to an ideal of archetypal or universal love is so strong that they may have difficulty finding a partner in real life.

As this sign and house are preoccupied with universal concerns, when Chiron transits through Pisces we would expect to see its themes manifest themselves within the collective, and indeed they do. Since the early nineteenth century every transit of Chiron through Pisces has seen a major war and featured issues such as the rights of black people and/or other socially oppressed groups. Racism and the abuse of human rights provoke strong emotions of guilt, fear, anger and sorrow in us. They are flagrant examples of everything that divides man from man and betrays our underlying sense of unity; they thus typify at a collective level the wound of Chiron in Pisces.

Chiron was in Pisces from 1861–9. During this period the American Civil War raged; the abolition of slavery was a contentious issue opposed by the Southern states, reluctant to give up the privileges it had brought them. Although the 13th Amendment to the Constitution (1865) freed the slaves, the legal equality of black people was shortlived.

Chiron was again in Pisces from 1910–18. World War I 'changed the face of Europe forever'; invasions and counter-invasions radically altered the boundaries of many countries. Thousands of men were disabled by noxious gas, used in warfare for the first time. The suffragettes were active in England, demanding the vote for women. Invasions, gas and mass suffering are all typically Neptunian themes congruent with Chiron in Pisces; the carnage of war bears a chilling resemblance to the bloody rites of the bull-god – the symbolic sacrifice of the phallic power of the male. War does this literally. The most recent transit of Chiron through Pisces (1960–69) saw the fiercest period of guerrilla activity in the Vietnam War. Countless young men were killed or maimed; many returned disillusioned or addicted to hard drugs; others disappeared without trace. Here also are the Piscean themes: unseen enemies, deception, sacrifice, disillusionment, drug addiction. In America the 'Peace and Love' movement was active, accompanied by music inspired by drug experiences; mass disillusion set in as the American Dream became the American Nightmare. Characteristically Piscean experiences of material and emotional chaos, insecurity and mourning are evoked on a mass scale through war. Imagine how many mourn the loss of one person, and extend that to the millions lost in these large-scale wars that occurred while Chiron was in Pisces: this gives a sense of the collective emotional experience generated by war.

Rhodesia declared unilateral independence in 1965, rejecting demands for voting-rights for black people. The United Nations retaliated by declaring it an 'illegal nation', and Rhodesia was progressively isolated by economic sanctions. It finally became Zimbabwe after fifteen years of war with unusual and clearly Piscean features. The UDI chart of Rhodesia shows Chiron conjunct Saturn in Pisces in the 2nd house: Chiron conjunct Saturn suggests isolation and the subtle erosion of guerrilla warfare (Chiron in Pisces); Chiron in the 2nd house here symbolizes suffering due to lack of material resources and entrenched values (Chiron/Saturn). Also appropriate to Chiron in Pisces, the grass-roots inspiration for this war came from the first martyr to the cause of liberation, a Shona woman named Nehanda who was executed at the end of the last century. She went to her death saying: 'My bones will rise again', and her spirit is said to have possessed a succession of mediums from that day until now. She is the national guardian spirit, an archetypal mother-figure in her wrathful aspect of righteous anger on behalf of her children. During this war, mediums provided practical assistance for guerrillas with their intimate knowledge of local terrain; they also consulted the ancestral spirits, who frequently foretold the

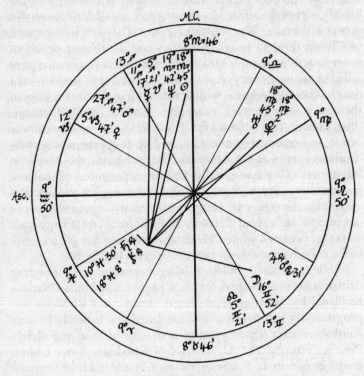

Rhodesia (UDI)

whereabouts of the enemy.[20] This rich interweaving of different dimensions of reality was expressed through songs that created political impetus through embracing Marxist ideology. The form was typically Piscean: during a *pungwe* (all-night session of ecstatic dancing and singing), mediums would become possessed and inspire people with spiritual commitment to the cause of liberation. Marx also has Chiron in Pisces, conjunct the Chiron of the UDI chart; it is square Neptune in Sagittarius, which is conjunct the Neptune in Sagittarius of the Zimbabwe chart. Marxism was used in a Chironian way, as a transitional philosophy, complemented in other dimensions by the activities of the spirit mediums.

This last transit of Chiron in Pisces also saw the culmination of the career of Martin Luther King. Chiron is prominent in his chart, and many people believe his death did even more than his life to mobilize national feelings of guilt (see pp. 246–8 for more information on his horoscope). Both he and President Kennedy were at their peak while Chiron was in Pisces, inspiring people in a characteristically Neptunian way, appealing to their idealism and need for a charismatic leader; they both embodied the *Zeitgeist* of Chiron in Pisces, like the two fish. Chiron is in the last degree of Pisces in the chart of President Kennedy, and it has been said that his assassination marked the end of an era. His reputation has been somewhat tarnished by discoveries of his connections with the mafia, his involvement with Marilyn Monroe and suggested connection with her death. As usual, with the 12th house, Pisces and Neptune, things are often not quite as they appear!

8 · Chiron in Aspect

The Inner Planets

Traditionally, the planets from the Sun to Mars represent the different spheres of our personal life, while Jupiter and Saturn relate us to society: Jupiter represents our desire for expansion and our philosophical and social aspirations; Saturn concerns form and structure, goals and ambitions. In the classic shamanic cartography mentioned in Chapter 1, these first seven planets represent the Middle Realm, bound by the laws of space and time. However, each of these planetary principles also has its numinous and archetypal level: it is no accident that the planets are named after gods and goddesses. For example, at a personal level Venus represents what gives us pleasure; however, behind our human instinct to beautify ourselves, attract others and thus to enrich our life, looms the figure of Aphrodite, with her awesome powers of both fertility and vengeance.

To summarize the relevant themes from Chapter 5, when Chiron aspects any planet up to and including Saturn, its principle may be wounded; it may be a blind spot in the psyche, where we do for others what we cannot do for ourselves. In addition, transpersonal experiences characteristic of a planet may open up, potentially bringing creativity, inspiration and originality, but perhaps also fear, crisis and pain. We can respond to this in a variety of ways ranging from total resistance to total 'possession', as described. An all-or-nothing, either/or pattern is common, and this split is the wound needing to be encompassed if the energies represented by the aspect are to be integrated into our lives. Where Chiron touches us we are wounded and can also wound; here we can heal, and are also naturally open to the transpersonal, to both its celestial and infernal dimensions.

The Outer Planets

Let us explore the outer planets in terms of the classic shamanic cartography described in Chapter 1. Chiron aspecting an outer planet in the horoscope brings the likelihood that at some point in our life we will encounter the realm it represents, often when the Chiron configuration is triggered off by a strong transit of Chiron or the other planet. Powerful events or inner experiences may overtake us: we suddenly enter another dimension of reality, stopped in our tracks, inspired and temporarily transformed. However, these realms are *timeless*, and although they may open to us, through dreams, twilight states or experiences of altered consciousness, the metaphor of the journey implies neither a progression from one realm to another nor a linear sequence of clock time: the journey is our life, in both its inner and outer aspects, and these experiences may take considerable time to integrate. Although there is the view that we evolve *from* the limitations of Saturn *to* the perspectives represented by the outer planets, this linear model is not borne out by observation of what happens in real life, and in my opinion may create further 'futile struggles' accompanied by guilt, frustration and betrayal of the requirements of the Saturnian principle: it is perhaps rather a question of *consciousness*.

The shamanic cartography provides a useful overall image within which this interweaving can be placed, as it addresses in a non-linear way the process of individualization. The outer planets not only represent collective issues but also they describe a terrain of inner subjective experience, *transpersonal* rather than personal, where universal motifs of the inner life are touched. However, as described in Chapter 3, this is often underpinned by unconscious experiences of extreme suffering dating back to the pre-verbal period of our life.

In this schema, Uranus can be seen as the celestial map-maker, representing our latent intuition of divine order. Without some semblance of a map, we may lose our way in the wilderness within. Ultimately, however, a map of our own unique inner world will evolve through the experience of the journey itself, rooted in the common archetypal themes encountered. Although this map is surely not the territory, and Uranus may err on the side of safe mental distance from deep emotional experience, none the less he provides perspective and understanding. In this sense, astrology is a Uranian discipline, an ancient and highly sophisticated map of the psyche that has survived translation into many different cultures over time. Uranus also represents the sudden onset of the initiation process and the rupture with the everyday world – the period of time outside society and the quality of mental illumination that may accompany it. Negatively, however, an overdose of Uranus can leave us ungrounded like Ixion,[1] bound to the fiery wheel of our insights and tumbling ceaselessly in the sky, out of touch with human life: we may think we understand everything but be tragically without the resources to live our vision. We may know our own horoscope inside out, but this does not necessarily enrich our life or mean that we have any real depth of self-knowledge.

Neptune represents the celestial realm of paradise with its deep feelings of unity, bliss, redemption from suffering, communion with cosmic beings and divine all-embracing love. Here, the experience of ecstasy pervades us; we are enraptured, overtaken and dissolved in an ocean of feeling. The obvious danger is that we may not want to return, or that, when we do, we feel confused, deceived and bereft, dreading the hard edges of the material world of separate forms, and perhaps longing to renounce the world altogether.

All life springs from the primeval waters that flow from the tree (of life) and gather at its base, waters which are limitless, an essential sea circulating through all of nature. These waters are the beginning and end of all existence, the ever-moving matrix that nurtures and preserves life. The World Tree, expressing its milky golden sap, denotes 'absolute reality', a return to the centre and place of origin, the home of wisdom that heals.[2]

Pluto represents the infernal realms which feed the roots of the World Tree. The word 'Tartarus', the deepest region of the Greek Underworld, has the same root as the word 'tortoise': in ancient Hindu mythology, the earth was said to be supported by the god Vishnu incarnated as a tortoise. Likewise, we may descend to

Tartarus in order that the tree of our new life may be deeply rooted. In the Underworld, the shaman meets the spirits of his ancestors: in psychological terms, here we meet and slowly come to terms with our particular psychological heritage and immediate family relationships. The shaman will meet various demons and malicious or destructive spirits: these may be personifications of our own unconscious anger, envy, greed, power drives, and so on, as well as positive potentials that may have turned upon us because we have refused to acknowledge them. However, at a transpersonal level, these Underworld experiences can be particularly fearsome and alien to us, as there are no images of an apparently angry and destructive countenance included within the traditional Judaeo–Christian pantheon for devotional purposes. Tibetan Buddhist deities such as Kalachakra or Yamantaka, or the Hindu Kali, are examples of such images; these figures and the Tantric images of sexual union from both traditions provide a transpersonal context for typically Plutonian experiences.

During the loss of innocence that features in this terrain we may feel ourselves to be roasting in a hell of emotional pain, subjected to tortures of various kinds: we may be tormented with unfulfillable desires; we may feel ourselves to be eaten alive, eventually to be re-membered and reborn to our forgotten selves. In Greek mythology, however, the Underworld also included the warm and pleasant Elysian fields, whose inhabitants lived in sensual bliss, free to be born again on earth whenever they pleased. The Underworld is also the realm of the instincts, and for many people these experiences foreshadow a reconnection with sexuality and creativity in a deeper way, as the 'cellular consciousness' of Pluto comes alive.

Hard and Soft Aspects

Hard aspects (0°, 45°, 90°, 135°, 150° and 180°) usually have a sense of pressure, conflict or urgency; struggle, dilemma, tension and opposition are common. However, with these aspects we also build strength of character and the ability to withstand conflict and achieve in the world. Hard aspects are more likely to manifest themselves overtly – in events or people who personify their qualities. On the other hand, soft aspects (60°, 120° and the so-called abstract aspects) express Chiron's attributes and themes in a more *qualitative* way, with a personal aura or sense of being rather than an actual life experience or event. Soft aspects flow easily, in a creative or destructive way, and, as they are less externally obvious, their tendencies may take time to detect and be difficult to manage consciously.

The Question of Orbs

In practice, it is useful to be flexible: using the system you were taught as a basis, judge which orbs seem appropriate for each horoscope on its own terms. Try the orbs you generally use for Saturn; take into account the strength of both Chiron and the other planet, and modify this if necessary to encompass the details of what clients might tell you about themselves and their lives.

Chiron in Aspect to the Sun

When Chiron is in aspect to the Sun, there is a wound to the solar masculine principle and thus our experience of individuality, 'soloness' and purpose. Our sense of being at the creative centre of our own world may be damaged, and we may make someone else the centre of our universe; we then promote their interests and help them to shine, basking in their reflected glory, living our Chiron/Sun aspect vicariously. We are able to foster the talents and self-expression of others, but may discount our own worth and then feel despair and envy. Lacking the sense of an inner personal centre, we could be especially prone to being taken over by archetypal energies, for good or ill. Se pp. 307–15 for an example of this in the horoscope of the Reverend Jim Jones.

Conversely, we may be charismatic, and shine brightly; we succeed in becoming the centre of attention, being loved and admired by many, but somehow we cannot recognize and enjoy it. In childhood, we perhaps lacked the experience of being at the centre of our parents' lives. Our parents may have been somewhat childlike themselves, needing validation of their worth from us, and thus we may have the wound of narcissistic isolation. If we were not sufficiently mirrored and validated for our uniqueness, we probably learned very early how to survive by delighting others, reflecting their aspirations, and being only that which pleased them. We may adopt many different personae, but feel estranged from ourselves: no matter what eminence we achieve, we feel phoney. Our false self is seen, while our true self may weep somewhere in the background. We could feel the need to display ourselves, and only feel real when on show; we may be over-sensitive to criticism or confrontation, which we seek to avoid with an exaggerated panache. On the other hand we may be afraid to shine, as our inner being has a painful history of not being accepted and validated: we look everywhere for a mirror, and see only our own reflection.

The Sun is the only heavenly body that casts a direct shadow on the earth; the full moon casts shadows but its more diffuse light is reflected from the Sun. This 'dark side of the sun' is relevant when Chiron aspects the Sun. It represents egomania, narcissism, a belief that one's purpose is god-ordained and therefore any means justify the attaining of it. With these aspects, we can become authoritarian, and desire to be in sole control of life and everyone we come into contact with; we may be wilful, inflexible, contemptuous and always need to be right. Coming face to face with this controlling, destructive and autocratic side of the masculine principle is often a difficult part of the journey of those with Chiron/Sun aspects. On the positive side, these aspects can signify the ability to achieve and to fight for what we want in life. We could have natural qualities of leadership, as people will warm to our sense of noble purpose. Some with Chiron/Sun aspects gather a following, but some become ardent followers of others, projecting their individuality onto them, emulating them and living in their shadow.

Women with Chiron/Sun aspects often lack confidence in their masculine side, and it may be difficult to embark on creative enterprises that require focus, goal-orientation and organization. They may live in the father's shadow, modelling themselves on his unconscious images and expectations of women. They are sometimes preoccupied in finding the 'right man', and this usually means one through whom they can live out their own masculine side, and from whom they can take their sense of identity, purpose and achievement. For example, a woman with Chiron opposite her Sun in Gemini married a man with Sun and Moon in Gemini; she was attracted to the mercurial wit and brilliance he displayed, which she could not feel within herself; later she bitterly resented him for it, and turned her sharp tongue on him. Jackie Kennedy has Sun in Leo in the 9th house, square Chiron in the 6th house in Taurus conjunct the North Node and possibly the Descendant; although a woman of style and individuality in her own right, she is perhaps even more famous for having been the wife of two extremely rich and powerful men, President Kennedy and Aristotle Onassis. When still a child, she reputedly told her father that she would marry the President of the United States when she grew up!

With Chiron/Sun aspects, the image of the father will be

coloured by Chironian themes. He may have been weak, ill, impotent, wounded, absent or insubstantial – or at least perceived in that light; he may also have been a wounding influence, violent and rough. Sometimes, however, the father is a spiritual mentor, guru and guide: he is supportive, wise and fosters individual growth. The son of such a man may have problems, feeling unable to compete, and perhaps even rejecting the positive attributes he has inherited; he may travel a long and circuitous route to reclaim them. Women with Chiron/Sun are sometimes groupies, projecting the image of saviour or healer: they pursue charismatic men, gurus, musicians or other public figures; they try to be their counterparts – the wounded woman, the damsel in distress or the wife of the great man. On the other hand they may see men as wounded; they may attract 'lame ducks' who need emotional or financial support, and who in turn wound them.

With Chiron in aspect to the Sun, we have a natural ability to reflect to others their sense of self, which is often the very thing we cannot experience inwardly ourselves. We may be magnetic and attractive, but perhaps also very lonely, if we allow ourselves to feel it. Men with this aspect sometimes feel responsible for healing or resolving something inherited from their father. Some have a gift for positive fathering, whether or not they have their own children; they could work with children, facilitate creativity or help foster individuality in others by discussing goals and objectives from a position of respect and emotional detachment.

Susan Atkins has Sun in Taurus in the 3rd house opposite Chiron in Scorpio, conjunct the MC in the 10th house; it is also square Mars and Saturn in Leo in the 7th house. Her father was weak, violent and an alcoholic. She became psychologically enslaved to Charles Manson, and was imprisoned for her participation in the ritual murder of Sharon Tate. Charles Manson has been described as the 'Son of the Terrible Mother'[3] and he symbolizes her 10th-house Chiron in Scorpio, as she was possessed by a Kali-like figure devoted to destruction. She wrote an autobiography significantly called *Child of Satan, Child of God*. While in prison she discovered that she had healing powers, and she now leads a ministry from within her cell; this expresses Chiron conjunct the MC, a healing vocation. She tells a poignant

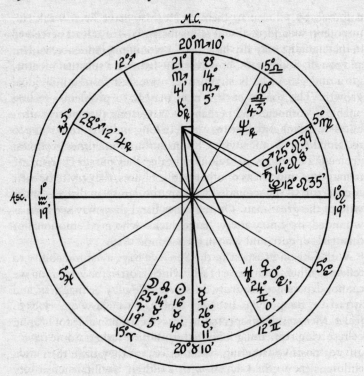

Susan Atkins

anecdote from her childhood: she saw a gigantic crucifix on a hill, which was dismissed as 'only imagination' by her parents. Later on, reading her Bible by candlelight, she went too close to the flame and a hole was burnt through it. This episode filled her with doom and foreboding, and she felt from that moment that there was a dire fate in store for her, a typical Scorpionic feeling. Chiron opposite the Sun in the 3rd house gives her an openness to the realm of imagination and transpersonal ideas. A book is a 3rd-house object; its burning and her subsequent conviction of doom express a tragic example of Chiron in Scorpio opposite a 3rd house Taurus Sun, an idea become literalized and self-destructive.

D. H. Lawrence, whose chart was previously mentioned

on p. 63 and p. 119, has Chiron in Gemini in the 8th house, square Sun and Jupiter in Virgo in the 11th house. He had a life-long conflict with his father, and spent his early days competing with his older brother William who was brilliant, athletic and 'animal-looking' (Chiron in Gemini, wounded by sibling rivalry). When William died, D. H. Lawrence was pushed by his mother (Chiron in the 8th) to take his place in the sun, so to speak. His father was a coal-miner, and Lawrence envied his wildness and freedom from the pressures of the educational system under which he had suffered (Chiron in Gemini). Lawrence's health was permanently undermined in puberty by long hours of travelling and pressure to succeed at school (Chiron in Gemini). Lawrence also expressed his Chiron/Sun conjunction through a fascination with the male physique, and strongly believed in the value of male brotherhood. Although he had a horror of homosexuality, he saw the avoidance of intimacy and physical contact between men as a crippling influence on society (Sun in the 11th). We can also see here the characteristic longing of Chiron in Gemini for the 'other twin'. Lawrence wrote about (Chiron in Gemini), and struggled to live, the very qualities that he rejected in his own father. A circle of admirers, usually women, often surrounded Lawrence (also typical of Chiron/Sun aspects), like planets orbiting around his Sun. True to the Chironian function of being a mentor or foster-father, he could be like 'a kindly gardener who had, very precisely, decided that you were to grow, and who, by that act, awakened in you the feeling that there was something in you which could grow'.[4]

A Chiron/Sun aspect is a powerful stimulus to the process of individuation. There has always been a connection between horses and the sun. The latter connection is 'due not merely . . . to the fact that the horse was the "vehicle" of the sun-god but because, through its swiftness, strength and activity, it was itself a symbol of the sun'.[5] We have seen that horses are important in many shamanic cultures, the symbolic means for magical flight or ecstasy. The initiatory cycle of the shaman includes a stage which Joan Halifax calls the 'solarization of consciousness', where we move from the periphery to the centre of our life. With Chiron aspecting the Sun, the healing of our suffering may come through the recognition of the wider context of life and a sense of our individual place in it, where 'the laughter of compassion wells up from the human heart'.[6] With Chiron aspecting the Sun, we are called upon not to shine for ourselves alone, but for the greater glory of God.

Chiron in Aspect to the Moon

When Chiron aspects the Moon, our relationship with mother is usually featured, and is often the source of deep wounds. She may have been emotionally inadequate to our needs: perhaps she resented motherhood and would have rather been doing something else; perhaps we felt rejected or abandoned at some critical stage. We may have assumed a mothering role very early in life, for a variety of reasons, but before we have received enough mothering ourselves. We may have mothered our mother, or looked after numerous siblings in a large family. Later we may become stuck in this role, becoming 'supermothers', for moving out of it would mean feeling the suffering, anger and emotional deprivation underneath. One person with the Moon opposite Chiron felt rejected by her mother, who wanted a son. She herself became a mother very young. After raising several children, she worked in old-age homes, looking after sick people. She tried her whole life to 'do it better than her mother', and went into a crisis after her first daughter sought therapy because of their relationship: her world crumbled when she realized that her daughter felt wounded by her, in spite of every effort to the contrary. At her Chiron return she courageously embarked on the task of rebuilding her sense of identity, including aspects of her nature that had been left out because of her strong identification with the mother role.

If you have Chiron in aspect to the Moon, you are probably more aware of the emotional needs of others than you are of your own; you instinctively know how to provide what others need in order to feel comfortable, but become resentful if you stop to wonder who is looking after you. The pressure of your unmet needs can make you manipulative, and go to great lengths to get the attention you are not able to ask for directly. You may seek out a mother-figure, hoping she will meet your needs without ever a word being spoken, just as you do for others. You probably attract to you those who need mothering, only feeling strong when in the role of caretaker. Perhaps you even feel you know what is best for others, and are surprised when they manage without you! Although you may have deep instinctive wisdom in this area, you also tend to be somewhat interfering; it is not easy for you to let others be or allow them to make their own mistakes.

Sometimes a woman with Chiron in aspect to the Moon may turn her good-mothering instincts outwards, and reserve her bad mothering for herself. She could have an open house, where all the neighbourhood kids go for tea and biscuits, or to get patched up if they fall and hurt themselves; she may work with children, or babies, or be concerned with maltreated or undernourished children. However, her own self-esteem is often low, and she works hard at maintaining the good-mother role to compensate, and thus prove her worth. This 'supermother' role also serves to protect her from directly facing the wounds she may have received from her own mother. Alternatively, with Chiron in aspect to the Moon, women sometimes reject the role of mothering, consciously feeling no maternal urges, finding it difficult to enjoy babies and young children, and having a horror of anyone becoming dependent on them. When the mothering instinct itself is rejected, blocked or wounded, it does not disappear, but becomes unconscious, able later to manifest itself in a larger-than-life way. Alternatively, women may become devitalized and drained as they narrow down their world to try to protect themselves from the bad mother 'out there'.

With this placement, sometimes a woman's mothering instincts are wounded to the point where she is either unable to have children or does not want them. Part of her individuation process could then be consciously to mourn this and to befriend the power of her own instincts, so that she does not become possessed by their anger at not having been physically fulfilled. Instead of shrivelling with bitterness, she may instead open herself up to a profound relation with the inner world of images – the non-rational and lunar side of consciousness which is a gift of this placement. Lunar consciousness reflects and illuminates the network of unseen connections that make up the web of life, in the form of feelings, subtle energy fields and images. Rather than being a superimposed system of ideas, lunar consciousness is subjective and intuitive, holistic and embedded in organic life.

The lunar goddess has both a bright face and a dark face, as we have already seen in the figure of Artemis. Her bright aspect reflects light in the form of caring for others and contributing to life by honouring the feeling element in situations; her gifts are ecstasy, holistic awareness and intuition. Her dark aspect, however, includes destructive irrationality in the form of militant subjectivity, a tendency to become swamped with emotional reactions to projections, and a resistance to order or discipline. Those with Chiron/Moon contacts may sabotage themselves through their own emotionality, and yet be unaware of their feelings. I am using these terms in the Jungian sense, where emotion is the discharge of energy that accompanies something emerging from the unconscious, be it a memory, a feeling, a thought or new idea. Feeling, on the other hand, is a conscious function which makes relatedness possible in the present, as well as a sense of valuing oneself and others. Often those with Chiron/Moon contacts are very emotional, and sometimes they accuse others of being unfeeling. They may also tyrannize others and spoil relationships with emotional outbursts; their emotionally demanding behaviour usually has its origins in early childhood; they are still reacting angrily to the pain of insufficient mothering.

Sometimes the wound of Chiron/Moon manifests itself in eating disorders, for we may try to take in good mothering in this way. For example, one woman has a bucket-shaped chart with Chiron focal in the 10th house conjunct the MC, both in Aquarius; Chiron trines Moon in the 5th in Libra, and is also quincunx Sun in Cancer in the 2nd house; Sun and Moon square each other. She was seriously overweight, and her body became a source of embarrassment. She became progressively more afraid to go out (Chiron in the 10th, as fear of the world); in particular, she hated men looking at her. When she realized the seriousness of her problem, her initial response was very Aquarian: she went on several weekend courses which addressed the problem of eating disorders, and as a result decided that she would make a career (Chiron conjunct MC in the 10th house) of helping women with similar problems. Meanwhile, her own weight problem remained intractable. She had Taurus rising, and when transiting Chiron was conjunct her Ascendant, she began in-depth psychotherapy. Eventually she did begin to lose weight as she confronted some of the deeper issues that were being expressed through it. Like Chiron, she had to surrender to the Underworld in order to be healed.

Men with Chiron/Moon contacts often remain painfully aware of the feeling life of their mothers, and are consciously or unconsciously eager to accommodate her and make her happy, even becoming the kind of man she would like them to be – perhaps like a substitute husband. They may become 'anima possessed', or dominated by moodiness, emotional manipulativeness and veiled or overt hostility towards women. Later in life, men with Chiron/Moon aspects are often found in partnerships where they play the mother role, whether it is a work relationship, a friendship or a marriage. They may also attract wounded women to them, or find themselves very aware of emotional suffering in others and want to do something about it. Having a strong contact with the feminine side of their nature, they may also be very creative. Robert Graves has Chiron conjunct the Moon in Libra; through his historical approach to myths he traced them back to their lunar roots in matriarchal times. An interesting example of a man who has this aspect is Dr Benjamin Spock, with Chiron in Capricorn opposite Moon in Cancer; he set out standards (note Chiron is in Capricorn) of infant care which influenced a whole generation of young mothers and their offspring, especially in America; one cannot help wondering if he was trying to out-mother his mother, as he vicariously inflicted upon millions of babies the same disregard for natural rhythms as he must have experienced from her.

Yet sometimes men with Chiron/Moon aspects appear to have no contact with their feeling and reflective side, except through women, whom they may seek to dominate and control. Then we see a macho man, whose masculinity expresses itself in a raw way without being tempered by any qualities from his feminine side. He may both idealize and denigrate women; in extremes, he may be violent and contemptuous. All this points to wounding situations in his early relationship with his mother. For example, Charles Manson has Chiron in Gemini in the 2nd house, trine Moon and North Node in Aquarius in the 10th; Chiron also

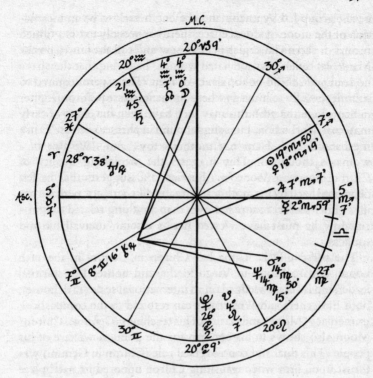

Charles Manson

$$♼ = ♂/⚷ = ♂/♆ = ♆/♃$$

squares a Mars/Neptune conjunction in Virgo in the 5th house and is quincunx Jupiter in Scorpio in the 7th house. He was the guru (Chiron) of a group called 'The Family' (Moon). His philosophy (Chiron) included the belief that he and 'The Family' would dwell inside the 'Mystic Hole' (Moon = Mother = Womb) in Death Valley, while the blacks and the whites would fight to the death in the cities; this fantasy expresses the warring opposites of Chiron in Gemini. He equipped dune-buggies with machine-guns to be the Horses (Chiron!) of the Apocalypse, and called himself 'Angel of the Bottomless Pit'. He had connections with an

occult group led by a woman believing herself to be an incarnation of the moon–goddess Circe; there supposedly exists a filmed
record of sacrificial orgies held at new and full moons (Chiron/
Mars/Neptune). Manson hated women, believing that they have
no soul and should be the slaves of men. They were required to
submit sexually to him anywhere and at any time (Chiron/Jupiter
in Scorpio in the 7th); this may well have been the effect of early
maternal deprivation. His songs abound in phrases such as: 'I am a
mechanical boy, I am my mother's toy', and, 'We live in a
woman's thought.'[7] This suggests the wounding quality of
Chiron aspecting Moon in Aquarius, and suggests that he felt
depersonalized by his mother and treated like a object; perhaps her
idea of her son was more her own than anything related to him –
certainly he must have viewed her as distant, unavailable and
soulless.

The present Dalai Lama has Chiron in Gemini in the 11th
house, square Moon in Virgo in the 2nd house. His spiritual
leadership is acknowledged on an international scale (11th house);
both Easterners and Westerners can respond to the compassion,
immediacy (Moon) and clarity of his teachings (Gemini). Chiron/
Moon also shows in his concern for the political welfare of his
people. This dual and controversial role (Chiron in Gemini) was
thrust upon him when transiting Chiron opposed its natal place
and squared his Moon: he witnessed the destruction of much of
Tibet's ancient cultural past when the Chinese invaded, and now
lives in exile (Chiron in the 11th house) from his homeland
(Moon). Chiron/Moon is also expressed in his unusual childhood: while still a baby, he was recognized as the reincarnation of
the previous Dalai Lama, and when only six years old began the
specialized and rigorous education (Chiron in Gemini) which
prepared him for his destiny.

Dr Miriam Stoppard has Chiron conjunct South Node conjunct Moon, all in Gemini in the 2nd house. Dr Stoppard is well
known to British TV audiences for her programme *Where There's
Life*, in which subjects of medical and psychological interest are
aired, usually by way of discussing actual life-experiences with
members of the audience. Her interviewing manner is warm and
motherly (Chiron/Moon) but simple and direct (Chiron in the

2nd house). She has a gift for enabling people to communicate (Chiron in Gemini) their personal feelings and life-experiences (Moon) with unusual candour, and in a way that touches and benefits the public at large; the message implied throughout is that it is healing to talk about painful things (Chiron in Gemini).

Mother Teresa of Calcutta has Chiron in Pisces opposite Sun in Virgo, both square Moon in Gemini. She won the Nobel Peace Prize in 1979 for her work in Bombay with destitute and homeless people, having been called by God to do so. Her life serves as a model of selfless compassion (Chiron in Pisces). Her prayers and meditations abound with lunar imagery – of feeding, nourishment – and speak of the needy: 'Christ is longing to be your Food. Surrounded with fullness of living Food, you allow yourself to starve . . . There is a great hunger for God in the world today.' She speaks of Christ coming 'in distressing disguise – in the hungry man, in the lonely man, in the homeless child, and seeking for shelter'.[8]

Chiron in Aspect to Mercury

When Chiron aspects Mercury, this principle is often wounded and we may then see 'supermercurial types' portraying the various archetypal figures associated with it. In her book on Mercury, Pam Tyler describes two faces of Mercury – ruler of both Gemini and Virgo. She associates the god Hermes with the sign of Gemini, and the ancient Egyptian god Thoth with the sign of Virgo. Let us briefly contrast these two.

When in the cradle, Hermes is already up to mischief: he steals Apollo's sacred cattle and, when discovered, charms his way out of trouble, setting the precedent for many of his later misdemeanours. He outwits his superiors with guile; he rebels and subtly evades. He boldly invites himself into the Olympian circle, and later earns the title of 'Messenger of the Gods', many of them being indebted to him for being rescued from various tight spots. He finds a way out of deadlock or potentially humiliating situations, and is frequently a key figure in the unfolding of the destiny of other gods, arriving in the nick of time with a crucial message, or clinching an important deal. To my knowledge, there are no stories in which Hermes himself is captured or punished; he usually manages to wriggle out of the consequences of his actions. Yet he is also the god of boundaries – the name Hermes comes from the Greek word *herma*, a pile of stones used in ancient times to mark the boundaries of property. Perhaps this paradox explains Hermes' mobility: he passes unhindered everywhere from the heights of Olympus to the depths of the Underworld.

Thoth, on the other hand, represents Ra (another sun-god), acting as his servant and scribe. He is the guardian and enforcer of the laws of Ra, the upholder and administrator of his justice. It was Thoth who intervened in the struggle between Osiris and his evil brother Seth, and cured them both of the wounds they had received. In his association with Virgo, Thoth represents control, discipline and the productive use of mental energy; he signifies the ability to withstand conflict, to encompass the duties of daily life with dignity, and thus to be productive.

`With Chiron in aspect to Mercury, however, there is another archetypal figure which frequently accompanies this aspect: the Trickster. Jung points out that the alchemical figure of Mercurius contains many typical trickster elements, and this ambiguous figure was also an important character in the palaeolithic world of myth and story. Although represented as a fool, a lecher and wily cheat, he is nevertheless a kind of culture hero credited with bringing to mankind skills such as metallurgy, the use of fire and the reckoning of time. Remnants of the Trickster may be seen today in the carnival figures of clowns, buffoons, devils, imps, griots (Africa) and Pulchinellos. These mischief-makers turn things upside-down, bringing chaos and disorder; they break the bounds of convention and taboo with celebratory delight.

The Trickster is thus a universal figure like the shaman, with whom he shares certain characteristics. He represents a form of consciousness still connected with the animal kingdom and the instincts; he can change shape at will into an animal or another human form. His energy is chaotic and amoral. The parts of his body can be autonomous. For example, he is said to be able to remove his anus and entrust it with independent tasks; his hands can fight each other, and his penis can grow long enough to cause perplexing problems! Useful plants are also said to originate from his penis, thus connecting the Trickster with the creative spirit and fertility (remember that Chiron is also credited with originating the medicinal use of plants). Thus the Trickster initially represents a chaotic, fertile and emergent consciousness. However, he is eventually pinned down and tortured; through suffering he grows in moral strength and pledges himself to serving humanity. In a sense, his progression from primitive daemon and *enfant terrible* to a figure made sober, wise and responsible through his suffering lies behind both the wily Greek Hermes and the sombre Egyptian Thoth, for the cycle of his development contains all these aspects, and it seems we forget his origins at our peril.

Psychologically, the Trickster seems to represent that within us which works in a direction contrary to our highest and most noble aims. He loves to see pride come before a fall, and is a natural antidote to the self-importance, pretensions and inflations encountered in the quest for consciousness and integration. The more we endeavour to reach our highest, to become godlike, to actualize our potential, the more this figure constellates quietly underneath, ready to trip us up at any point should we dare to forget the chaotic origins of our hard-won sense of order, personal integration and consciousness. The Trickster is at work when annoying synchronicities, lapses of memory, misconnections and misunderstandings prevent us achieving goals dear to the ego. He can reduce to a shambles the most carefully ordered pattern of meaning, plan of action or contrived self-concept, as he especially resists being controlled, grounded, or owned. If we become too 'civilized', we may be inviting trouble from the Trickster, who will compensate for our pretensions by quickly showing up the emptiness of our façades and collective adaptations.

In his essay, 'On the Psychology of the Trickster Figure', Jung takes the somewhat linear view that 'the trickster is a collective shadow figure, an epitome of all the inferior traits of character of individuals'.[9] Joseph Campbell has this to say in response:

Such a view, however, is presented from the ground of our later 'bounded' style of thought. In the palaeolithic view from which this figure derives, he was the archetypal hero, the giver of all great boons, the fire bringer and teacher of humanity.[10]

On a personal level, people with Chiron in aspect to Mercury are nobody's fools, and they see through pretences. Like the Trickster, they may enjoy putting people down with a well-placed comment that pierces the façade. Equally, they sometimes envy the clarity, panache and sophistication of others. They may find themselves taking the brunt of wounding remarks, but usually they enjoy being the one who refuses to join the bandwagon, the one who always finds the fly in the ointment. They may have a gossip-columnist attitude, always seeking out the juicy story that tarnishes the bright picture painted by others. Hedda Hopper, adept at 'minding other people's business', has Mercury in Gemini semisquare Chiron in Cancer.

With Chiron in aspect to Mercury we can be powerful and sometimes compulsive communicators either through non-verbal means such as music or mime, or through the traditional Mercurial pursuits such as writing, speaking, journalism, or teaching. Perhaps we want to challenge people into awareness and self-reflection, or feel we have important things to say; we may have a nose for controversy and enjoy stirring it up! Some people with Chiron in aspect to Mercury have a flair for languages; Maria Callas has Chiron trine Mercury, and learned several languages fluently in a short time. A sinister example of Chiron/Mercury is found in the horoscope of Joseph Paul Goebbels, with Chiron conjunct Mercury in Scorpio in the 4th house. As the official propagandist of Nazi Germany he helped Hitler to power, for a while controlling the entire German media network. His Chiron/Mercury in Scorpio here indicates the control of others' thoughts through disseminating wounding and irrational ideas. When the Nazi regime fell Goebbels committed suicide with his entire family. With Chiron in the 4th his identification with the 'Fatherland' was so deep that he did not survive its 'wounding'.

Those with Chiron/Mercury aspects often have a sharp intuitive mind, which, if permitted to express itself, may show great brilliance and originality of perception. The minds of these people operate in a direct and instinctive way, untrammelled by stale concepts and prejudices. They have the ability to get to the heart of the matter, and may be good mediators or debaters. They enjoy contentious issues, and can usually be relied upon to come up with original views and surprise solutions; they often have a knack for stating the obvious which everyone else is missing. Individuals with Chiron in aspect to Mercury may be very good at helping others to clarify their thoughts, and to foster people's ability to communicate.

Communication often takes non-verbal forms with Chiron in aspect to Mercury. For example, Meher Baba, the 'silent mystic' has a T-square with Chiron in Virgo opposite Mercury in Pisces, both square Pluto and Neptune in Gemini. After a realization which occurred when transiting Chiron was in Pisces, opposing his natal Chiron and conjunct his Mercury, and Saturn was transiting Pluto and Neptune in Gemini, Meher Baba went into lifelong silence. During this time he profoundly touched many people through his silent presence, facilitating healing and inspiration (Chiron/Mercury). He would write out simple phrases expressing his experience of the Absolute in which he dwelt. When he entered the silence, his natal Saturn was opposed by Chiron – a suitable image for retreating behind a wall of silence.

Chiron/Mercury aspects are also common in the horoscopes of famous musicians. Jimi Hendrix, Pablo Casals, Yehudi Menuhin and Maria Callas all have Chiron/Mercury contacts, and also have to their credit a highly original technique (Mercury). They have the ability to invoke in the listener an awareness of transpersonal levels of reality. In Maria Callas's chart, there is a grand trine in fire signs: Sun conjunct Mercury and the Ascendant in Sagittarius, both trine Chiron in Aries and Neptune in Leo.[11] She also has Chiron square Pluto, and she played Medea in Pasolini's film of that name. Chiron appears in the opening scene, half horse and half man; later he appears as two fully *human* beings. Far from this being progress, however, Chiron now feels desecrated. The Centaur must not be civilized out of existence, but must be allowed to continue living inside the human and inspiring him. We are told: 'His logic is so different to yours that it would be incomprehensible to you.' This is perhaps the logic of Chiron/Mercury, the Trickster.

Some people with Chiron/Mercury contacts experience difficulties at school. Their flair for communication may lie not so much in the verbal and rational field, but in areas which address the feelings or the intuitive and non-rational side of life. Others feel fear and turmoil when trying to commit their thoughts to paper or to express them in words. Their own thoughts may lie hidden beneath a state of mental chaos, which may at first be frightening as it refuses to be forced into any logical mode. With Chiron in aspect to Mercury, the thinking process is still closely connected with its chaotic origins; the irrationality of the Trickster lurks close by and may scare us off using our minds creatively – although, if we take the risk, the results are often quite extraordinary. William Blake has Chiron conjunct Venus in Capricorn in the 6th house sextile Mercury in Scorpio in the 5th.

His writing is a good example of someone able to communicate visionary experience in words; many find quite incomprehensible his florid and subjective writing, which includes dark and prophetic visions (Mercury in Scorpio in the 5th house).

On the other hand, some people with Chiron in aspect to Mercury have a gift for clear logical thinking and an ability to create order from a welter of sense impressions and information. They have penetrating minds, and study obscure or esoteric subjects. For example, Walter Koch, who originated the system of house divisions used throughout this book, has Chiron conjunct Mercury in Libra in the 1st house (Chiron in the 1st is the innovator). He was a researcher and gifted intellectual with an astonishing memory; after being wounded in the leg during World War I he subsequently wrote prolifically about astrology. Michel Gauquelin, another famous researcher, has Chiron in Taurus in the 10th house, very near its discovery degree and opposite Mercury in Scorpio in the 4th house. He began to examine the fundamentals (4th house) of astrology, at first with the aim to debunk or wound them (Chiron opposite Mercury in Scorpio). However, his meticulous research provided statistical evidence which led him to become more and more interested; his work is controversial, challenging basic concepts but also providing a fertile source of categorized data for researchers. Developing the Thoth side of Mercury may be difficult but rewarding for people with Chiron/Mercury. Fear of inner chaos may almost paralyse the minds of some with this placement, rendering them unable to communicate their own experiences, but able to write technically or scientifically about things separate from them. Thus Chiron/Mercury people are found doing work which is typically Virgoan in nature – researching, categorizing, ordering.

With Chiron in aspect to Mercury, we might have a good ability to withstand mental conflict and embrace paradoxes without finding them disturbing; our awareness of incongruousness and appreciation of the absurd may be very well developed. We could have a zany, acerbic sense of humour, not hesitating to speak the truth, regardless of who gets humiliated in the process. We can wound with our humour if it conceals a fear of deep feelings and personal intimacy. There are no sacred cows with

Chiron/Mercury. Anything may be the subject of a witty remark or a simple but penetrating comment. Like Hermes, humour can release emotion and break deadlock; it helps us to relax and see ourselves in our folly. Several famous comedians have Chiron/Mercury contacts, and their humour often contains social or political comment. Chiron/Mercury humour can be very serious, intent on producing awareness, educating people and mocking the customs, prejudices and institutions which make up our society. For example, Alan Alda has Chiron in Gemini in the 5th house, trine Sun conjunct Mercury in Aquarius in the 1st house. Alan Alda plays a doctor in the famous television series *M*A*S*H*, a black comedy set in an army unit during the Korean War. The series does not proselytize, but through the pathos of black humour brings awareness of the inhumanity of war. This is one typical Chiron/Mercury approach: not to come on heavy, but to foster consciousness through trickery!

Chiron in Aspect to Venus

With Chiron in aspect to Venus we may have the gift of seeing beauty where others do not notice it and of finding value in what they dismiss as ugly or worthless. Our values are intensely personal. We adhere to them with great tenacity, and our Venusian preoccupations can even assume philosophical or political dimensions: we might campaign for women's rights, racial harmony, or be an enthusiastic supporter of the arts. We quest after someone or something of great beauty and value, or perhaps for wealth, glamour or lasting romance. With this placement, we often meet people who already seem familiar to us; perhaps we feel we have known them in other lives, and may even have some idea of the details. I have met several people with Chiron/Venus aspects who had intractable problems in a relationship that were only resolved by taking this perspective; with these planets in aspect we are often opened to other dimensions of consciousness through painful relationships with others. We find inspiration and discover our next steps in life through intense and synchronous meetings with people who bring new ideas, rich interpersonal encounters, suggestions, insights or business contacts. However, we might not realize that we in turn do just that for others, and remain unaware of how much we are appreciated by them. The most important relationships in the lives of those with Chiron in aspect to Venus are frequently those which bring artistic inspiration or personal growth, rather than those which lead to marriage or child-rearing.

With Chiron in aspect to Venus, we are very sensitive to disharmony between people, and may become involved in others' disputes and take them personally, even if they have nothing to do with us. Perhaps we unconsciously feel responsible for bringing love and harmony into life! This may have roots in early childhood situations: we may have assumed the role of peace-maker and mediated between warring parents, siblings or in-laws; we may have been under pressure to side with one parent against the other in a divorce or separation. Later on, we engage in futile struggles to resolve the unresolvable in relationships – we may have to learn to give up trying. It is often difficult for us to endure conflict, as we may be striving after a level of harmony which is unrealistic and impossible to attain. Alternatively, we could stay in situations of almost intolerable interpersonal conflict, hoping eventually to bring harmony and reconciliation, but wounding ourselves in the process.

With Chiron/Venus aspects, we may experience a baptism of fire in our first intimate relationships; if we do not learn to stand for our own values, we establish a pattern of always accommodating others – a pattern which usually has its roots in earlier difficulties. People with Chiron in aspect to Venus sometimes follow someone else's path and take on their values and artistic aspirations. For example, one man had a Chiron/Venus conjunction the 10th house in Libra, conjunct a Libran MC; he had a history of relationships with women who had careers in various branches of the arts. He invariably ended up following suit: he became a photographer when he was in a relationship with a photographer, and worked in the theatre when he was living with an actress. This had its origins in his relationship with his mother, who had given up a promising career as a singer in order to raise a family, and hoped that her son would follow in her footsteps into a career in the performing arts.

Chiron aspecting Venus often brings a genuine ability to open others' capacity for relationships and to touch them deeply. This quality usually comes with maturity, however, and initially we might struggle with an idealized or distorted picture of what relationships are about. Perhaps we require others to be more open with us than we are willing to be with them, or we see people as mirrors of ourselves and find differences hard to encompass. Although we long for interpersonal harmony, others may find us oppressive; if we are oblivious to the impact we have on others, we will be unable to handle the repercussions. Sometimes incurably romantic, we experience isolation and disappointment when real life falls short of our refined ideals. Perhaps we feel betrayed by friends or lovers, when in fact it is our own idealism which betrays us with impossible standards of harmony: we quest after unattainable people, enjoying the bitter-sweet pain of emotional dramas, impossible situations, tragedy and unrequited love. As Robert Johnson puts it: 'One of the great paradoxes of romantic love is that it never produces human relationship as long as it stays romantic.'[12] If we ignore difficult feelings in the name of creating harmony or a 'perfect relationship', emotional disasters often follow.

For those with Chiron/Venus contacts, relationships bring their major lesson in life. There is often difficulty with the darker side of relating, with its sexual competition, emotional manipulation and underground power struggles. However, their journey will usually take them into these areas, and holding on to innocence may result in their becoming vulnerable to being exploited emotionally, sexually and financially. Underneath their considerable Venusian charm, tact and diplomacy, those with this placement are adept at getting their own way, knowing how to manipulate others' feelings and even set people against each other; they can be very controlling and contrive to dominate relationships by subtly refusing to compromise.

With Chiron in aspect to Venus we may be drawn to the 'beautiful people', and envy those who are wealthy, glamorous or famous for artistic achievements. We could become deceived by the external trappings of Venus, and part of our quest may be to reconnect with our capacity for sensual pleasure and rediscover our need for authentic relationships, rather than seeking out or living up to images. We could be somewhat vain and obsessed with our physical appearance, feeling uncomfortable unless we are 'dressed to kill': close friends or lovers never see us in disarray, and we find signs of ageing very upsetting. Perhaps we secretly enjoy provoking envy in others, and use our beauty, artistic gifts and magnetic sexuality as weapons. On the other hand, however, we may be unable to appreciate our own talents or beauty, regardless of what others say. We may fear the envy of other people, and may feel deprived of the Venusian gift for enjoyment of the realm of the senses. With Chiron/Venus contacts, the painful abuse or neglect of our gifts can eventually lead us to see physical beauty, pleasure and artistic abilities as divine gifts to be cherished and shared.

The story of Psyche and Eros is one whose themes often appear in the lives of people who have Chiron/Venus contacts. Psyche is a young woman of such dazzling beauty that people worship her instead of the goddess Aphrodite, who becomes angry and jealous. In spite of her beauty, however, Psyche is lonely and unfulfilled. After an oracle predicts that she will never find a mortal husband, amidst much sorrow and mourning, Psyche resigns herself to a death-marriage. Instead of the expected disaster, however, she finds herself borne aloft by the wind and carried to the palace of Eros, where she is treated with gentleness and servants see to her every need. She spends idyllic nights with her lover Eros, but he always departs before dawn, as she is forbidden to see him in the light of day. Psyche has two sisters who are deeply envious of her beauty and her new-found glory. Eros warns her about their destructiveness and counsels her not to be influenced by them. However, when they visit her magnificent palace home, they sow the seeds of mistrust and fear, convincing Psyche that her beloved Eros is a dangerous and ugly monster, and that she must somehow contrive to see him in the light. One night, overcome with curiosity and worry for her own safety, Psyche shines a lamp on Eros when he is asleep, planning to kill him. What she sees is not a monster, but a man of such exquisite beauty that she is intoxicated and throws herself upon him with consuming passion. However, some drops of hot wax from her lamp fall upon Eros, waking him, and thus her transgression is revealed. Eros flies away, with Psyche desperately clinging on to him; she falls to earth, alone, to see her lover vanish upwards without her. Eros takes temporary refuge with his mother Aphrodite, who is enraged by his love for Psyche, and casts him out. Psyche wanders in suicidal despair, and is eventually brought to the house of Aphrodite. She decrees that she must embark on a quest to prove her worth, and sets her some seemingly impossible tasks to accomplish. With assistance from various helpful animals, Psyche does accomplish all the tasks, including a perilous journey to the Underworld, and is reunited at last with her lover Eros.

The contrast between the noble, mournful and innocent Psyche beset with painful trials and the powerful, vengeful and envious Aphrodite underpins this myth. It is Aphrodite who both causes

Psyche's suffering, but, in the guise of Psyche's jealous sisters, she is paradoxically also the one who stimulates the quest for consciousness. Psyche endures a period of trial and suffering for the sake of renewal of her relationship, and gains through it her wholeness. Aphrodite represents the negative aspects of matriarchal consciousness, opposed to individual relationships with men – an envious mother goddess who refuses to release her son and brooks no competition from other women. Psyche's helpers are always from the animal kingdom, and this symbolizes the gradual loss of her innocence through the assimilation of the instinctual side of her nature. The destructive envy of Aphrodite is overcome in this way; only then can Psyche reclaim her right to individual love. [13]

These contrasting characters often appear in the lives of those with Chiron in aspect to Venus. Sometimes a woman with Chiron/Venus contacts has had difficulties with an envious mother or sisters. Growing into womanhood and creativity may be so fraught with fear that this transition is never made, and she may opt for a sad innocence instead; acknowledging her Aphrodite side, her own sexual competitiveness and desire to be centre stage may be difficult but is important. A mother unaware of her own envy may become mentally or physically ill as her daughter approaches the threshold of puberty; she may play the role of being hard done by and show so little pleasure in anything the daughter feels that sexuality, sensual pleasure and enjoyment of life are taboo because the mother does not have them. Daughters of such mothers grow up unconscious of their sexuality, but very attractive to men; they often attract unwelcome sexual advances, which cause embarrassment, anger, fear and indignation.

Psyche's suffering is for the renewal of relationship at a more conscious level than it was before. Likewise, suffering through relationship may be a dominant theme in the lives of people with Chiron/Venus contacts. We need to discover and acknowledge the purpose of this suffering, however, or we may become entrenched in the role of the victim. Through the trials of the darker side of human interactions, we feel a loss of innocence, but may thus grow in our individual sense of identity, and gain in compassion and consciousness. The intoxication of being in love with love and then coming to earth with a bump is also a familiar experience for those with Chiron in aspect to Venus; they may cling relentlessly to their illusions like Psyche clinging on to Eros as he disappears into the sky. They usually suffer more than once the repercussions of making someone else the centre of their universe; when the person leaves, they have to rebuild their lives from scratch, undergoing a painful period of inner trials, like Psyche.

Men with Chiron/Venus aspects may, like Eros, fly off at the first sight of a woman who wants to be an individual in her own right. They may seek out pliable, self-effacing women, only to be confronted later on with the full might of an emerging Aphrodite! Somewhere in the lives of men with Chiron and Venus in aspect, there is usually a powerful, magnetic and sensual woman. The relationship could be one of mutual wariness or of passionate involvement and admiration. She is often kept at a safe distance as friend and confidante rather than lover. Likewise, if you are a woman with Chiron and Venus in aspect, you may wonder why men keep their distance although you know yourself to be attractive enough! A man with Chiron and Venus in aspect usually has good style, taste in clothes, an eye for beauty (his own and others), and likes to be seen at the best places. If your man has Chiron/Venus, wear expensive perfume and take care of your appearance; let him know your Aphrodite side is there, but don't scare him off by overdoing it! Above all, do not mother him. Men with Chiron in aspect to Venus have a deep appreciation of feminine beauty and often make wonderful partners for women who aspire to be both self-sufficient and deeply feminine as well. Their own artistic and feminine sides are often well developed, making them gifted and artistically creative. For example, a man with Chiron in Capricorn in the 6th house square Venus in Libra in the 4th was from a poor family, and was mocked for his rather feminine physical appearance. Later he became a teacher of Physical Education, and an accomplished sculptor in stone. His Venusian sense of rhythm and beauty was engaged in his work (Venus aspecting Chiron in Capricorn in the 6th). To his students he emphasized enjoyment, grace, health and beauty rather than competition (Chiron/Venus). His interest in sculpture is expressed by Chiron in Capricorn in the 6th, an earthy sign in an earthy house traditionally concerned with crafting material.

An example from history illustrates some further Chiron/ Venus themes. All the members of the first family to establish a mission in the area of Africa that became Rhodesia have close Chiron/Venus aspects in their horoscopes.[14] From the social and moral context of the time and their involvement with missionary Christianity over several generations, we can make an educated guess that the world of sensual enjoyment, raw instinctuality, creative self-indulgence and other Venusian joys was vigorously denied. They carried the collective wound of unrelatedness to the instincts (Chiron/Venus), the pressure of which drove them to 'darkest Africa', where they met their 'other halves', projected on to the black people whose souls they were trying to save. Characteristic of Chiron/Venus, they imposed their values (Venus) and religion (Chiron) rather than engaging in a truly mutual exchange. Robert Moffat, the father of the first family, has Chiron in Virgo trine Venus in Capricorn and square Mercury in Sagittarius. He was a robust and idealistic man who wrote voluminous daily journals (Chiron/Mercury) in the form of letters to his wife (Chiron/Venus), including detailed descriptions of his encounters with the notorious Ndebele warrior chief Mzilikazi. Over time a curious bond grew between these two men of such extremely different cultural, racial and personal backgrounds. This is an example of a Chiron/Venus relationship which made history: treaties were signed and permission granted for the establishing of the first mission station. See the horoscope of Dr Ian Player in Chapter 11 for another example of a Chiron/Venus relationship whose ripples spread into a global context. Interestingly, Robert Mugabe also has Chiron exactly conjunct Venus in Aries, trine Jupiter in Sagittarius. As Prime Minister of Zimbabwe (formerly Rhodesia), Mugabe initiated an official government 'policy of reconciliation' (Chiron/Venus). This has had the effect of providing an inspirational backdrop for the creation of a new multiracial state, but initially led to various abuses in the name of unification. Other features of his leadership express the 'bridging' qualities of Chiron/Venus: his political values are neither exclusively Marxist nor capitalist, and traditional African culture is being revalued alongside Western education and technology.

Chiron in Aspect to Mars

With Chiron in aspect to Mars, we may have been wounded by negative and destructive expressions of the Mars principle in our early environment. If the home environment was like a battlefield of open or concealed warfare, we perhaps decided: 'I'll never be like that.' Then we grow up dreading that the destructiveness may once again erupt, become over-cautious and throw out the baby with the bath-water, suppressing our own capacity for positive self-assertion, healthy expression of anger and desire for conquest and mastery of our life. With Chiron/Mars aspects, if we grow up afraid of confrontation and unaware of our own anger and wilfulness, we could frequently fall foul of others' aggression.

If we are carrying a burden of angry feelings from past situations where we could not get our own way, whether it was appropriate or not, we might also be carrying an exaggerated sense of our own destructiveness, and control ourselves carefully in order to protect others from it. We then tend to pass the buck or give away our power in a manner described by the signs and houses surrounding our Mars/Chiron aspect, only to fight with whoever did take the initiative. For example, with Mars in Libra square Chiron in Cancer, we could descend into feelings of helplessness (Chiron in Cancer) to avoid personal confrontations or making decisions (Mars in Libra); we fight back by sulking (Chiron in Cancer) and refusing to co-operate (Mars in Libra). Thus we may actually control situations by not taking action, by not expressing ourselves or making decisions. This passive aggression in turn attracts aggression from others, and as the 'injured party' we can genuinely be at a loss to know why. In retaliation, we may cultivate the art of annoying and provoking others, subtly or directly.

If our Mars capacity for self-assertion, direct action and rising to challenge is wounded, we may find it difficult to know what we want and tend to become inert, passively aggressive and resentful. We could become ill as a way of controlling others, as an outlet for our unexpressed anger, or to defuse situations in which negativity has escalated because we have not taken a stand or expressed our feelings. Our symptoms will affect body functions and organs which are ruled by Mars: we get fevers or become anaemic; we get hot rashes and headaches, our muscles feel weak. Yukio Mishima, the Japanese writer who committed ritual suicide, has Chiron conjunct Mars in Aries; whatever the religious or philosophical reasons for his suicide, it serves as an expressive image for those whose Chiron/Mars aspects have been turned against them.

People with Chiron/Mars contacts sometimes inadvertently ignite the fuse of unexpressed anger in others. They stand back with astonishment and watch their friends, lovers or work-partners get angry, unreasonable or even violent. Some people with these contacts have a knack of keeping their own hands clean, as it were, and if you are in a relationship with someone who has a Chiron/Mars contact, don't be surprised if you often get angry! If you have Chiron in aspect to Mars, it may be useful to learn how unconscious aggression, wilfulness and destructiveness works, both in yourself and others, as you will probably encounter it.

The opposite is also common, where the lives of people with Chiron/Mars contacts seem full of positive action, discipline and energetic achievement. I would associate Ares, the god of war with this aspect; he also represents blood-lust, uncontrolled aggression, enjoyment of destruction and the desire to provoke conflict. The goddess Athene, however, twice managed to overcome him in battle. As she represents, among other things, the ability to mediate in conflicts and to reflect before taking action, this suggests something important for those with Chiron in aspect to Mars. A little reflection may go a long way if you have these planets in aspect.

In the life of Cecil Rhodes we find what is perhaps a compensation for the feeling of having no right to exist that often underpins Chiron in the 1st house, ruled by Mars. His Chiron is in Capricorn, and makes a great many aspects including a quincunx to Mars. His exploitiveness and greed for territory were perhaps his struggle to gain a substitute for the primary sense of being

(Chiron in the 1st house); he strove to make himself immortal through conquests to honour Queen and Country (Chiron trine Pluto and Uranus and Pluto in Taurus in the 4th house). A country was named after him (Rhodesia), and thus culminated his search for confirmation of his existence. He met his downfall through one Princess Radziwill, an unstable and psychic woman (Chiron/Moon in Cancer in the 7th), who had been in the secret service of Bismarck and pursued Rhodes relentlessly. Rhodes talked freely to her about matters of state, although he knew that she was a correspondent of French and Russian newspapers. Having laboured nobly for the Empire, he came perilously close to betraying it – a situation congruent with Chiron in the 1st

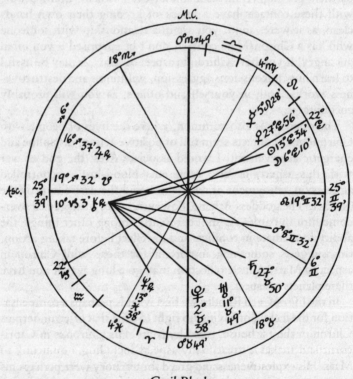

Cecil Rhodes

house in Capricorn aspecting Mars in Gemini. She forged his signature on bills (Chiron in Rhodes's 1st house here symbolizes someone trying to steal his identity!) and created a financial scandal (Chiron/Pluto in Taurus) which tarnished Rhodes's reputation and caused him harassment over several years. Some biographers suggest that the stress of all this weakened his health and contributed to his death. Typical of Chiron/Mars, Rhodes was always a controversial figure, but with Chiron in Capricorn he would indeed have been deeply wounded by damage to his public image.

If we look closely into the lives of those with Mars/Chiron contacts who are known for their positive Martian qualities of forthrightness, leadership and dynamism, we often find relationships in which they are indulged like babies; on the other hand, they may habitually vent the negative side of Mars on someone, browbeating a wife or lover with extreme petulance, moodiness or overt cruelty. Cecil Rhodes provides an example of this. His Chiron/Mars qualities are obvious: he exercised supreme control over those under him; he made no attempt to conciliate his enemies; with his resolutely inflexible will and intense patriotic loyalty he worked for the aggrandizement of the British Empire. He was an ardent admirer of the Roman Emperor Marcus Aurelius (note Chiron opposes Sun in the 7th house), and was particularly impressed by his writings on the enduring nature of human achievements (Mars in the 6th house quincunx Chiron in Capricorn) as opposed to the transient nature of human life. Rhodes collected a bodyguard of adventurous young men around him, whom he treated with ruthless authority; he demanded great personal sacrifice from them in terms of pandering to his every whim. However, one observer describes Rhodes as a 'great baby', incapable of being left to himself.[15] Between the first and second conjunctions of his Chiron return, Rhodes died of a dropsical condition with enlarged blood vessels which interfered with his breathing; Mars (also associated with blood) is in Gemini, which rules the lungs. His epitaph poignantly expresses Mars/Chiron: 'So little done, so much to do.'

This illustrates the compulsive doing which is often the bugbear of those who have Chiron and Mars in aspect, where the

Chironian theme of 'futile struggles' may be particularly relevant. If you have a pattern of restless and compulsive doing, which does not lead to your feeling fulfilled and productive, but which over-extends your resources and leads to frustration and even illness, it might be useful to ask yourself the question 'What am I *really* trying to do?' With Chiron/Mars, you could discover that your *unconscious* goal is a potentially self-destructive one, a futile or impossible endeavour that is best left alone. Examples of this attitude are: 'If only I could do something *totally* original, then I would be noticed', or, 'If only I could become rich and powerful then my father would envy me.' The themes of wanting to be the first, best and only, or an attitude of 'I'll show them' are often interwoven here with a desire to punish others. Unearthing hidden fantasies of omnipotence and grandiose conquests may mean you have more choice to redirect or perhaps tame this energy, instead of being compulsively driven beyond your limits and then having to deal with the repercussions. Ross and Norris McWhirter, twin brothers who started the *Guinness Book of Records*, have Chiron in Aries trine Mars in Leo: it would be interesting to know how many of the people listed in it for their bizarre conquests also have Chiron/Mars aspects!

People with Chiron in aspect to Mars have a powerful creative energy which can be wild, wilful and ruthless; although they may achieve a great deal, they can also be merciless and care nothing for others' feelings. They have an instinctive understanding of competition, knowing how to bring down rivals and enemies by exposing their weaknesses; they can easily inflict wounds on others' self-confidence and make them feel disempowered. People with this aspect who do express powerful qualities of leadership and disciplined will in military, sporting or physical achievements are usually controversial figures, like Cecil Rhodes. Or Winston Churchill: he has Chiron in Aries in the 7th house opposite Mars in Libra in the 1st house. Opinions about his contribution to history differ: some regard him as the hero who helped save Western civilization from the scourge of Nazism with his heroic conquests made against all odds; others think of him as an arrogant and aggressive warmonger. Note Chiron is in the 7th house, where we often meet our shadow projected on to others; on a personal level, Churchill was perhaps battling with his own shadow.

Most of us with Chiron in aspect to Mars are not destined to become famous leaders like Rhodes or Churchill, or infamous for our violence like Susan Atkins, Charles Manson and the Reverend Jim Jones, who all have strong Chiron/Mars aspects (their horoscopes are discussed elsewhere in this book). Nevertheless we do carry this powerful energy with its potential for creation or destruction, and part of our journey through life will be the struggle to come to terms with it. While her Chiron/Mars sesquiquadrate aspect was being stimulated by a Pluto transit, one woman with Chiron sesquiquadrate Mars had frequent dreams about hordes of *berserkers*. These fearsome Norse warriors were said to become possessed by battle frenzy and destroy everything in their path. This woman had previously identified herself as someone who was efficient, always on the go and doing something creative – both a supermother and career woman; this transit brought a shift of perspective and the abandoning of conquests which in retrospect did not seem to matter so much and had become a burden to her.

If you have Chiron in aspect to Mars, you may have to get used to not being liked by everyone and sometimes making enemies, as people could also project their own unconscious aggression on to you. If you are to express the energy of this aspect in a positive way, you will need to have a strong sense of self-worth, as on your path through life you are likely to encounter opposition, surreptitious or overt hostility and competition from rivals. You need to discover what you truly and deeply want and go after it – which may be difficult if you are someone who needs confirmation from others, or if you tend to get swept along in a tide of activity which turns out to be meaningless for you in the end. Indeed, one of your lessons may well be to honour your own capacity for achievement, positive action and appropriate decisions. You could have the gift of being able to confront others directly and with feeling about thorny issues, and thus to open up new possibilities and dispel evasion and confusion in relationships. You have a gift for empowering other people, helping them to clarify what they want, to formulate their life direction, and mobilize their energy towards success. In other words, you can help those who have problems with their own Mars.

Chiron/Mars aspects are sometimes difficult for a woman to handle. The figure of the Amazon looms large here and may cause difficulties in relationships with men. She may become identified with what she can achieve, or feel compelled to compete with men for the sheer conquest of it, and earn herself the reputation of being a 'ballbreaker' in the process. Conversely, by devaluing or castrating her own ability to achieve, a woman with Chiron in aspect to Mars may attract men who show the negative face of Mars in brutality and violence. Claretta Petacci was Mussolini's mistress and was executed with him; she has Chiron in Pisces square Mars in Gemini. Her Mars conjuncts Mussolini's stellium of five planets in Gemini, which includes his Chiron and his Mars. She played siren, muse and inspiratrice (Chiron in Pisces) to his Mars; her own 1st-house Mars perhaps expressed itself mainly in her obsession with Mussolini, which began when she was still a child and led to her death.

Men with Chiron/Mars may feel their masculinity is somehow wounded. The brutish, competitive and aggressive Ares is a figure representing masculine qualities that contain a great deal of vital energy and can turn very nasty indeed if banished to unconsciousness.[16] Men with Chiron/Mars may mask their sensitivity by becoming macho; alternatively, they could seem docile, refined and cultivated, and attract to themselves powerful women who take charge. Woe betide a woman who falls into this trap, as she may find herself on the receiving end of an onslaught of unconscious hostility, and the fight will be on! Men with Chiron/Mars contacts often have to build from scratch an inner sense of their masculine power, finding the middle ground between the opposites of brutishness and emasculation – which is no mean task.

With Chiron in aspect to Mars, activities such as competitive sport or trials of physical endurance often provide a release for these powerful instinctual energies. Building good musculature could help both men and women hold this energy and direct it towards positive achievements, rather than allowing it to turn sour, backlash and attack their own sense of confidence. Those with Chiron/Mars contacts often thrive when they put their considerable energy behind someone else or an impersonal cause. Their enormous vitality could lead them to overdo things, however, and they often have difficulty regulating their energy. When Chiron/Mars contacts are functioning compulsively, people put excessive effort into everything, and turn simple tasks like making a meal into a Herculean labour!

Roberto Assagioli has Chiron in Gemini in the 12th house, conjunct Cancer Ascendant; it forms a grand trine with MC in Pisces and Mars in Libra in the 5th house. Assagioli was the founder of Psychosynthesis, a synthesis of different esoteric and psychological approaches to the psyche, whose techniques feature the use of the will. He wrote *The Act of Will*, which suggests the need to align the personal will of the personality with the transpersonal will of the higher self. This is often an important consideration for those with Chiron in aspect to Mars, who by nature are out for themselves and the achievement of their desires. If this principle is wounded, we may be forced to find a wider collective or transpersonal perspective within which to operate. Indeed, with Chiron/Mars contacts, our own personal desires are often blocked and thwarted until we find a way to link them with the deeper concerns of humanity at large.

Chiron in Aspect to Jupiter

People with Chiron/Jupiter contacts often have messianic tend-encies, the nature of their message being indicated by the signs and houses involved: they are great seekers after an ever-elusive enlightenment, panacea or ultimate truth. Jupiter rides Chiron like a hobby-horse, off on his mission, keen to enlist as many fellow-travellers as possible. However, with a Chiron/Jupiter aspect, we could have big hopes or grandiose aspirations, but avoid human life in the areas covered by the aspect; like Pro-metheus, punished by Zeus, we usually have to submit to great suffering there. If an inner conflict escalates we may be unable to contain it, and our pain may prompt us to dedicate ourselves to global causes. However, as ordinary mortals with Chiron/Jupiter aspects, we are unlikely single-handedly to stop the arms race or end world famine; we may instead be called upon to recognize the inner pain we have invested in these causes. For example, if we have abused and ignored our own animal natures, we could become vociferous Animal Rights campaigners; if we are inwardly divided against ourselves, we might follow the anti-Apartheid bandwagon; if we are afraid of our own sup-pressed aggression, we might protest about the violence on our streets.

I am not suggesting there is no value in committing our sense of injustice to a collective cause. However, as working astrologers, from time to time we may encounter someone with a Chiron/Jupiter contact who harbours some such dream or is on a trip which has escalated out of all proportion and is asking for help. Although a down to earth approach may stave off disaster, the issue can perhaps also be seen as a valid *symbolic* expression of the person's religious instinct, indicating the *inner* path of integration which the psyche is trying to follow. Some are destined to enact or fulfil their self-appointed mission; others may be called upon to sacrifice it for the sake of their own wholeness. However, it may be more appropriate to discuss the possible symbolic meaning than to give advice, for no matter how well meant, we may thus merely collude with the client's Chiron/Jupiter pattern of seeking an external spiritual authority. To quote D. H. Lawrence:

I have outlived my mission and know no more of it . . . the teacher and saviour are dead in me; now I can go about my business, into my single life . . . I wanted to be greater than the limits of my hands and feet, so I brought a betrayal on myself . . . for I have died, and now I know my own limits.[17]

The loss of a cherished vision or mission is often part of the life-journey of those with Chiron/Jupiter aspects, as with Chiron in Sagittarius or the 9th house.

Sometimes, with Chiron/Jupiter, our capacity to symbolize and internalize meaning is itself wounded; we enact inner issues in a concrete way which at best leaves us feeling drained and empty and at worst may cause emotional or financial catastrophe. On the other hand, with Jupiter in aspect to Chiron, we could experience quests, journeys, and pilgrimages that are immensely productive of healing and inner growth. The crucial factor is our willingness to reflect deeply on our experiences, to balance our expansion with enough stillness and introversion where some inner synthesis (Jupiter) can be reached. If we let Chiron/Jupiter run away with us, we are in danger of leaving a trail of unprocessed life-experience behind us, becoming ungrounded and losing our humanity. On the other hand, if we affront Jupiter we could become chained like Prometheus to the feeling of self-betrayal and denial of our vision and inner truth.

People with Chiron/Jupiter contacts often have some extraordinary saving grace crop up in their lives: some new factor will enter a situation just when all seems lost. On the other hand, the wound of betrayed faith in God is frequently found. With Chiron in aspect to Jupiter, we may secretly feel special, favoured and beloved of the gods. With this attitude, we can initially win a lot of good things in life with our firm inner belief that we deserve them, but rage and indignation follow the rude awakening to our mortal limits. Misfortune may hit us hard, as we are unprepared: our unbounded optimism turns to despair and the belief that we are hounded by bad luck when things fail to work out as ideal. 'Pray to Allah but tie up your camel', is a Sufi saying which addresses this. With Chiron/Jupiter, however, we have an astonishing ability to bounce back from illnesses, personal tragedies and crises of faith.

Where Chiron/Jupiter aspects are found we tend to overdo things and to experience the extraordinary. We are very alive to the archetypal level of life in these areas, but sometimes also prone to excess, fanaticism and messianism. Ordinary life and simple truth can be lost, and we are prone to exaggeration in these areas of life. Lord George Byron had Jupiter conjunct Chiron, both in Gemini, in the 12th house. The florid emotional excess of his writing (Gemini) is certainly 12th house in character, more archetypal than personal. For those with Chiron aspecting Jupiter in Libra, for example, relationships cannot be ordinary, but become a means to connection with realms of higher consciousness or an experience of social or cultural expansion. With Chiron aspecting Jupiter in Cancer or the 4th house, our home and family or our roots and national origins may be almost deified.

One woman, whom I will call Brenda, has Jupiter in Leo in the 10th house, squaring Chiron in Taurus in the 7th; Jupiter also rules her Sun and Moon in Sagittarius. She wanted to work in the healing field, but had difficulty finding the right channel. Brenda became obsessed by David Bowie, whose Chiron is exactly conjunct her Scorpio Ascendant, and whose Jupiter opposes hers. She even moved to England to be near him, as she felt he was healing her; her move had the typical Chiron/Jupiter qualities of pilgrimage and literalization. This fantasy relationship (Chiron in the 7th) provided Brenda with an archetypal framework for her to explore her own inner world. She was interviewed for a book about the psychology of the relationship between stars and fans, and the interview was broadcast. Ironically, what began as a vicarious living of her own Jupiter in Leo, with its need for social prominence, fame and adoration, led to a measure of notoriety as 'the fan of the great man'. Chiron/Jupiter has a very strong capacity for devotion, as her story illustrates.

Those with Chiron/Jupiter often enjoy taking risks and tempting fate. Zeus was sometimes said to have been the father of the three Fates, who executed his decisions. Earlier versions of the myth, however, put supreme authority in the hands of the Fates themselves. With Chiron/Jupiter contacts, we may have a sneaky feeling that *we* are the final arbiter of our own destiny – which gets us into difficulties when we overstep our limits! We could, however, tend to play God while also testing life to see who is really in charge of what; we long for the boundaries which we cannot provide for ourselves.

Chiron/Jupiter aspects often signify a capacity to teach and inspire others, and to assist them in the process of finding meaning in their own lives. We may have a gift for reaching an overview of situations, being able to bring out the best in people, their true hopes and aspirations. Some people may enjoy our positive outlook on life and our trust in its bounty. Sometimes, however, Chiron/Jupiter signifies the wound of too much optimism: we could come from a family or a culture where any sign of depression or sadness is immediately dismissed, banished with positive thinking or jollied out of existence with some distraction. Before we have learned to value our darker side, we might play a brittle 'superJupiter' role in order to prevent ourselves and others from seeing our pessimistic, moody and depressive side, which sees neither meaning nor hope and has no comforting perspective of philosophical expansiveness. The Chironian and the temple of Zeus sharing the summit of Mount Pelion are an evocative image here. There may be a manic-depressive element in Chiron/Jupiter people, where depression alternates with periods of elation and enthusiasm.

Chiron/Jupiter aspects sometimes indicate a wound to our sense of hope, optimism and confidence in the bounty of life's possibilities. As children, our expansive feelings of generosity and optimism may have been crushed and thus have gone underground. Our parents may have had big hopes that were dashed: perhaps they lost fortunes or felt dogged by bad luck. We may have been cautioned against being too happy and carefree – their religious framework may have been too repressive and severe for our Jupiter to feel truly at home. They may have been atheists with no religious tradition. In this case, we carry the accumulated unconscious and suppressed religious aspirations of our ancestors. We could then find ourselves compelled to undertake a long search through various perils and extremes. The tendency to externalize is very powerful with this combination, and it often takes repeated disillusionments for those with Chiron/Jupiter aspects to be able to rediscover their inner spiritual authority. Krishnamurti has Chiron retrograde in Libra in the 8th house, square Jupiter in Cancer in the 4th house. He was 'discovered' as a child in India, and brought up by the Theosophists to be their future Master. He dramatically rejected this inflated and imposed sense of identity (Jupiter in the 4th), and formulated instead a philosophy (Jupiter) which looks deeply (Chiron in the 8th) into the nature of conflict itself (Chiron in Libra), and encourages people to rely on their own inner source of guidance (Jupiter in the 4th house). Ironically, and perhaps not surprisingly, he still became a spiritual guide for many people.

With Chiron/Jupiter, we could be obsessed with finding 'higher meaning' in the areas covered by the houses and signs in which the two planets are placed. Our intuition is strong, and we may have intimations of the future but also have difficulty bringing these possibilities or lofty ideas into form. Chiron spends part of its orbit between Saturn and Jupiter, and this perhaps symbolizes a perspective (Chiron) which can honour both the form (Saturn) and the meaning (Jupiter) without confusing or doing violence to either. Jung has Chiron in Aries, opposite Jupiter in Libra. His insights and approach to depth psychology came largely through his own experience (Chiron in Aries), were formulated through his intuition (Chiron/Jupiter), and led to conflict with his mentor Freud (Chiron/Jupiter in Libra). He wrote a great deal about the alchemical basis of the transference relationship (Jupiter in Libra) and its transformational possibilities. He articulated a 'religion' of individual inner meaning (Chiron/Jupiter) – a process of internalizing religious symbols once contained within external religious forms.

D. H. Lawrence has Chiron in Gemini in the 8th house square Sun/Jupiter conjunct in Virgo in the 11th house. Although this side of him is perhaps less well known, D. H. Lawrence nurtured the typical messianic fantasy of founding an élite religious order, a colony he called Rananim. In retreat from the world, its members would undergo personal transformation and rebirth (Chiron in the 8th), and then return to the outside world to foster new growth and 'seed the sterile ruins of Western civilization' (Jupiter in detriment in Virgo). He began recruiting people in earnest when transiting Chiron was in his 5th house, square its natal place, and opposite his natal Sun/Jupiter conjunction. Of this enterprise, Cecil Gray, a wealthy musician and snob, said the following:

The idea of spending the rest of my life in the Andes in the company of Lawrence and Frieda filled me with horror – the combination of the mountain heights and psychological depths was more than I could easily contemplate. Apart from anything else I was already weary and sceptical, sick and tired of his dark gods, sensuous underworlds, and all the rest of his literary 'properties'. I accused him of allowing himself to become the object of a kind of esoteric female cult, an Adonis, Attis, Dionysus religion of which he was the central figure, a Jesus Christ to a regiment of Mary Magdalenes.[18]

This very Saturnian view may be Gray's chief claim to immortality, as he seems to have lurked in Lawrence's shadow.

D. H. Lawrence originally wanted to go into the Church, but was put off by the restrictive religious morality instilled into him by his mother. As a child he would pray for his father to be converted to a chapel man or die (see the section on Chiron in aspect to the Sun – p. 191. The Rananim community may be seen as an enactment of his unresolved issues with his own family (community = family); his feeling of not belonging prompted him to imagine his own place where he could invite others to belong; note he talks of 'rebirth', not 'enlightenment', and this is congruent with Chiron in the 8th house. His rejection of European civilization is perhaps an externalization of his passionate attempt to break free from the strict Protestant ethics which severely repressed his own instinctual life in childhood. Here is his personal credo:

I want to put into the world again the big old pagan vision . . .[19] My religion is a belief in the blood, the flesh as being wiser than the intellect. We can go wrong in our minds. But what our blood feels and believes and says, is always true. The intellect is only a bit and bridle. What do I care about knowledge? All I want is to answer to my blood, direct, without fribbling intervention of mind, or moral, or whatnot.[20]

Note the Chironian juxtaposition of blood and intellect, and the poignant fact that Lawrence was unable to father children himself (Chiron square Sun). In this sense he could not answer to his own blood, although he certainly did so through his words. Typical also of Chiron/Jupiter is his struggle to formulate a unique personal philosophy. With these planets in aspect, we may be compelled to find a philosophy of personal meaning that befits our own life-experience; the comfort of belonging to the collectively accepted religion may be denied us, and this is both our wound and our challenge:

I intend to find God: I wish to realize my relation with him. I do not any longer object to the word God. My attitude regarding this has changed. I must establish a conscious relation with God.[21]

This illustrates yet another common Chiron/Jupiter theme, where we tend to play God (or Goddess) and then suffer dereliction: we inflate and deflate. With Chiron/Jupiter, through acknowledging our deep need for an inner source of wisdom and guidance for ourselves, we can perhaps eventually relinquish these extremes and find the Inner Teacher speaking quietly within.

Chiron in Aspect to Saturn

As described in Chapter 5, Chiron's relationship to Saturn implies the breaking down of boundaries and the possibility of a different attitude to the question of the limits necessary for human life. Individuals with Chiron/Saturn aspects will react to this process of transformation in a variety of ways, but initially there is usually an either/or to contend with. Either we have too much Saturn: we are rigid, fearful and judgemental of ourselves and others; or we do not have enough: we feel depressed, insecure and unable to function in the world. In addition, with Saturn in aspect to Chiron, father looms large. Here we meet the more severe and forbidding forms of the archetypal Father – one face of Saturn – usually first personified by the actual father. However, Chiron/Saturn issues involve different levels: the personal, the ancestral, the collective and the archetypal. In reality these themes overlap and interweave, as illustrated in Chapter 11 in the charts of Dr Ian Player and the Reverend Jim Jones; here, however, I will describe them separately.

On a personal level, Chironian themes are usually seen in the relationship with the father. He may have been physically or mentally ill, weak or lacking in some way, in need of healing or redeeming; he could also have been a petty tyrant. If we have grown up with a wound in the Saturnian area of limits, boundaries and structure, we will feel deeply insecure; perhaps our rebelliousness was not checked in a healthy way, or we suffered an authoritarian and strict upbringing. Either way, we could become old before our time, and be very serious from a very young age, having had to be our own father for one reason or another. The father can also be the one who wounds, persecutes or dominates, leaving a legacy of fear and hatred in the child. Similar to when Chiron is in Capricorn, people with Chiron in aspect to Saturn often grow up rejecting their father; they may flee far from his neediness, his violence, or the overpowering restrictions he may have imposed, only to discover that this 'father' follows them everywhere – in relationships with authority-figures and in personal relationships. In struggling to be different, we may be living our father's unlived potentials, unconsciously trying to redeem him by fulfilling his unrealized ambitions or unconscious desires. With Chiron/Saturn contacts, if a woman's primary emotional bond was with her father, she may later fixate on men who appear quite different from her father, but who on closer inspection may be seen as her father's unconscious self; she may marry a man exactly like her grandfather or even great-grandfather. Alternatively, she may rebel and become an 'Amazon', seeking personal achievement and emotional independence. She may reject men, knowing only relationships that 'come to nothing', as they are modelled on her relationship with her father.

The father issues suggested by Chiron/Saturn are usually wider in scope than the personal father, often involving our psychological inheritance over several generations – our collective patterning – and eventually the archetypal principle of Father. If you have Saturn and Chiron in aspect, it may be helpful to examine your family-tree to discover the life-patterns and psychological characteristics of your father's side of the family. You might discover, for example, that you are blindly following an inherited ancestral path which could lead to disaster and failure; you could be creating life-structures based on choices made generations ago, thus unwittingly following in your father's footsteps. With Chiron/Saturn aspects some people feel that their purpose is to redeem a negative inheritance from the father's side of the family: there could be burdens, responsibilities or family skeletons in the cupboard which do not go away. Some people will struggle with these all their lives; others will have the opportunity (usually a transit involving Saturn or Chiron) to let go and recognize that the past cannot be undone. On the other hand, we can also inherit positive qualities: feeling connected with the aspirations and values of our forefathers may bring considerable comfort and feelings of inner support. The theme of ancestral continuity and a creative relationship with our extended past is important with Chiron/Saturn contacts: it deepens our feeling of participation in history and belonging in time (Saturn).

The archetypal presence behind Chiron/Saturn aspects is often initially a judgemental and condemning male figure, like the negative side of Yahweh in the Bible. This god watches over us, lest we fall into error and sin, and if we do he punishes us. Concepts such as original sin, the fall of man into disgrace and exile from paradise due to the waywardness of womankind, and so on, may bite deep into the sense of self-worth of those with Chiron/Saturn contacts. If creation itself is deemed blame-worthy, we will need to be redeemed and saved from our 'wickedness', and will constantly engage in self-justification. We must then cast blame in order to appease our sense of outrage and retrieve the fragments of our self-worth; others must be punished so we can remain righteous. This scenario of judgement and blame, if not enacted externally, may go on internally in the minds of those with Chiron/Saturn aspects: they may damn themselves and/or their creations. In the myth, Saturn swallowed his children for fear that one would eventually overthrow him. When Chiron is in aspect to Saturn, this theme is frequently met: our control mechanisms work overtime, resulting in agonizing periods of creative sterility, depression and fear. However, unlike Uranus/Saturn aspects or transits, when Chiron is in aspect to Saturn, the possibility exists of encompassing rather than trying to get rid of this: compassion and grounded creativity may follow, like the Golden Age of the early days of Saturn's rule.

Chiron/Saturn contacts often indicate a strong super-ego which criticizes and belittles, heaping scorn on everything we try to do. This voice is often unconscious and projected on to partners, parents, society or any other suitable hook – we then do battle with this external authority. Its effect can be paralysing, leaving us depressed and unable to enjoy life or foresee anything better. Prompted by our wounded sense of inner worth, we may become the 'nice guy' and take our cue from others. We could become preoccupied with appearance, prestige, success and status, but take our sense of structure and identity from our pro-fession, from organizations, societies or institutions. The anger that accompanies our struggle to shed this burden of guilt and unworthiness may wreak havoc in our internal and external lives. Order, discipline, law, responsibilities, place in society, the ability to achieve and create through perseverance and overcom-ing obstacles are some of the areas where difficulties may appear.

With Chiron/Saturn aspects, our relationship with the entire physical realm could be difficult: we may experience sudden disasters, sickness, failure and feelings of being crippled or impotent in the areas of life represented by the houses and signs involved. It is important, however, to bear in mind what lies underneath: repeatedly trying to get things working again is often doomed to fail if the underlying issues of self-judgement and lack of self-worth are not gradually brought to light with compassion.

With Chiron aspecting Saturn, we have a combination of extreme vulnerability and brittle defensiveness, finding it difficult to allow feelings of emotional need; we perhaps never approach others without full emotional armour-plating, although when alone we feel painfully vulnerable and long for this to be seen. We can appear aggressively self-sufficient, capable and independent but experience periodic collapse: of ambition, capacity to work or inner sense of coherence. A Chiron/Saturn contact may mean difficulty with imagining that things could be any different; this can even become a self-fulfilling prophecy. In this case, there are usually highly-charged issues connected with the personal father involved. For example, one young man with Chiron conjunct Saturn in Pisces repeatedly failed exams and spoiled career-aptitude tests, although he was known to be intelligent. His father was uneducated, drank a lot, was sullen and uncommunicative; he had left home when his son was still young. The young man was trying to be like his absent father over whom he still unconsciously grieved (Chiron in Pisces), and thus he was resisting any further education.

The expression 'laager mentality' will be known to anyone interested in South African politics, and is sometimes descriptive of Chiron/Saturn aspects. In South Africa, pioneers would pull their wagons into a circle each night to protect themselves from wild animals and hostile black tribesmen. Today hardline Afrikaners, descended from these pioneers, believe their god-given duty and responsibility to the world is to preserve the white race intact from contamination by other races: hence apartheid. (See pp. 320–25 for the horoscope of South Africa). Hendrik Verwoerd has Chiron in Sagittarius, conjunct Saturn in Capricorn, both in the 12th house; Saturn is conjunct the Ascendant, and Chiron is also opposite Neptune in Cancer in the 6th house. Verwoerd, as Prime Minister from 1958 to 1966, enshrined and institutionalized this belief, although it was already operating in practice. Ian Smith has Chiron in Aries in the 4th house sesquiquadrate Saturn in Leo in the 9th house. As the last Prime Minister of Rhodesia, he held out against world opinion through a bloody guerrilla war for fifteen years before independent Zimbabwe was created. He had polio in his youth, and the left side of his face is paralysed; he certainly resisted 'changing the face' of his country (4th house). Also characteristic of the positive side of Chiron/Saturn, he did not flee after his defeat, but remained to serve in the government for a further seven years.

Margaret Mead was born a few days before Verwoerd, and her Chiron configuration shows how differently the same themes can be expressed in two different lives. She also has Chiron conjunct Saturn in Capricorn in the 12th house, with Saturn conjunct her Capricornian Ascendant. She was an anthropologist who became almost a cult figure with her studies of primitive tribes – a suitably Chironian subject. Although her work has recently been partially discredited, doubts being cast upon the objectivity of her research (Chiron in the 12th house), her descriptions of sexual freedom combined with moral responsibility certainly tantalized public imagination (Chiron in the 12th). Regardless of the 'objectivity' of her research, she certainly gave form (Saturn) to the collective longing (12th house) to redeem the 'primitive' within. She portrayed a 'Golden Age' of healthy and spontaneous expression of the instinctual self (see Chapter 11 for further consideration of this Saturnian theme).

When Chiron is in aspect to Saturn, we usually must encounter our own inner fear, rigidity and contempt for others as well as our inherited or collective attitudes of repressiveness and ultra-conservatism; we might feel deeply ashamed when these qualities are first discovered inside ourselves. We could try and palm them off on others, deny them or feel righteously indignant; we blame the government, the flu, or our horoscope as we struggle against the oppressor within. However, if this can be honestly included as part of our make-up, without making it worse by demanding change and transformation, we may find it bestows a measure of inner freedom and a feeling of being much more at home in the world of form. In the words of Kahlil Gibran: 'And if it is a despot you would dethrone, see first that his throne erected within you is destroyed.'[22] Although we might be saddled with a 'tyrant' subpersonality, it is still possible to recognize that this is not all of who we are, to carry it with humility and thus not to oppress others with it. If you have a strong Chiron and Saturn aspect, a look at Blake's painting of Nebuchadnezzar could perhaps help you see this aspect of yourself with some humour and compassion.

Sometimes, we meet a person with Chiron and Saturn in aspect who has a relaxed and natural sense of authority. This is not authority by virtue of wealth, status in society, profession or achievement: it is rather the hard-won dignity of someone who has faced the depths of his or her own soul, its darkness and despair as well as its hope and joy, who has emerged with a sense of wisdom and acceptance of life, and who is willing to carry considerable responsibility. Chiron/Saturn aspects may eventually bring the gift of a deep acceptance of incarnation: the Wise Old Man or Woman may in time emerge from what once was a painful wound. This figure respects tradition and limits but does not identify with them; wisdom is gained through the discipline of full participation in life rather than withdrawal from it. He or she is truly both in the world yet not of it.

Chiron in Aspect to Uranus

When Chiron aspects an outer planet, it acts as a mediator or bridge, potentially enabling the qualities of the outer planet to be expressed in a powerful way in our life, for good or ill. However, the intense pressure of the aspect could also drive us into pre-occupations which widen our horizons too far; we become too concerned with the larger picture, collectively or spiritually, and neglect the demands of our individual life. One way or the other, we will need to come to terms with the powerful collective issues and also the transpersonal consciousness represented by the Chiron aspects.

There were about forty exact Chiron/Uranus oppositions between 1952 and 1989, and this period has been fraught with many typically Uranian trends and events. Since the end of World War II there has been much social and ideological turmoil; revolutionary subcultures of all kinds have sprung up in many countries; terrorism has become widespread; the issue of individual rights has become a focus of controversy, protest and sometimes militant activity; minority groups of all kinds have fought for their right to exist and express themselves. The discoveries of the New Physics exploded the myth of solid reality, and rejection of materialism led many people to drop out of the established (Saturn) mainstream of society. In true Uranian fashion, better options were sought and alternative life-styles were tried, often based on communal models. Social ferment has ranged from escapism and passive rejection of the system to violent attempts to force change, overthrow the old order and challenge prevailing attitudes.

In the individual chart Chiron in aspect to Uranus often heightens the desire for freedom from constraints, especially in relationships. People with this aspect are often 'superUranian', apt to make sudden changes and cut off relationships and careers in mid-stream; they could also be prone to unexpected and often unwelcome events happening to them; they love new ideas and want to try new ways of living, perhaps feeling compelled to break through limitations and to stand out in the crowd. George Sand, who was Chopin's lover, has Chiron as part of a T-square, it is in Capricorn in the 10th house, opposite Sun in Cancer in the 4th, both square Uranus in Libra in the 8th. She was a highly individualistic woman who dressed in men's clothes when this was unheard of. Chiron/Uranus people have a strong belief in individualism, as long as it is their own! They may be intolerant of others' ideas; although believing in freedom of speech and thought, they may be blissfully unaware of the contradictions in their behaviour. They may feel an urgent need to make a mark, to be remembered above all as an individual, whatever they may or may not have achieved. They want their individual life to mean something in the overall scheme of history, and are often pre-occupied with social and political issues.

Even those who are more introverted and less inclined to become directly involved in social or political issues will quietly seek out the unusual, the bizarre, and follow paths going counter to collective norms; they will sometimes have close friends or enemies who are very obviously Uranian. Edgar Allan Poe has Chiron conjunct Sun and Mercury in Aquarius, square Uranus conjunct the North Node in Scorpio. He wrote macabre and intriguing stories (Chiron/Mercury) that often have an unex-pected twist at the end. *Tales of the Unexpected* is one of his most famous collections – appropriate for someone with Chiron/Uranus! People with Chiron/Uranus contacts can be brilliant and original thinkers; they are iconoclastic and challenging, and often perceive situations with penetrating clarity; their laser-beam mind may make others feel uncomfortable, as they often survey life from a position of distance and detachment. Their wound may be a lack of connection with their personal feelings, as well as the disillusionment felt when life fails to live up to their ideal plan.

One feature of the Chiron/Uranus combination is the con-viction that anything can be changed; nothing is sacred, and traditions may be seen merely as restrictions to be dispensed with. The French poet Charles Baudelaire had Chiron in Aries in the 8th house, square Uranus in Capricorn in the 4th house. His sensual and psychological excesses eventually led to his death from syphilis (Chiron in the 8th house). He transgressed boundaries of every kind; his poetry inverts the sentimental or bloodless aesthetic, glorifying instead the depraved, the perverted and anything which society rejects. Note the Chironian theme of siding with the outsiders, the self-destructive 8th-house quality of his quest, and also his challenge to current notions of acceptability (Uranus in Capricorn).

Chiron/Uranus people may indiscriminately rebel against external restrictions, and yet paradoxically be resistant to deep inner change. Creative introversion may be difficult, as they are often restless in their search for something new and different. Some have an uncanny ability to incorporate the unexpected without flinching or being thrown off course; they may thrive on change and usually experience plenty of it, whether or not it is consciously sought. They often go out on a limb and courageously try new things, even in the face of ridicule or lack of support from others. However, they might have difficulty admitting to their mistakes; they can also be brittle and inflexible, unable to change course and flow with the tide of necessity. The true creative capacities of people with Chiron/Uranus usually come to the fore once they have found and accepted their own internal criteria of limitation and discipline – in other words, when they have a sound relationship with their own Saturnian principle.

The urge to improve the world is often strong with Chiron/Uranus, and this echoes the story of Prometheus. If we strive too hard for the power of individual choice, freedom and consciousness, without also paying our respects to the gods from whom we steal, we may suffer the painful inability to manifest anything of our individuality. In the words of Oceanus, Chiron's father-in-law:

> Oh my unhappy friend,
> Throw off your angry mood and seek deliverance
> From all your suffering . . .
> . . . your plight is the inescapable
> Reward, Prometheus, of a too proud-speaking tongue.
> You still will not be humble, will not yield to pain;
> You mean to add new sufferings to those you have . . .
> You are a far more prudent counsellor of others
> Than of yourself.[23]

Chiron aspecting Uranus often brings difficulties with authority. However, our rebellion, and indeed our wound, may be an inability to accept a higher authority than our own personal choice. Whether that higher authority is seen as the police, our parents, God, or indeed the demands of our own psychological growth, part of our journey may involve learning to distinguish between an attitude of healthy, creative challenge and a wilful, indiscriminate sense of rebelliousness, which perhaps lingers from adolescence. Considerable frustration may result when our Uranian drive for freedom repeatedly causes disaster instead of actualizing the creative change that is hoped for.

Our quest will involve finding a way creatively to embody our individuality in life. Some people with Chiron aspecting Uranus take time to reach a workable relationship with the unavoidable Saturnian limitations of life in the world, trying everything possible to avoid bowing down to any kind of authority. Others awaken later on in life to Uranian promptings: marriages disintegrate, children are abandoned, new love affairs and new careers are started as these individuals experiment with their new-found urge for freedom. They may be quite unstoppable, and go to extremes trying to break through previous limits; illness may then provide the brakes on the system running out of control.

People with Chiron/Uranus may be quick to detect hypocrisy in others, but blind to their own hypocrisy. One person, for example, felt so contemptuous of the society in which she grew up that she rejected it entirely and joined a spiritual community isolated from the mainstream of society. Although she had played Uranus as regards the old order, she was unaware that her true individual self was equally imprisoned by the new rules and restrictions which she had taken on; she pursued her new way of life with unflinching zeal and self-righteousness. Those with Chiron/Uranus may think freedom is to be attained by rejecting or overthrowing structures 'out there', seeing the lack of individual freedom as a problem of society. They are perhaps more than most inclined to search for an alternative framework of political, social or esoteric ideas in which they feel at home.

People with Chiron/Uranus are very sensitive to collective ideas and susceptible to their influence. They may react emotionally to *unconscious* ideas, which only lose their charge once the ideas and the emotion are separated. For example, a woman with Chiron opposite Uranus was a clairvoyant by profession, and she dreaded social occasions where she might meet new people; she feared that men in particular would be cynical and contemptuous when they discovered what her profession was; she would become inwardly enraged to such a degree that she herself became hostile, sometimes before any such conversation had occurred. Eventually she realized that she was in fact reacting to the unconscious collective idea that clairvoyant women are witches – dangerous women who belong on the outskirts of society. She had been making human men the bearers of this wounding idea, not giving them a chance to be different from what she expected; in this way she was dehumanizing them as she in turn felt dehumanized by them. Other highly charged Uranian ideas concern individual rights, political beliefs and ideals, social causes, as well as systems of personal growth.

If you have Chiron in aspect to Uranus, part of your journey may involve discovering such internalized collective ideas, which have a wounding or dehumanizing effect, especially in relationships. It may also be useful to examine critically the attitudes and belief systems, whether religious, social or political, which formed your mental environment when you were growing up. With a Chiron/Uranus aspect, you may really be struggling for *mental* freedom. To attain that, however, you may have to work hard to grow beyond these thought-structures. Reacting emotionally and rejecting them does not work if previous conditioning has not been dismantled through conscious awareness being focused on it. To go beyond our mental limitations means examining our own thought-processes, which demands great discipline.

Both Robert (already mentioned on p. 213 in the section on Chiron/Venus) and Mary Moffat have Chiron conjunct Uranus, in Leo and Virgo respectively: this reflects the strength of their convictions and their desire to enlighten people with 'God's word'; they were indeed agents of change. They had a daughter, who was also called Mary. She was born only three days after Baudelaire, and their lives are interesting to compare. Both

Baudelaire and Mary have Chiron in Aries, amongst a stellium of two planets in Pisces and five in Aries, all square Uranus in Capricorn. Mary married David Livingstone, the famous missionary and explorer, a suitable partner indeed for a woman with such an Arian emphasis, square Uranus! Her father's Chiron/Uranus midpoint conjuncts Mary's North Node, symbolizing his Chiron/Uranus issues carried forward and incorporated into her destiny. We can see the similarity in theme between what Mary lived out externally and what Baudelaire experienced internally . . . Mary constantly exposed herself to the dangers of the unknown, venturing where no white woman had been before, believing she was 'bringing light to the Dark Continent'. Baudelaire explored the 'Darkest Africa' of the senses in an inward and typically 8th house way; he shone light on the wild denizens of the underworld of his own psyche.

When Chiron and/or Uranus activate each other by transit, you may experience extraordinary expansion of mental consciousness which may be difficult to integrate; at these times, you might see and understand the map of your life and be awed by its organic symmetry. These visions may stay with you throughout the rest of your life, and may cause pressure for you to follow or obey what you have seen, and anguish in case you make the wrong decision. Perhaps it would be a useful analogy to compare these Chiron/Uranus visions to the aerial view seen when flying over your life, as in an aeroplane: you cannot stay up there forever, as embodied human life is lived on the earth. Coming down is not 1 ally betraying this vision, for the aerial view remains. Part of your journey may be to trust that someone up there (Chiron/Uranus) is seeing it for you, so you can descend and live your human life knowing that even if you sometimes feel lost, this too is part of the journey. Pure Uranian visions tend to take the form of: 'If I were a perfect being I could . . .' However, Chiron/Uranus encourages us to include our imperfections, wounds and limitations.

The gifts of Chiron/Uranus include the ability to give birth to the new without indiscriminately rejecting the old, a powerful intuitive sense, a capacity for compassionate detachment from emotionally laden ideas and situations, and a deep understanding of the process of creative thinking. Chiron/Uranus expands our thinking beyond the either/or attitude to new and more organic ways of thinking. 'Energy follows thought' is a well-known principle of esoteric philosophy which Chiron/Uranus instinctively understands, knowing that unless our patterns of thought are changed at the very deepest level, any change in behaviour is but a fragile pantomime that disintegrates under stress.

Chiron in Aspect to Neptune

People with Chiron and Neptune in aspect often have remarkable access to the world of dreams, imagination and fantasy; they may never have lost this child-like connection that for many of us does not survive education, growing up and the demands of life in the material world. These realms are experienced as utterly real, perhaps more so than solid external reality, and therein lies the wound of Chiron/Neptune: the gift and the liability of a natural sense of the unified reality from which the world of form derives and to which it eventually returns. Here, what we think or feel or want is as real and tangible as anything else, and may personify itself in dramatic form in our imagination. It could be difficult for us when worldly reality intervenes and shows us that our imagination is not magically omnipotent, does not necessarily correspond with what is 'out there', and that our longings will not necessarily be fulfilled just because we feel them strongly.

With Chiron/Neptune contacts, limits, exclusiveness or boundaries that prevent this merging could make us feel victimized or become angry, depressed and confused. Conflict is particularly threatening and wounding, as it highlights the reality of separateness, and we may find it difficult to stand up for ourselves and our personal needs. A common Chiron/Neptune response to interpersonal conflict is tearful collapse and feelings of being unable to cope. Those with Chiron/Neptune aspects often idealize or depreciate themselves and/or others, employing the hysterical defence of playing victim and 'poor me' if they sense imminent confrontation; they may assert themselves by well-timed displays of emotion, vulnerability or physical weakness; they are not above playing mad in order to avoid uncomfortable situations. Conversely, they are sometimes easily deceived, and tend to be easy prey for people intent on deceiving or exploiting them; they may not see danger until it is too late.

The dissolving of the illusion of duality is often a feature of the Chiron/Neptune experience, but to allow our individual life to melt into chaos is to literalize this. We might periodically experience floods of emotion and feel our solidity is being washed away; we then feel stripped of our hard-won sense of individual identity and ability to cope in the world. Before we have reconnected with the inner sense that All is One, our desire for unity may express itself in bouts of drinking, in confusion, self-destructiveness, lack of responsibility in worldly affairs, and other classic Neptunian difficulties. Chiron/Neptune urges conscious recognition of this desire, for we cannot embody these energies in an appropriate way if we are unconscious of what their compulsions represent; we will probably instead be taken captive by them and swept away.

Discrimination between fact and fantasy often takes a long time to develop, and our spiritual longings are usually contaminated with a regressive desire to return to an undifferentiated state of bliss and avoid adult responsibilities. Chiron/Neptune contacts, however, do bring the pressure to embody Neptune in our life. Some with this aspect may find themselves drawn to fields where the imagination is important, such as the world of film, television or theatre; others will draw upon the world of inner images for their painting or writing; yet others will work in the Chironian fields of healing and teaching. One way or another, Chiron/Neptune demands a suitable form through which it can either be expressed or at least held in our hearts as an inner truth which infuses and sanctifies our daily life, rather than allowing ourselves to be dragged into an imaginary never-never land where we languish, drained of vitality.

People with Chiron/Neptune aspects absorb moods and feelings from the environment without realizing it, and will quickly become tearful in the presence of anyone holding in their own sadness. This can extend further, into the realm of collective emotion. As a striking example of this, a woman with Chiron in Pisces trine Neptune in Scorpio found herself crying inexplicably for hours, having images of chaos, graves and people screaming and dying. When later she turned on her television, she discovered that while she was experiencing this, a bomb had been detonated in Northern Ireland at a Remembrance Day service, killing and wounding many people. Immediately she saw this, her mood changed and she was able to let go of the experience.

Some painful personal feelings that she was trying to stave off had become contaminated with this flood of collective feeling, had escalated and overtaken her; it was only when she shed the identification with collective suffering that she found her own personal feelings underneath. However, with Chiron and Neptune in aspect we may in time be able to express what is unspoken and not yet felt by others in a creative way, without suffering ego–disintegration in the process. Thus we can help others regain their sense of connection with themselves and with life as a whole, serving the principle of Neptune in an individual-ized way. With enough discrimination and ego–stability, Chiron/Neptune people can be genuinely mediumistic, with finely tuned perceptions of other levels of reality and an ability to use this for the good of others.

With Chiron in aspect to Neptune, we might try and deal with this sensitivity by isolating ourselves. Although periods of such isolation are healing and refreshing, if we remain unconscious of why we need it, we could sink into feelings of powerlessness and identification with the outsider, the scapegoat or the victim, retreating into a world of fantasy and refusing to engage with life. In this fantasy world we perhaps see ourselves as healers and redeemers, and fear of our imagined power increases our impotence in daily life. Alternatively, we could retreat into iron–clad defences, and vigorously fend off anything which threatens to dissolve our control over our lives; we may become cynical and emotionally impoverished, or sceptical and hostile towards anything mystical or intangible. One person with Chiron conjunct Neptune in Libra in the 10th house remained a resolute disbeliever in anything magical, occult or inexplicable, although he worked in a successful publishing company (10th house) specializing in books on these subjects, and hence had many friends and business associates (Chiron in Libra) involved in Neptunian activities; he acted as a bridge (Chiron) between them and the public at large (10th house). Here again is Chiron doing for others what he cannot do for himself.

Often, however, Chiron/Neptune people are irresistibly drawn to the occult, to experimentation with drugs, and to techniques of consciousness–expansion which involve ecstasy and loss of boundaries. While these experiences are natural to, and characteristic of, the Chiron/Neptune path, they are fraught with danger, and may further weaken an already fluid ego-structure. While people with Chiron/Neptune aspects might believe they use drugs for sacramental or self-exploratory reasons, there is usually also an element of escapism and desire permanently to inhabit these realms in order to avoid suffering the separateness affirmed by our senses. Timothy Leary, whose horoscope is examined in Chapter 11, has Chiron stationary direct in Aries in the 4th house trine Neptune in Leo in the 8th. His famous personal credo of 'Turn on, tune in, drop out' was described in the book *The Politics of Ecstasy* – a Neptunian title indeed!

One young man with Chiron conjunct Neptune in Libra in the 6th house became a Buddhist monk, took vows of celibacy (Chiron in the 6th), and worked in a refugee camp in Asia. He showed great strength when witnessing appalling suffering, but by the time he returned to Europe, he was ill with several undiagnosable symptoms (Chiron in the 6th) which left him weak, mentally confused (Neptune) and unable to eat. He refused to acknowledge the reality of his symptoms, let alone consider that they might be trying to tell him something; he denied personal pain on principle, believing the personal ego and the body to be an illusion. He spoke only in philosophical tenets, and I had an eerie feeling that there was 'nobody home'. As transiting Saturn and Pluto were both conjunct his Chiron/Neptune at the time, I imagine his condition may have escalated into a life-or-death situation. When Chiron aspects any of the outer planets, we may be fated to live its themes in an extreme form. However, for most of us, Chiron/Neptune means that our heartfelt conviction of cosmic oneness asks somehow to be allowed to exist alongside our separate individual life. Embracing this paradox is not easy, and we will frequently feel driven to sacrifice one or the other.

Chiron/Neptune people often have a strong charismatic presence, an aura of loving acceptance which attracts people who are suffering, in pain or in need. However, this can degenerate into a situation of 'power over', mutual delusion, psychic vampirism and exploitation, where one person plays saviour and the other becomes the one who eternally suffers and is in need of redeeming.

The urge to redeem, to pour ourselves forth in sympathy, to heal and give comfort, may have to be contained and resisted if we are to honour the deeper needs of others and ourselves. However, once our regressive and misplaced sacrificial tendencies have been confronted and we have embraced our own pain, Chiron/Neptune contacts may mean the capacity for deep compassion, unconditional love and profound acceptance of ourselves and others as they truly are, faults and all. Perhaps this Neptunian feeling quality is indeed essential to the process of dissolution and change, for without it, 'transformation' is merely another futile struggle to live up to impossible dreams of ourselves, which deepen our wounds and prevent healing from taking place.

Neptune can be envisaged as the One within, throughout and containing the Many. Like all Neptunians, individuals with Chiron/Neptune seek oneness, needing to find some unified spiritual context behind the duality of life in the world. The Chiron/Neptune sense of unity is an emotional sense rather than an intellectual precept or philosophy; it is inclusive and thus seeks not to rise above material life with disdain, but ultimately to embrace it with loving acceptance. Unlike the Uranian vision, it is not concerned with individual potential or complex and inspiring systems of cosmic order. It is rather an oceanic feeling of participating in the unfolding cosmos or of being engulfed in the primordial sea of being.

All men are caught in an inescapable network of mutuality, tied in a single garment of destiny. Whatever affects one directly affects all indirectly. I can never be what I ought to be until you are what you ought to be, and you can never be what you ought to be until I am what I ought to be.[24]

Martin Luther King has Chiron trine Neptune in Virgo, and this inspired statement encapsulates the challenge of Chiron/Neptune: to find a way of being that honours both the reality of the oneness that lies behind the different forms of life and also the requirement for the personal boundaries and limits necessary for human life in the world. For 'being what I ought to be' also involves caring for *myself* as an individual, as I am not separate from the rest of humanity. Ignoring my individual needs could be a misplaced sacrifice, as described previously in Chapter 5 and also in the section on Chiron in Pisces and the 12th house.

The Chiron configuration in Martin Luther King's horoscope is as follows: Chiron is in the 1st house in Taurus, conjunct Jupiter and the Ascendant in Taurus, square Mercury in Aquarius in the 10th, trine Neptune in Virgo in the 5th house; it is semisquare both Moon in Pisces in the 11th house, and Mars in Gemini in the 2nd house. The Sabian Symbol for his Chiron degree is especially interesting: 'A cantilever bridge across a deep gorge.' Rudhyar interprets this as:

The conquest of separativeness through group co-operation. The person who has suffered deprivation and loneliness can give new substance to his

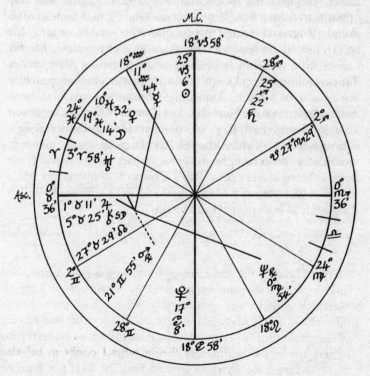

Martin Luther King

or her emotional life by participating in a collective project. All great evolutionary challenges imply the overcoming of basic difficulties. A step ahead must be taken, yet an abyss confronts evolving man.[25]

Chiron is also at the midpoint of Mercury/Jupiter, and this describes his power as an orator. His most famous speech had the refrain: 'I have a dream . . .' This dream (Chiron/Neptune) was an ideal of racial equality and liberation from prejudice; he came to embody (Chiron in the 1st house) this dream, especially for oppressed black people in America; indeed he stands for all humanity as an example of hope (Chiron conjunct Jupiter) and practical idealism (Chiron in Taurus conjunct Jupiter, trine Neptune). When he made this speech transiting Chiron was at 12°57' Pisces, conjunct his Moon and Venus in Pisces; it was also opposite transiting Sun, Venus, Uranus and Pluto, which were all in early Virgo and the first three conjunct his natal Neptune. This speech indeed expressed a Neptunian moment in time. Martin Luther King was shot in the neck when transiting Mars was in Taurus (ruling the neck), and about 30' past an exact conjunction with his natal Chiron. Transiting Chiron was just 0°12' into Aries, quincunx natal Neptune. The Taurus MC of his supposed assassin, James Earl Ray, is conjunct Martin Luther King's Chiron within 1' of arc. Although Ray claims he was the innocent victim of a conspiracy, he made his impact on the world (10th house) through this event. Ray's Chiron is conjunct his MC, therefore also conjunct Martin Luther King's Chiron: he sealed King's fate as both prophet and victim.

Chiron in Aspect to Pluto

Major learning experiences for Chiron/Pluto people feature typically Plutonian themes such as sexuality and the use or abuse of power, personal and collective destructiveness, deep and complex emotionality, transformative experiences and the ability to regenerate oneself. Once they have come to terms with the destructive potential of this aspect, Chiron/Pluto people are often able to channel powerful healing to others; they may have a conscious experience of the realms beyond physical death and develop a deep instinctive understanding of the laws of Pluto. These laws are not only concerned with our individual bodily survival, but also with the will of the 'body of mankind', of which we are part.[26] It is perhaps when we refuse to recognize this, taking the power of life and death into our own hands that Pluto's destructiveness is unleashed. The Chiron/Pluto experience is of life and death as two sides of one process; it reminds us that in the end we have only our own souls to answer to, and that the will of the unfolding universe works through us, with or without our conscious participation.

In shamanic terms, we 'meet our demons' in the areas of experience suggested by the houses in which Pluto and Chiron are placed, and they are described by the signs involved. For example, those with Chiron conjunct Pluto in the 10th house in Leo may meet potentially destructive situations in their professions; these in turn may involve projections of their own unconscious feelings of envy, rage, jealousy and greed; Leonine 'demons' may show egomania, self-centredness and narcissim; as this conjunction is in the 10th house, the early relationship with the mother is implicated.

Whereas Plutonians usually have an ability to see the hidden dark side of life, some people with Chiron in aspect to Pluto have a blind spot here, and are unable to detect or deal with destructiveness in themselves and others. They may over-estimate others' power and be affected by unconscious envy or aggression directed towards them or which they themselves feel. Chiron/Pluto

people can become tense or emotionally reactive without knowing why; they initially mistrust their instincts about people,
attributing all good to others and all bad to themselves, or vice
versa. Often, however, their intuitive sense turns out to be
correct: the Chiron/Pluto journey involves reconnecting with
and learning to trust these deep instincts. Then those with these
planets in aspect can 'see in the dark': they have an uncanny sense
of self-preservation; they can sense trouble and therefore have a
knack of avoiding disaster, and an ability to react instinctively
and creatively to danger. For example, a friend of mine was quietly
enjoying a romantic dinner with a man who has Chiron quincunx
Pluto when he suddenly rushed out of the restaurant, overturning
his chair and spilling his wine. It transpired that a motorcycle had
crashed into his car which was parked in the next street, out of
earshot. He arrived in time to take the motorcyclist to hospital.
The incident astonished him as much as my friend, and he could
only describe what happened as an overwhelming physical compulsion which propelled him outside to his car; at the time
transiting Mercury opposed Chiron, and the Sun was squaring his
Pluto, both within a few minutes of being exact.

Chiron/Pluto people are often irresistibly drawn towards
situations that promise danger, excitement, sexual power and
financial or emotional intrigue. They secretly relish the fires of
intense experience, testing their phoenix-like abilities to rise again
from catastrophe. The thrill of a moth heading into that same old
flame is familiar to many with this aspect! But this is also an
addiction which Chiron/Pluto eventually urges us to resist,
understand and let go of. Rather than invoking Pluto to the
surface to wreak havoc in our lives, Chiron/Pluto bids us let go,
to be ourselves transformed by dying to our old ways of being and
immature attitudes of omnipotence or belief that: 'It will never
happen to me.' With maturity Chiron/Pluto people can feel the
peace and quiet confidence which comes from having faced a
great deal of emotional pain; death becomes an ally rather than an
enemy to be vanquished or with whom we take our chances.

People with Chiron in aspect to Pluto often have difficulties
with intimate relationships, which degenerate into power struggles if too much emotional vulnerability threatens to open up.

They are often secretive about their true feelings, and may become sexually promiscuous to ensure they remain emotionally unattached and therefore in control. Through this, they may unconsciously be seeking to heal deep wounds in their early relationship with their mother. This may drive them on relentlessly, always feeling unfulfilled and getting progressively more angry, until perhaps a severe crisis will force them to internalize this process, when they may at last receive the healing they need from the archetypal Mother of All.

People with Chiron/Pluto often have great emotional depth and penetrating insight into others. Once able to encompass their own emotional wounds, they are capable of great loyalty in relationships; nothing shocks them, as they see and accept the very worst in themselves and others. Chiron/Pluto initiates transformation through acceptance of *what is*, at the deepest level. The emotional reserve shown by many Chiron/Pluto people sometimes conceals a fear of their own unexpressed or imagined anger and destructiveness; they may silently say: 'Keep away for your own good', but also hope that you won't, as they long for their fears to be proved groundless. In extremes, Chiron/Pluto people may be tormented by feelings of responsibility for others' negativity over which they have no control, and feel their personal will paralysed by these fears. In psychology this is called a negative inflation, and masks the extreme vulnerability felt by people who have lacked positive containment from their mother at a very early stage of life. Their response to this early wound may be a deep-seated but unconscious conclusion that they are being punished for being a bad person; thus they make themselves the 'aggressor', identifying with the bad mother. Later on this 'badness' must be kept hidden, and it is then difficult for Chiron/Pluto people to bring anything to light, to express themselves or be creative, as they feel what is within them to be essentially bad. Regardless of the quality of the mothering received, Chiron/Pluto people often feel themselves well and truly to have fallen from grace, sharing this tendency with those who have Chiron in aspect to Saturn; the concept of original sin can be uncomfortably real for them.

Plutonians often have a strong power drive; people with

Chiron/Pluto aspects might have spent their youth in unchallenged omnipotence, going their own way regardless, and ruling the roost with storms of outrage; later they may have a tremendous drive to transform the areas of life represented by the houses and signs involved. If the urge to change and regenerate people and situations is compulsive, it may bring misery, guilt and emotional disaster. Consciously acknowledging power issues and putting them into appropriate perspective is important with Chiron/Pluto aspects, for if they are repressed they bring self-destructive situations, negative relationships and even suicidal feelings.

Some individuals with Chiron/Pluto aspects have a powerful contribution to make to the collective. For example, the first black African Attorney-General of Zimbabwe has Chiron in Scorpio square Saturn and Pluto in Leo; he has worked to transform the existing Roman Law system (Saturn) to encompass important aspects of African tribal law. However, those with Chiron/Pluto aspects can be dominated and exploited by powerful individuals, and need to struggle free, thus learning at first hand about the nature of power, its use and abuse. Experiences of powerlessness, helplessness and extreme vulnerability are all too familiar to Chiron/Pluto people; but they may eventually come to feel, in the very cells of their bodies, that life survives and they are part of it, 'alive' or 'dead'.

Sometimes, when Chiron aspects Pluto, there is a wound inherited from the mother's side of the family: there may be mental or physical diseases, difficult psychological patterns or family issues involving power and wealth. As with Chiron/Saturn, it may be useful for Chiron/Pluto people to study their family-tree, especially on the mother's side – although women on the father's side of the family also represent images of the feminine which have a deep influence. Individuals with Chiron/Pluto are often forced to come to terms with a powerful inheritance, be it positive or negative. Unknowingly, they could be driven to bring fulfilment and healing to their mother and sometimes her ancestors, perhaps by manifesting their unlived potential or by unwittingly following their life-scripts. Women who represent positive images of feminine strength could be discovered within the heritage, providing positive inspiration and healing. .

One woman with Chiron trine Pluto in Leo in the 10th house remembers saying to herself at quite a young age: 'I'm going to be different to the women in my family if it's the last thing I do.' The women in her family were mainly subservient, unfulfilled and without any opportunity to express independent creativity. However, she literalized this drive by having an abortion, not wanting to be subservient to a man and child; to her dismay, she then repeatedly sabotaged other creative endeavours, thus actually following the dreaded pattern. When transiting Chiron opposed the midpoint of this Chiron/Pluto, she turned from struggling to become a more individualized woman *against* the ancestral pattern to doing it *on behalf of* her foremothers, invoking the support of her ancestors by this shift in attitude: she began to co-operate with the pattern of her fate rather than fight it.

In many African religions the ancestors play a crucial role. As mentioned in Chapter 1, the network of family relationships extends beyond physical death; the dead are included by the living as part of life, honoured with ceremonies and consulted for material and spiritual guidance. Most importantly, perhaps, they comprise a protective membrane around the living, shielding them from direct exposure to the world of archetypal energies beyond. In shamanic terms, we need the protection of our ancestral spirits if we are called to encounter the deeper layers of the psyche. In psychological terms, this means deep reconciliation with our family inheritance; even if actual relationships are beyond repair we can still work with the inner images represented within the family, as they remain alive within us, like internalized ancestral spirits. On a physical level, our ancestors carry our genetic inheritance; their psychological patterns and archetypal propensities represent the interface between the personal and the collective layers of the unconscious. Chiron and Pluto both cross over the orbit of their neighbouring inner planet; this process of interpenetration, like blood circulating through the body, can bring healing to relationships within the ancestral fabric even after death.

Whether we think literally of the spirits of the dead, or psychologically of parental imagos perhaps does not matter as much as our attitude to what lies beyond human life. The psychological perspective may bring the comfort of feeling that we have explained something and can therefore deal safely with it – we ward it off by attributing it to one complex or another. An encounter with the spirits of the dead, however, will provoke a fear and awe perhaps more appropriate to Pluto's realm than smug and sophisticated understanding. In our culture we are cushioned from the reality of death, but Chiron/Pluto people need to examine and transform this antiseptic collective attitude in themselves, or they may become morbidly obsessed with death and afraid of life. Many shamanic initiation rituals have at their core an experience of facing death, literally or symbolically. Likewise, many people with Chiron/Pluto come close to death through illness or emotional crises at least once in their lives, or experience the loss of those close to them at an early age. Our first realization of death is often shocking, but with Chiron/Pluto, there may be a specific trauma connected with it. For example, a woman with Chiron at 29°57′ Gemini in the 8th house, semi-sextile Pluto at 0°1′ Leo in the 9th house first encountered death as a young child when she saw a frozen mouse. She left it under a hedge, expecting it to thaw out and scurry off. When it didn't, part of her froze in pained bewilderment (Chiron in Gemini). This memory itself lay frozen for about forty years; when it finally thawed, much further grief was released: her mother died when she was eleven and she had never fully mourned this loss, as her very first experience of death was still unprocessed (Chiron in the 8th house).

Sigmund Freud has Chiron as part of a T-square, in Aquarius in the 3rd house, squaring both Pluto in Taurus in the 7th and his Scorpio Ascendant. For Freud, the unconscious was a repository of repressed instinctual drives (Chiron/Pluto) and socially unacceptable aspects of oneself. His analytical methods (Chiron in Aquarius in the 3rd) sought to reconnect the patient with original traumatic situations or repressed feelings, a typically literal Taurean view. With this fixed T-square involving Chiron and Pluto, however, Freud's work amounts to a head-on encounter with the Underworld. In London, the Freud Museum is situated in the house where Freud lived the last period of his life. His consulting-room is exactly as it was when he saw patients there and typifies the atmosphere of Chiron/Pluto healing. It is dark, still and silent, crowded with statuettes, paintings, icons and artefacts of ancient civilizations, especially Egyptian and ancient Greek. Notwithstanding Freud's denial of the intrinsic nature of the religious instinct, I found this room permeated with reverence for the 'dark gods' (to borrow a term from D. H. Lawrence, who was himself influenced by the writings of Freud).

Finally, let us track the current Chiron/Pluto cycle, from the last conjunction to the next one. Chiron was conjunct Pluto in Leo

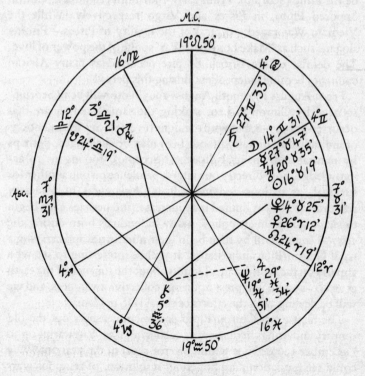

Sigmund Freud

from June 1941 to May 1942, during which time genocide was occurring in Europe under the Third Reich. The astonishing organization and secrecy required for this unprecedented campaign of extermination were as typically Plutonian as the goal itself. Hitler's 'Final Solution' was supposed to rid the world of the scourge of the Jewish race – a monstrous image of Chiron/Pluto in Leo, where only the pure solar hero, here meaning someone from uncontaminated Aryan stock, was deemed worthy to survive and rule the world. By early 1947 Chiron was in Scorpio, squaring both Saturn and Pluto in Leo, remaining within orb of the square to Pluto until October 1948. Still in shock, millions of people were trying to resume some semblance of normal life, perhaps realizing that somehow life would never be the same (Scorpio). From early 1961 until early 1966, Chiron opposed Pluto, in Pisces and Virgo respectively. While the Vietnam War raged – typical of the duality of Pisces – Piscean slogans such as 'Make Love Not War' spoke of the power of love. The demise of the British Empire occurred as many African countries became independent during this period.

From August 1992 until August 1993 Pluto will be in Scorpio, squared by Chiron in Leo, making the same fixed square that occurred in 1947–8, but with the signs reversed. Separatist notions of individuality or nationhood (Leo) may be challenged, perhaps by natural and financial disasters (Scorpio), forcing us to acknowledge more directly our interdependence on one another for survival, as nations and individuals. Awareness of planetary resources (Pluto) as limited may increase, and perhaps even begin to shape government policy; many individuals born during the 1947–8 square will by then be in their mid forties and carrying a natal Chiron/Pluto inheritance. It will be interesting to see who appears on the world stage. Doubts about the survival of the earth as an eco-system will press upon our collective awareness, and we will be dealing with the effects of the AIDS epidemic.

The next exact Chiron/Pluto conjunction ushers out the old century and brings in the new: it occurs in 11°24' Sagittarius on 30 December 1999, and is within orb for most of the year 2000. We could see escalation, and hopefully resolution, of religious wars and doctrinal conflicts (Sagittarius). Both Northern Ireland and

South Africa come to mind. The 1801 chart for the UK has Chiron at 3°42′ Sagittarius, and Pluto at 5° Pisces; therefore this transiting Chiron/Pluto conjunction will affect both, also marking its Chiron return. The MC of South Africa's chart is at 8°14′ Sagittarius, involving also a T-square comprising the Sun, Pluto, Chiron and the Nodes and the Ascendant/Descendant axis (see p. 322 for the horoscope of South Africa); undercover involvement (Pluto) of foreign powers (Sagittarius) is suggested, and perhaps a breakdown of the structure of society (10th house). Interestingly, the last Chiron/Pluto conjunction in Sagittarius occurred during a significant phase of South African history, which was characterized by intensive expansion (Sagittarius) into the interior by settlers connected to the Dutch East India Company. The first major clashes between the Boers and the Bantu occurred only a few years later, in 1779. The Dutch Reformed Church was closely associated with the Company, and at this time no other Christian sect was allowed freedom of worship. The early Boers believed themselves to be descendants of Shem, while black people were descendants of Ham.[27] In the Old Testament, Noah cursed the people of Canaan, the biblical descendants of Ham, with the words: 'He shall be his brothers' meanest slave.'[28] This biblical justification allowed slavery and exploitation to co-exist with piety (Chiron/Pluto in Sagittarius).

An obvious danger with Chiron/Pluto in Sagittarius is the collapse of meaning and loss of hope on a wide scale, which in turn makes people prone to fanaticism, religious persecution and dehumanizing 'spiritual fascism', of which the above example from South African history serves as an illustration. We may also see an outbreak of prophecies of the end of the world. Let us hope, however, that Chiron/Pluto in Sagittarius will bring a renewal of personal meaning through a re-examination of such 'religious' attitudes. The timing of these conjunctions perhaps symbolizes the possibility of a synthesis (Sagittarius) of old and new (Chiron) in many areas of life. Interest in ancient religions (Pluto) could become increasingly widespread as people instinctively realize that to embrace an appropriate archetypal context might enable them to survive and prosper both as individuals and as a species. In the Alice Bailey system, the Earth is the esoteric ruler of the sign of Sagittarius, and perhaps this conjunction will underline in an unequivocal way the need to make reparation to the Earth and to revise our attitudes before it is too late.

Chiron in Aspect to the Moon's Nodes

The Nodes are a polarity by house and sign, and although one end may be weighted by natal aspects, or stimulated by transits, the overall life development suggested by the Nodes occurs through a cyclic exchange between them. Briefly, the North Node represents uncharted territory where we must struggle, exercise our will and make choices. It feels unfamiliar and uncomfortable, but applying ourselves to this area of life-experience and learning its lessons bring considerable returns in terms of well-being and satisfaction. By contrast, the gifts, qualities and issues represented at the South Node are already familiar and usually manifest themselves without undue effort. There we find our karmic inheritance, whether we think of this as family patterns or past lives or both; it is also our line of least resistance, where we retreat when the going gets tough. Although we can rest and creatively withdraw at the South Node, if we hide there we may feel impoverished and fraudulent. We often need to release and let go of whatever the South Node represents, or put it in a form symbolized by the North Node and bring it forward. Chiron's themes appear most directly when it conjuncts or squares the Nodes. Although any aspect can be of significance, and should be considered in the Chiron configuration, this section is confined to comments about the square and conjunction.

When Chiron squares the Nodes, individuals may feel blocked by their wounds and limitations; they stumble over the same issues (suggested by Chiron's house and sign placement) every time they try to go forward in life. They often have a strong sense of destiny which will not let them rest. For example, one woman had Chiron in the 11th house, squaring her North Node in the 2nd house and South Node in the 8th; she wanted to be a body-therapist, but had a highly paid job with considerable political influence as a trade-union official (11th house). Although she completed a massage training, and felt her true vocation to be in the area of personal transformation (8th house) through healing the body (2nd house), her attachment to having 'revolutionary' power in the eyes of the collective (Chiron in the 11th) made it difficult for her to change careers, when she knew that if she worked as a healer it would be in relative obscurity. She eventually did give up her old job and in time came to express her 11th-house Chiron in Cancer in another way by teaching massage to groups of people (11th house); her speciality was helping people to reconnect with their feelings (Chiron in Cancer).

With Chiron squaring the Nodes, our limitations and wounds need to be included in our self-concept and idea of our purpose in life; any attempts to forge ahead by trying to exclude them result in crisis. Our whole idea of self-actualization may need to be re-examined, perhaps transformed from an achievement-oriented and one-sided idea of 'spiritual progress' to one which addresses the whole person. For example, a man who had spiritual pretensions of which he was initially unaware ran therapy groups; he had Chiron in the 4th house in Libra, squaring the North Node in Cancer in the 1st house and South Node in Capricorn in the 7th. He blamed his wife and family (Chiron in Libra in the 4th) for holding him back; he eventually left them, only to find that he felt so emotionally insecure (Chiron in the 4th house) and depressed that he was in fact no better off.

The lives of people who have Chiron conjunct either Node strongly reflect Chironian themes. They may embody one of the figures from the myth, living out the role of teacher, wise person, healer, mentor, saviour, victim, sufferer, wounded one, wounder, acolyte, devotee or apprentice. For example, Gandhi has Chiron conjunct the South Node in Aries; he embodied and personified his philosophy of non-violent revolution (Chiron in Aries can signify passive aggression) even though it cost him and thousands of others their lives. Laurens van der Post has Chiron conjunct the South Node in Aquarius in the 4th house; he is a typically Chironian figure who has bridged different cultures and had enormous impact on collective thinking. People with Chiron conjunct either Node may have a strong sense of vocation in Chironian fields such as teaching or healing; alternatively, they may have intimate relationships with therapists, priests, people who are ill or physically or mentally handicapped, or who represent in some way the mythic images and themes in the story of Chiron. For example, Jane Roberts has Chiron conjunct the North Node in Taurus, part of a stellium consisting of Chiron, Moon, Sun, Jupiter and North Node all in Taurus. Jane Roberts was a medium through whom an entity named Seth spoke; numerous books of teachings were compiled from his addresses. She writes that she would often receive his communications when doing practical chores (Chiron in Taurus), although later these became formalized sessions.

When Chiron is in hard aspect to the Nodes, if its themes are not lived consciously, perhaps through commitment to a personal quest for consciousness or following a healing vocation, they usually manifest themselves anyway, and can even take over the person's life in a negative way. For example, one person who had Chiron conjunct North Node in Capricorn in the 7th house alienated many of her friends; she often adopted a false tone of wisdom and benevolence without realizing it, giving unsought advice and making people feel patronized and therefore irritated. In fact, her father had been a teacher, and, although she secretly felt a vocation in this direction, she had determined not to follow in her father's footsteps, as they were in perpetual conflict – a typical Chiron in Capricorn issue.

Karen Ann Quinlan has Chiron in Capricorn in the 2nd house, the apex of a T-square also involving Venus in Aries in the 4th house opposite Neptune in Libra in the 10th. She went into a coma in 1975, when transiting Chiron was exactly conjunct her Venus. During the following ten years before she died, she lived the myth of Chiron literally, unable either to die or be healed; her T-square is also poignantly suggestive of the story of Sleeping Beauty.[29] When she finally did die, Mercury was exactly opposite her Mars in Sagittarius in the 10th house, a transit perhaps symbolic of Prince Charming awakening her to a new life beyond the physical realm. During the first year of her coma, she was on a respirator; her parents fought and won a historic court case, gaining permission to turn it off and allow her to die. The legal system was challenged (Chiron/Node in Capricorn); the right to refuse unwanted medical intervention and die a natural death became a controversial issue as the publicity surrounding the case grew. However, when the respirator was legally switched off,

Karen Ann did not die for a further nine years. At the time of her death Chiron was in Gemini, opposite her Sagittarian Ascendant; her chart shows an interesting novile of transiting Chiron to her Uranus in Cancer in the 8th house, traditionally associated with death. Rudhyar describes the novile aspect (40°) as 'a period of tribulation and interior formation',[30] like the archetypal forty days in the wilderness; Michael R. Meyer says the novile is 'subjective or unmanifested growth'.[31] We will never know what she lived in her inner life during those years.

If those with Chiron conjunct either Node are unable or unwilling to take seriously their inner life and the urge for individuation, including both their gifts and their wounds, they sometimes unleash great destructiveness, becoming 'the one who wounds'. Alternatively, they may compulsively try to 'heal' situations, to make things better, always attracting people who need to to be validated, redeemed or healed; they can also become identified with the victim, or become a scapegoat or outsider. Hitler has Chiron conjunct the North Node in Cancer in the 9th house, opposite Moon/Jupiter/South Node, all conjunct in Capricorn in the 3rd house. His Chiron/Node highlights his philosophy (9th house); his genocidal mission may be seen as a philosophically rationalized (Chiron in the 9th house) enactment of the anti-Semitism lying deep within the European collective psyche. He strove to 'heal' and safeguard his own race (Chiron in Cancer) by eliminating another one. Hitler's own ancestry is uncertain, but recent research suggests that his grandfather was possibly Jewish, or that Hitler may have believed he was.[32] Thus his attempt to exterminate the Jews can also be seen as an escalation (Chiron/Jupiter) of his desire for personal vengeance on his entire family, in whose hands he suffered brutal treatment as a child (Chiron/Moon). On an archetypal level, however, Hitler has been virtually mythologized (Chiron/Jupiter) as the Antichrist. Note that the last exact Chiron/Pluto conjunction in Leo, in mid-July 1941, occurred in the 9th house of Hitler's chart, barely 1° off his MC; this is a macabre indicator of his Plutonic 'vocation'. In 1938–9, when his Chiron return occurred, Pluto was just moving into Leo, and thus squaring his Taurus sun. The Chiron return can be a time of profound connection with one's true sense of vocation, of dedication to a path which will preoccupy the rest of one's life. As we will see in the next chapter, with significant points on the Chiron cycle, the positions of other planets are also an important influence. In this case, Pluto called and Hitler answered.

Those with Chiron conjunct either Node frequently become ardent devotees of a guru figure.[33] Breaking away from such an attachment may prove difficult for them, if not impossible. Often the experience goes sour under the weight of unresolved parental issues, and they may turn vehemently against their former beliefs and spiritual principles. Although at first people with this conjunction might have a pressing need for an external figure to help them connect with their inner source of guidance, eventually they will usually be forced to find their own way.

On the other hand, people with this conjunction can be naturally charismatic, and attract to themselves a following; the shadow side of this is being unable to take advice, suggestions or guidance from anyone, to their cost. One woman with Chiron conjunct the South Node in Gemini in the 3rd house spent most of her adult life as a teacher; when Neptune opposed this conjunction by transit, she sold all her belongings, gave up her job and joined a spiritual community. After a long and intense involvement with the guru and preoccupation with her own spiritual journey, she found herself with no money and little inclination to make her separate way in the world. Her Chiron return brought some hard lessons, as she was forced to do menial clerical work (3rd house) in order to survive financially.

Chiron in Aspect to the Angles

Finally, when Chiron aspects either the Ascendant/Descendant axis or the MC/IC axis, or both, it behaves rather like Chiron actually in those respective houses, especially if forming a hard aspect to the respective cusps. For details of this, refer to the appropriate sections of Chiron through the houses. If Chiron is in soft aspect to either axis, it is often a helpful aspect highlighting the creative possibilities of the houses involved. In either case, the affairs of the houses in question will be coloured with typical Chironian themes, and Chiron will seek expression through those areas of life.

9 · Kairos: Transits of Chiron

And if in the changing phases of man's life
I fall in sickness and in misery
my wrists seem broken and my heart seems dead
and strength is gone, and my life
is only the leavings of a life . . .
then I must know
that still I am in the hands of the unknown God,
he is breaking me down to his own oblivion
to send me forth on a new morning, a new man.

D. H. Lawrence, 'Shadows'

As we have seen, Chiron's *process* stimulates the unfoldment of our individuality and its expression in life. Its characteristic *space* is the opening, threshold, link, bridge or doorway; its characteristic *time* when in transit, to both its own natal place and to other planets, may be described by the Greek word *kairos*. Kairos was the personification of opportunity, and had his altar on Olympus.[1] Hence, the word means an opportunity, the right moment, when the timeless or eternal realms intersect with our clock or Cronus (Saturn) time; the archetypal nature of an experience may suddenly reveal itself, releasing a process which was previously frozen or stuck; a dam may give way, enabling the river of our life to continue flowing. *Kairos* is the 'aha!' experience, which may unlock the door to insights and new possibilities. However, this may be experienced by the ego as a wounding attack and, as we shall see below, we may at first meet the experiences of Chiron transits by defending ourselves against them and blocking them out.

The Chiron Cycle

Because Chiron's orbit is very elliptical, it spends much longer in some signs than others – as much as seven or eight years in Pisces and Aries, and only about two or even less in Virgo and Libra. Hence, its cycle cannot be conveniently divided into approximately equal quarters like the Saturn cycle. The Chiron cycle strongly stimulates our journey of individuation, and this may or may not sit comfortably with the needs of the Saturn cycle; it represents at one level the stages of growth of our ego-bound self and the assimilation of the past, and at another the integration of this into viable and/or collectively approved forms. The first square of Chiron to its own natal place may occur anywhere between the age of about five (Chiron in Leo/Virgo/Libra) and about twenty-three (Chiron in Aquarius and Pisces).

If you follow the Chiron transits through your own life, you will see that they often correspond to major turning-points, crises, events or life-experiences which leave a deep mark, and which may permanently influence the course of your life. Issues left unresolved and hopes once abandoned may return at the next turn of the spiral, perhaps allowing their integration in a new form; old wounds may open up and seek healing, and unfinished business from the past may make an unwelcome appearance. The tone of the Chiron/Chiron cycle is one of awakening, rebalancing and intensification of our commitment to life; it represents a series of opportunities to realign inwardly with our deeper nature, and perhaps also a realization of how this seeks to manifest itself in the outer world. In this way we may often catch hold of a thread of personal meaning running through the Chiron cycle, which *deo gratias* culminates at about the age of fifty in a sense of rebirth, new life and wider purpose at the Chiron return.

Let us consider four points of the Chiron cycle – the major 'hard' aspects it makes to its own natal place: the waxing or first square; the opposition; the waning or second square; the conjunction or Chiron return. These are the most obvious points with which to reach an overview of the Chiron cycle, as they are more likely to manifest themselves in observable events and experiences. It can also be revealing to cast charts for the exact moment of the transit you are studying: there will be one or three, depending on how many exact transits Chiron makes. What this shows is the *kairos* of the transit or series of transits. Given that the doors to the timeless realms are opened, this moment may make a powerful impression upon us, and may therefore also describe the nature of the ingredients which repeat later on at the next turn of the spiral. Other key transits that may be occurring at this time will form part of the overall quality of that moment. This is illustrated by the horoscope examined at the end of this chapter. As a brief example, one woman had Pluto conjunct the Ascendant during her first Chiron/Chiron square, and all subsequent points of the Chiron cycle were coloured with Plutonian themes, including the death of three people close to her and dramatic changes in her personal appearance and self-concept.

If the first Chiron/Chiron square occurs very early in life, before the first Saturn/Saturn square, it is likely to be marked by trauma and unhappiness; the resulting acceleration of psychological growth is often then stabilized through physical illness. The hard aspects on the Chiron/Chiron cycle often also correspond with an opening to the transpersonal, when wider spiritual realities impinge strongly upon us. Therefore, the earlier the first Chiron square, the more difficult these experiences will be to digest and integrate, as they will often have underlying them an experience of deep woundedness. These transpersonal experiences, positive and/or negative, may lie dormant for many years before their core can be approached consciously and their inner meaning understood, perhaps awaiting the Chiron/Chiron opposition or an outer planet transit to a key part of the Chiron configuration. During subsequent Chiron transits, to itself or other planets, the same illness pattern may recur, or similar life-situations will be met; the same psychological ingredients will constellate in a different form, but carry the same meaning.

The first Chiron/Chiron opposition often very clearly intimates something about the purpose and meaning of a person's life and will often echo life-events or even physical symptoms from the period of the first Chiron/Chiron square. Both the opposition and the second square may also provide an opportunity for healing wounds to the instinctual nature. A reconnection with sexuality and the life of the senses frequently accompanies Chiron transits; this provides an opportunity to rebalance the 'upper' and 'lower' parts of our nature, and thus to mitigate one-sidedness which may have developed through life or which is intrinsic to our nature.

The final Chiron/Chiron square is potentially a very creative time, as by now we may have more maturity and understanding of ourselves, more sense of our place in life. However, if we have mostly lived within inherited and/or collective Saturnian structures and not taken seriously the life of our own soul, it may be a very painful time. Past betrayals of the self may have to be mourned and let go of; we may need to confront inwardly our apathy, intransigence and lack of responsibility for our inner being. The response to this pain is often to begin in earnest the quest for self-discovery, pursued with all the intensity stemming from a recognition of time wasted and opportunities lost.

At the Chiron return, if we have not already done so, we begin orienting towards death, the end of our physical life on earth. The half-way point of life has passed. Women will bear no more children, and have usually been through the menopause within the previous few years; the demands of their mothering role will have changed as their children become more and more independent. The Chiron return poses the question: 'What am I going to do with this last part of my life?' Often material relating to previous points on the Chiron/Chiron cycle will emerge again, for redigesting and placing within the overall life-structure in a new way. Once again sickness, depression and an inner confrontation with the self may occur; this time it often has as its purpose the integration of the entire cycle, an inner reviewing and restructuring, in order that the essence of it may be carried forward into the last part of life.

If a personal sense of connection with the numinous has not yet been found, denial and fear of death may invite the insidious and draining experience of meaninglessness. However, for many people, the Chiron return brings a very real sense of participation in the overall process of life as a whole, resulting in conscious commitment to their individuation and spiritual life. In traditional Hindu society, there are clearly demarcated stages of life:

only when a man has fulfilled his social responsibilities as husband and householder may he renounce the world and become a *sadhu* – a contemplative, or a monk in a religious order. With fifty years of life-experience, a person may be well equipped to intuit the overall pattern of meaning within their life, and to embark on a new cycle of self-discovery.

The first two Chiron/Chiron aspects, especially if they occur early in life, frequently accompany experiences of being wounded by others, being a victim of one's parents, siblings, schoolteachers and other authority figures. From a psychological point of view the experiences of our first few years irreparably affect our subsequent development. However, from an astrological point of view, the ingredients of these experiences are already written by the hand of fate. Life itself is mysteriously enlisted in the enactment of the scenarios whose script is written in the horoscope, which in this view represents and describes the portion of the infinite which we have been given to work with, willingly or otherwise.

The Chiron return invites us to take up the challenge of our life in this way. If the resentment, anger or blame for the pain caused by earlier wounding situations has not yet been acknowledged and fully felt, it may now erupt in bitterness, illness, despair and depression. However, there is often strong motivation for renewal at this time; we may feel that this is a last chance. However, as Gibran poignantly writes, this is not without its difficulties, for:

Not without a wound in the spirit shall I leave this city. Long were the days of pain I have spent within its walls, and long were the nights of aloneness; and who can depart from his pain and his aloneness without regret?[2]

People who have been very close to death often report experiencing a review of their whole lives, monumental in nature, sometimes occurring within the space of only a few seconds of earth time; digesting further implications of this may take years. This process of life-review often happens spontaneously during the last part of the Chiron cycle, most intensively when transiting Chiron is about 6° or less from its first exact conjunction with natal Chiron. During this period, many synchronous phenomena may occur that reconnect us with the past; they come to jog the memory, perhaps asking for something to be reconsidered, fully felt, reflected upon, understood in a new way, or indeed permitted into consciousness for the first time.

During this time, it may be beneficial to ensure that we have enough solitude – time to reflect upon, and perhaps to mourn, the ending of the Chiron cycle and welcome the last years of our life, to process and digest the past sufficiently so that it can become like compost, ensuring the fertility of the forthcoming period. Hopes and dreams which can no longer be fulfilled in their original form may need to be sacrificed, as the energy invested in them will be needed elsewhere if renewal is to follow. The second Saturn return, at about the age of fifty-six, follows on the heels of the Chiron return, thus representing an opportunity to ground the inner process of the Chiron return in a new form, to manifest its meaning in a concrete way in our life. However, if we have too much undigested life-experience by this time, too much unfinished business that we are unable or unwilling to confront, psychological contraction, narrowness and physical decline may quickly follow the Saturn return.

For example, a woman approaching her Chiron return wanted to begin painting again, something she had enjoyed as a child, but which she had not done since. To her disappointment, she found herself feeling very blocked, inhibited and not really enjoying it. She had natal Chiron in late Taurus, conjunct Sun in early Gemini, both in the 5th house. In discussing the wider context of her life, she expressed guilt that she had not provided her husband with a son. He had longed for a son, but she gave birth to two daughters. This preyed upon her, in spite of her Gemini mind trying to be rational about it. Her Chiron in Taurus was manifesting itself in dogged literalness, a frequent expression of this placement. When she did some imaginal work on the kind of son she wished she could have had, he was, predictably, symbolized by this Sun/Chiron in the 5th house. He would have been 'physically beautiful, practical and witty, and skilled in some branch of the arts' she said. Her guilt gradually faded once she was able to take this longing symbolically; she began to look forward to giving birth to the son she had always wanted in the form of her own creativity which had not yet had an opportunity to come out and play (Chiron in the 5th house).

Vertical and Horizontal Growth

Let us consider the symbol of a cross, taking the horizontal and vertical axes to represent two different kinds of growth: the *horizontal* axis of growth concerns our relationship with the world and other people, and the outer forms of our life; the *vertical* axis of growth is represented by the image of Chiron and mainly concerns *inner* self-discovery and the progressive linking of all levels from the instinctual through to the spiritual. If early relationships within our family are too negative, disturbed or tenuous, early transits of Chiron may correspond with the 'normal' development of life being arrested or aborted altogether. This is like the wound in Chiron's animal half, which may interrupt the maturing process of the *instinctual* life: our basic survival instincts, our sexual desires and associated courtship rituals which lead to mating and reproduction of the species and later nurturing and educating the young.

Transition Rituals and Transits of Chiron

In many 'primitive' cultures, these important thresholds of psycho-biological life were honoured with rituals, celebrations and initiation ceremonies. In this way, these societies addressed both the vertical and horizontal axes of growth, by the provision of a mythical context within which these crucial psycho-biological developments could take place and by the participation of the whole community in the event. Even today amongst the Shona of Zimbabwe, for example, every phase of life is honoured by ceremonies that include the ancestral spirits; the continuation and development of the biological aspects of human life are themselves a process regarded as holy, as something to be celebrated.

By way of contrast, few people in Western cultures benefit from such rituals of transition; those that remain have by and large long ago lost their numinous meaning. It was formerly the custom for Christians at puberty to receive confirmation into the fellowship of the Church, the 'Body of Christ'. Until recently this included taking vows to renounce 'the World, the Flesh and the Devil', and these words are still used in some Churches. Thus, at the vulnerable time of newly-emerging sexuality, many young men and women are 'initiated' into a religious allegiance which encourages the repression of their vitality and emerging individualized life.

During puberty an opening to the transpersonal dimensions of life often occurs. Prompted by the burgeoning fertility within the body, powerful images inspire people, and a religious sense opens up as, sexually and archetypally, we become aware of the 'other'. Indeed, it seems that during important stages of psycho-biological transition such as first menstruation, marriage, home-making, birth of the first child, and so on, the psyche needs and will seek out a transpersonal context within which the experience can be contained. Hence, images that enter the psyche at these times may have a profound effect on the rest of our life, even if unconsciously. In the absence of transition rituals containing appropriate transpersonal images that celebrate with joy the emerging womanhood or manhood of a person, the archetypal images dominant within the collective will enter. For many people in the Western world, this will be the Judaeo-Christian framework, with the attendant brutalization of the instincts. As an alternative, in recent decades, film-stars, rock-stars, or public-hero figures have become for many young teenagers the carriers of powerful archetypal images; embodiments of Ares, Dionysus or Aphrodite provoke hysteria, emulation and adoration. In the absence of any overt ritual of transition, however, the young psyche is left without guidance, to process the powerful emotion released as best it may.

A transit of Chiron, then, may accompany the interruption of the natural psycho-biological development. The direct route of expression is closed, and the process spirals on to another level. As progress is now fuelled by blocked instinctual libido or life-energy, development may be speeded up, intensified, and may then result in the inflated manifestations of Chiron that we have already met. For example, a woman whom I shall call Laura had Chiron in Capricorn in the 2nd house. She felt emotionally rejected by her father, whom she found cold, stiff and excessively formal; he became progressively more so as she developed sexually. With Chiron in Capricorn, this cut deeply. During her thirteenth year, transiting Chiron conjuncted her Venus in Pisces in the 4th house. Laura was musically talented, and since the age of eleven had put a great deal of energy into practising the piano and the violin. After school, she went to a music college; her first Chiron/Chiron square occurred during her second year, when Laura became very depressed and sought help. She felt desperately lonely and longed for a boyfriend; she felt unable to join the general rough-and-tumble of competing for partners. Although very attractive physically, she had no confidence in her beauty, a typical manifestation of Chiron in the 2nd house.

During a therapy session, Laura discovered that she had a hidden fantasy that no man would be able to resist her if she played music with him. As all her sexual energy was invested in her music, her diligent practising was actually dedicated to sharpening her powers of seduction. Then, when she played music with men who did not succumb to her (unconscious) fantasy of being irresistible, she at first tried harder, practised more, and eventually became inexplicably depressed. Chiron had transited her Venus during puberty, when her need for affirmation of her emerging womanhood was intense. It was during this time that the feelings of rejection took root. The feelings were unconscious at the time, congruent with Venus in Pisces in the 4th house. All the anger, and the determination to get her father's attention, that is, to 'seduce' him, went into her music. At the first Chiron/Chiron square, the issue emerged into consciousness. The projected self-image and/or fantasy sense of sexual omnipotence is frequently found with Venus/Chiron aspects, and here its disembodied expression in her music is typically Piscean/Neptunian. Laura unconsciously saw herself as a Neptunian siren-like figure, luring men to her with her music.

Here is an example of energy blocked at an instinctual level, continuing to function powerfully, but in a more indirect way. Laura was fortunate in that this emerged into consciousness only a few years later before too much pressure had built up, and hence the Chiron/Chiron square brought her the opportunity to redo this missed threshold and let go of her need for sexual validation from her father. Others are not so fortunate and may continue in a one-sided way, developing into apparently brilliant or successful people; later, however, the wounded instincts may rise up and clamour for attention, bringing sickness and chaos in their wake.

Repression of the Sublime

We may also suppress the spiritual and transpersonal intimations which come during Chiron transits. As Roberto Assagioli has pointed out, it is not only our sexual and instinctual drives which can be repressed; many people suffer from the 'repression of the sublime'.[3] Many children are highly attuned to intuitive perceptions of other dimensions; for example, they have imaginary playmates who may be more real to them than flesh-and-blood people, and their dreams and experiences of the twilight zone between sleep and waking may also be totally real. If parents are not able both to validate these experiences and to help the child to begin discriminating different levels of reality, these experiences may be suppressed through being greeted with scorn or rationalizations. Later, we may be afraid of the world of the non-rational, and also perhaps tend to be taken over by it.

Transits of Chiron to Other Planets

Traditionally, transits have been described in language implying that the slower moving planet 'acts upon' the other one. A transit of, say, Saturn to natal Venus, will be experienced as Venus being 'done to' by Saturn, where one's capacity for enjoyment is dampened, life is dull, relationships lose their magic, and so on; positively, artistic projects could find form and become grounded. This is analogous to the scientific view of matter consisting of particles acting upon one another. However, if we take another viewpoint, where matter consists of waves of energy, transits can be seen as an interrelationship of dynamic forces. We may still feel 'acted upon' by transits, but from a Chironian point of view, if there is a willed surrender to the process, there may be an experience of the interrelatedness of two planetary energies; this may still express itself in events unique to our individual life, but we have a sense of participation in the process. This is summed up in the words of Dane Rudhyar, who said that 'it is not the event which happens to the person, but the person which happens to the event'.[4]

Wounding or Healing of the Other Planetary Principle

If transiting Chiron conjuncts our natal Mars, we may experience hostility from others, but may also become aware of our own disowned aggression and suppressed drive for independence and achievement. The specific details of the experience usually correspond to the house and sign placement of both Chiron and the other planet. For example, if the Chiron/Mars transit mentioned above occurred in the 4th house in Gemini, then the experience might well take the form of arguments and discord (Chiron/Mars in Gemini) within the domestic situation. The emotional charge accompanying the event, however, might echo encounters in childhood with an aggressive father (Mars in the 4th house); we might encounter our own need to be right (Mars in Gemini), and so on. A wounding experience which occurs during a Chiron transit is often a repetition of a previous situation, and hence an opportunity for healing, a chance to do things differently, to gain insight and perhaps to exercise some choice.

The life-experiences and qualities represented by the planet which transiting Chiron aspects may be healed, released, or brought to life for the first time. One woman, who had not had any sexual relationships with men for some time, experienced a major awakening during a transit of Chiron conjunct her natal Venus; she had two or three lovers in her life at one time, a new and exciting experience for her. Both wounding and healing may come via other people during Chiron transits. In psychological terms, one part of the archetypal pattern associated with Chiron is projected on to another person, who then becomes an agent of Chiron. We may meet embodiments of our own Chiron or of the planet which it is currently aspecting. For example, when transiting Chiron in Gemini crossed over the Ascendant of a woman whose natal Chiron was in Libra in the 5th house, she had two consecutive affairs with men who both had Sun in Libra: transiting Chiron in Gemini of course brought two healers! Through these two relationships, she experienced an awakening of her Geminian Ascendant, with the Venusian overtones of her natal Chiron in Libra. She felt renewed pleasure in cultural activities such as visiting galleries, and going to the theatre; she also began to enjoy beautifying herself and going to the sauna, indulgences she had never before allowed herself. Both men were intellectual types who stimulated her mind (transiting Chiron in Gemini); she recaptured some sense of joy and spontaneity, long since lost through a painful marriage (Chiron in Libra in the 5th house). Although both affairs were typical short-lived 5th-house encounters, she gained much self-confidence and felt quite renewed afterwards.

Typical Healing Experiences

Chiron transits frequently bring a strong activation of the urge to individuate, which in turn stimulates major changes in life-style and personal orientation. Following a physical and/or emotional crisis, we may seek help for the first time; a significant teacher or teaching may cross our path, and we may also have strong learning experiences described by the aspect in question. Eventually a renewed sense of personal meaning and/or realization of vocation may be found as we reconnect with a sense of purpose in life.

Within the crisis we experience, we often have the opportunity to redo a missed threshold of maturation. The Chiron transits of Laura, described above, are an example of this. We are frequently starkly confronted with the oppositions and conflicts within us. The rebalancing of one-sidedness may be dramatic or subtle; it may be welcomed, but we might also find it threatening, if it involves becoming familiar with repressed, unwanted and destructive aspects of our own shadow, or indeed if it means positive changes which we find difficult to accept.

Various kinds of transpersonal experiences, positive or negative, may accompany the experience of suffering and healing. Any of the transpersonal domains as described at the beginning of Chapter 8 might open up to us, bringing a shift in perception, a 'breakthrough in plane', followed by an experience of 'hierophantic realization' – an appreciation of the underlying unity of all life beyond the dualism which we normally call reality. This kind of experience promotes healing, and the denial of it may be behind our symptoms of illness.

The experience of illness, as well as the death of someone close to us, will confront us with the frailty of our mortality; the acceptance of death itself brings healing to our attitude to life, just as Chiron's own healing followed his journey to the Underworld. After significant Chiron transits, people who have had difficulty 'being here' often realize with poignancy the transitoriness of life on earth, and feel renewed enthusiasm and sense of commitment.

Activation of the Mythic Themes in the Story of Chiron

Like any other planet, when Chiron is strongly active by transit, we may see striking examples of the mythic themes taking form in individual lives. For example, a man with Sun in Aries opposite Chiron in Libra took up archery and horse-riding at his Chiron opposition; he obsessively poured money, time and energy into these pursuits, which were totally at odds with the rest of his life. As the transit waned, he awoke as if from a dream which had cost him a small fortune to pursue, and began to ask himself what he was really doing. With Chiron opposite an Aries Sun, his core sense of individual malehood felt wounded for lack of a male role model; his father had died when he was five years old (when this opposition became exact by solar arc). Although he longed to be a macho and heroic figure, he also had Neptune in Libra, widely opposite his Sun and conjunct Chiron; he was very sensitive to the moods of others, eager not to hurt their feelings, and his own sense of boundaries was not very strong. Mars, the ruler of his Sun sign, was in Cancer; he often found himself in dependent relationships, and was vulnerable to being manipulated by women; although angry about this, he felt powerless to change it. The Chiron opposition brought an upsurge of masculine Arian self-assertion which seemed to have nowhere to go in his life, and hence it expressed itself compulsively in this mythical form. With natal Chiron in Libra, however, he began to realize that his challenge was to relate from a position of equality. This meant first becoming familiar both with his own regressive desires (Mars in Cancer) that resulted in subtle emotional bondage to others and robbed him of his power, and also with his under-ground desire to dominate others (Chiron in Libra opposite Sun in Aries).

A woman with Chiron in late Gemini, opposite a Sagittarian Ascendant, had only developed one breast at puberty; she thus embodied physically the image of the Amazon, and also had a rare and potentially fatal allergy to horses. When transiting Chiron was in early Gemini, conjunct her South Node and opposite her 12th-house Sagittarian Sun, she became intensively involved in both giving and receiving healing. She went to a retreat-centre in the country, and after a few days realized it was also a stud farm, and that she had been surrounded by horses with no ill-effects. Over the next few years circumstances forced her to become financially independent for the first time in her life, and thus to draw upon the Amazon part of her nature. She started a successful local newspaper, launched exactly on her Chiron return (Chiron in Gemini), which proved to be both creatively fulfilling and economically viable. Congruent with the Chiron return, it was also a community-orientated project aiming to create a network of people exchanging resources, services and skills. During the transit of Chiron in Gemini, her undeveloped breast actually began to grow: in other words, the Amazon within was awakened and began to function.

Transits of Chiron and the Image of Shamanic Initiation

During transits of Chiron, it may be useful to bear in mind the archetypal pattern of shamanic initiation as previously discussed, as it provides a mythic context for what is happening in our life, which itself may facilitate the deepening of our experience, allowing the process to unfold with our conscious participation. The sequence of illness or crisis, rupture of our current life-situation followed by a journey to the Underworld, a period of suffering and death followed by renewal and return may sound rather dramatic. However, anyone who has ever had a head-cold and gone to bed for a day has experienced some disintegration and renewal! The intensity of this pattern varies from a subtle progression of change which may go almost unnoticed but nevertheless enriches our life, through to periods of major disruption, breakdown and potential deep transformation of the personality and purpose in life.

Viewing even minor crises in the light of this image may enable the Inner Teacher to communicate with us; this may provide an opportunity for rebalancing our lives, for clarifying a problem, for letting go and getting a better perspective. To the extent that we are able to take this seriously and allow the process of withdrawal, introversion and return to unfold, we also open ourselves to the help, guidance and inner transformation which are there for the asking. In addition, any stations of Chiron that may occur during this period are times when a great deal of healing energy is on offer.

Transits to Natal Chiron

Sometimes when natal Chiron is transited by another planet, it will bring a recapitulation of a situation connected with Chiron's sign and house position. For example, a woman had Sun in early Scorpio, widely conjunct Chiron; during the year when Pluto had been conjunct the Sun by transit, her father died; later that same year she divorced her husband. A few years later, when transiting

Pluto was exactly conjunct natal Chiron, her beloved cat died, very close to the anniversary of her father's death. This opened the floodgates of unfinished grieving, for both her father and her husband. She had been agonizing about whether or not to have a child, and was also feeling very sterile in other areas of her life. She was unable to claim her fertility on any level in her own life, as she was still tied to her father with the bonds of unfinished grief. Here Pluto's transit to Chiron accompanied a 'repeating situation', another death, which enabled healing to flow.

Progressions Involving Chiron

If Chiron is in a close aspect to any natal planet and progresses to exactitude, Chironian themes will colour the life of the individual for many years, and will manifest themselves in the area of life indicated by the houses involved, and in a manner congruent with the signs involved. Progressions of inner planets to natal Chiron will be effective for about one year, depending on the speed of the progressed planet, and will form part of the overall life-context of that year. However, if aspected by the progressed Moon, the aspect will manifest more obviously for the duration (about one month). Likewise, if the progressed MC or Ascendant should make an exact aspect with progressed or natal Chiron, Chironian themes may be very strong during this time: I have seen many examples of people who changed careers while their progressed MC was aspecting natal Chiron, and often into Chironian professions.

Chiron in the Horoscope of a Visionary

Finally, let us look at Chiron transits in the life of a rare person who submitted totally to the transpersonal levels of what opened up during some key transits, and was fated to bring this to a creative conclusion. In the horoscope of Bernadette of Lourdes, Chiron is at 0°51' of Virgo, therefore in exaltation, in the 4th house. It sits at the point of a 'finger of God' or yod for-

St Bernadette of Lourdes

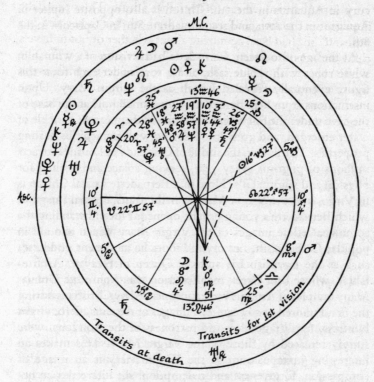

TRANSITS – noon positions

First Vision	Death
11.2.1858	16.4.1879
☉ 22° ♒ 31'	☉ 26° ♈ 17'
☽ 24° ♑ 14'	☽ 0° ♓ 8'
☿ 26° ♑ 56'	☿℞ 27° ♈ 43'
♀ 18° ♒ 21'	♀ 27° ♉ 16'
♂ 16° ♏ 49'	♂ 21° ♒ 8'
♃ 4° ♉ 53'	♃ 4° ♓ 27'
♄ 22° ♋ 49'	♄ 8° ♈ 17'
⚷ 12° ♒ 37'	⚷ 7° ♉ 33'
♅ 25° ♉ 39'	♅℞ 0° ♍ 17'
♆ 21° ♓ 16'	♆ 8° ♉ 59'
♇ 4° ♉ 31'	♇ 26° ♉ 23'
☊ 19° ♓ 6'	☊ 29° ♑ 43'

mation, quincunx both Uranus in Pisces in the 11th and Mercury in Aquarius in the 9th. Chiron is also opposite Jupiter in Aquarius in the 10th, and sesquiquadrate Sun in Capricorn in the 8th.

At the age of fourteen, Bernadette had a vision of a woman in white robes with a blue sash, and a rose under each foot; this figure eventually revealed herself as the Virgin Mary. Upon instructions from her, Bernadette dug a small hole at the base of the cave under the hill where the figure had appeared; a trickle of water emerged, and grew into a spring with miraculous healing properties. To this day, the shrine of Our Lady of Lourdes attracts millions of pilgrims every year, seeking solace and healing for physical and spiritual ills. Note that Bernadette's natal Chiron is in Virgo, and the Virgin Mary was the transpersonal image to which Bernadette's young psyche opened. Notwithstanding the somewhat effete images of the Virgin Mary which abound in popular Catholicism, her mythic roots lie in ancient goddesses such as the Egyptian Isis and the Queen of Heaven, Astarte-Ishtar, whose later Greek manifestation was Aphrodite Urania. Many temples of Artemis were appropriated by Christians during the first hundred or so years AD. Images of Artemis, fierce virgin huntress, fertility goddess and patroness of the Amazons, were simply replaced by those of the Virgin Mary. This makes an interesting juxtaposition, as the Virgin Mary is an image of compassion, forgiveness and redemption; she intercedes on behalf of mortal sinners and her womb gives birth to the incarnating Christ.

In Bernadette's chart, her North Node is found in Sagittarius, the sign ruled by Chiron; it is also conjunct the position of the Galactic Centre (24°41' Sagittarius at that time), which symbolizes the religious nature of her destiny and her role as a channel for energies coming from a higher order of reality. Natal Jupiter in the 10th opposite Chiron in the 4th also gives a strong religious sense. Jupiter is the transpersonal or esoteric ruler of Aquarius, and therefore strongly placed; here it also symbolizes a spiritualized version of mothering (10th house). Bernadette cared for the many (Chiron/Jupiter expanding the horizons), instead of the few children she might have had herself. Natal Uranus in Pisces in the

11th house here symbolizes an individual response (Uranus) to the spiritual longings (Pisces) within the collective at large (11th house); the healing and redeeming qualities of this vision are described by the sign of Pisces, ruled by Neptune. Chiron in the 4th house symbolizes the poverty and deprivation which characterized Bernadette's childhood, when her basic needs were often unmet owing to misfortune, illness and famine; as a young girl, Bernadette looked after her brothers and sister while her parents went out to work, although she herself was in poor health. Mercury in Aquarius in the 9th house symbolizes attunement with archetypal realities. Chiron sesquiquadrate her Capricornian Sun in the 8th house perhaps represents a block in the expression of her sexuality, which may have contributed to opening her up strongly to other dimensions. Through her inner union with the transpersonal image of the Virgin Mary and her expression of the vision it contained, she brought healing and grace to many people. On a personal level this also suggests Chiron opposite Jupiter in the 10th house, a larger-than-life mother-figure to which Bernadette turned; at a transpersonal level the Blessed Virgin called upon her in turn.

Looking at the transits for the day of her vision, we see that Chiron is in Aquarius in the 9th house, 1°3′ from an exact conjunction with her MC. Dane Rudhyar describes the abstract meaning of the MC as the final revelation of the purpose of our destiny, where, having died the ego–death of selfishness and been fulfilled in understanding (9th house), mastery is visited upon us in order that the work of our destiny can be made manifest for all to see. He describes a 'birth of light', whereby the transfigured personality becomes an agent of the larger whole which is his birthright; he is an *avatar*.[5]

Many of us will no doubt find Rudhyar's description a little difficult to relate to, preoccupied as we are with our 10th-house issues as representing our parental complexes and struggle to find our place in the world. Nevertheless, the truth of Rudhyar's vision is demonstrated by the lives of those who, like Bernadette of Lourdes, were fated to fulfil their soul's purpose in a direct and uncompromising way for the benefit of the spiritual heritage of mankind.

Continuing to examine the transits for the day of the vision, we see that Chiron is conjunct both Venus and Mercury in Aquarius; it is also within 45′ of the midpoint of Bernadette's Mercury/Venus. Venus is the transpersonal or esoteric ruler of her Gemini Ascendant; thus, planets representing both levels of the Ascendant are being transited by Chiron, which suggests a *kairos*, as described above, a bridge between eternity and the human world. Here, the event heralded the sacrifice of exclusive human and sexual love relationships that might have led to child-bearing and a normal life as a woman. Transiting Venus is 1°35′ from an exact conjunction to Neptune in Aquarius in the 10th house, echoing the same theme: the sacrifice of personal love in order to be a vessel of spiritual renewal for the collective. On the day of the vision, this natal 9th-house Venus sat at the apex of a T-square, formed by an opposition of transiting Mars in Scorpio to transiting Jupiter conjunct Pluto in Taurus. From a psychological perspective, in a chart such as this with so many elevated planets in Aquarius and Pisces, one can well imagine that an irruption of these Taurus/Scorpio energies, often primitive and explosively sexual, when focused on Venus in Aquarius could only be transmuted into a visionary experience, a divine union.

Transiting Mars is also 3°9′ from an exact square with her natal Neptune, and transiting Neptune is 1°28′ past the exact conjunction with natal Mars, thus repeating a combination of planets that often suggests loss of physical vitality, the weakening or refining of instinctual drives in favour of spiritual aspirations. Bernadette indeed became ill after these visions, with symptoms of a typical Mars/Neptune kind, including fever (Mars), temporary paralysis (Mars/Neptune) and weakness (Neptune). Mars/Neptune also describes the storm of controversy and confusion which flared up: Bernadette was interrogated by the Church authorities; rumours of miraculous healings (to which she made no personal claim) were disproved; and the newspapers said she was simply mentally ill. The Sun was conjunct her natal Neptune within 2°25′ on the day of the vision; the symbolic centre of that moment keyed in to her personal life via Neptune, for which the Sabian Symbol is: 'A large white dove bearing a message.'[6] In Christianity, the image of a white dove often symbolizes the presence of the Holy Spirit in portrayals of the Annunciation. In addition, doves were sacred to the goddess Aphrodite, and Neptune is considered as a 'higher octave' of Venus (Aphrodite), being concerned with transpersonal love in contrast to the more personal love that Venus represents.

We find transiting Mercury 7' away from exact conjunction to her natal Saturn in Capricorn, in the 9th house. The 9th-house Saturn in Bernadette's chart symbolizes her capacity to bring a powerful vision (9th house) into manifestation (Saturn). This Saturn also suggests the stern Judaeo-Christian god that sees Woman as the bearer of the evils of the flesh. If Mercury as messenger of the gods was acting on behalf of the god Saturn, the message must have been something like: 'It's the Virgin Mary or nothing' – no to the body and yes to the spirit. At any rate, through total submission to her experience (a gift of Chiron in Virgo), she subsequently enriched the lives of millions of people.

These visions of the Virgin Mary lasted for about three weeks, during which time more and more people gathered to watch Bernadette in her enraptured state, and to partake of the healing waters. During this time, several of the transits mentioned above became exact. Transiting Mars squared Neptune exactly, and Chiron crossed over the MC, here symbolizing the fulfilment of a healing destiny; additionally, Mercury moved to conjunct its own place, then Venus, the MC and finally Neptune, acting as 'messenger' to all these planets. The Sun conjuncted Jupiter, and also opposed her natal Chiron, restating the visionary quality of those two planets in combination. On 25 March 1858, when Mars in Sagittarius in the 6th house exactly squared natal Chiron, the figure in Bernadette's vision proclaimed herself to be the Immaculate Conception. Conception is a rather Martian event; here, Chiron/Mars symbolizes a conception on another level, an impregnation by the Spirit, the white dove of the Annunciation, the Sabian Symbol for Bernadette's Neptune. She was also entrusted with secrets which she refused to divulge, even to the Pope. This expresses her Chiron/Sun aspect, where she obeyed her inner authority even at the risk of defying the established authority of the Church. The visions were endorsed as genuine in 1872, when transiting Chiron opposed Bernadette's natal Chiron.

The transits for 16 April 1879, the day of Bernadette's death, are equally interesting, in the light of the above image. On this day, we find transiting Chiron conjunct transiting Neptune, both in Taurus and conjunct her 12th-house cusp. This Chiron/Neptune squares both her natal 9th-house Venus and Mercury in Aquarius, also prominent in the transits for the day of the vision. It is also in the same degree as Jupiter was on the day of the vision. Neptune looms large again; its characteristic themes of personal self-sacrifice, redeeming compassion and attunement to the spiritual longings of the collective are irrevocably woven into her destiny. The midpoint of her natal Chiron/Neptune is 25°23′ Scorpio; on the day of the vision, transiting Uranus in Taurus was opposite this midpoint within 4′; on the day of her death transiting Pluto was conjunct transiting Venus, exactly 1° opposite this same point, also aspecting her Saturn/Uranus midpoint (27°46′ Aquarius), a Chiron-sensitive point as described in Chapter 5. This sequence suggests first the apotheosis (Uranus) of the Neptunian figure of the Virgin Mary, and then Bernadette's death upon completion (Pluto) of her appointed destiny. On the day of her death, transiting Sun and Mercury are conjunct, squaring natal Saturn. Considering Mercury as the messenger of Saturn, as suggested above, maybe this time the message was something like: 'Message delivered. You can come Home now.'

Transiting Uranus is found within 43′ of exact conjunction to her natal Chiron, and just after midday the Moon opposed this point. The link between body and spirit, which we might suppose was already somewhat tenuous, was finally severed. Transiting Mars was conjunct natal Neptune, here signalling the final dissolution (Neptune) of physical vitality (Mars); this Mars/Neptune combination also featured in the vision chart. Bernadette's third Jupiter return had just occurred: with transiting Jupiter opposite natal Chiron, her visionary capacities perhaps expanded beyond the capacity of her physical vehicle to contain them.

Bernadette experienced her first Chiron/Chiron square at the age of only five; in the intervening years, before her vision of the Virgin Mary, Chiron had opposed her natal Mars, Uranus and

Pluto, and later squared them. When Chiron opposes a planet by transit, wounding events often occur; the agent of wounding is 'out there', and one identifies with either the victim or the healer aspect of the figure of Chiron. Wounding experiences of the nature of Mars, Uranus and Pluto at such a young age could certainly prime a little girl to become identified with the figure of the victim or the healer. In addition, during the year when transiting Chiron was square her natal Uranus in Pisces, her father lost the sight of his left eye in an accident; when transiting Chiron was conjunct her Sun, he lost his job and the family became increasingly poor; eventually they could not pay their rent and lived in a disused shed which had been abandoned as unhealthy and unfit for habitation. This is certainly a poignant symbol of Chiron in Virgo in the 4th house, a placement which focuses on the father. These conjunctions of transiting Chiron to Bernadette's Sun and Saturn in Capricorn manifested themselves outwardly as the misfortunes experienced by her father, which led to suffering and hardship for the family. In psychological terms, however, these transits suggest that the development of her ego and inner sense of security and structure might also have been wounded, leaving her more open than usual to the transpersonal. Bernadette was apparently a sickly child and backward in her physical development (Chiron in Virgo). In the light of these early Chiron transits, the sacrifice of her personal life and her subsequent early death perhaps seem destined.

At first, sceptics were quick to point out that these visions occurred only four years after Pope Pius IX officially proclaimed the doctrine of the Immaculate Conception, suggesting that the entire affair had been fabricated by the Catholic Church to give substance to this. However, in 1909, when transiting Chiron was in Aquarius and posthumously conjunct Bernadette's natal Jupiter and Neptune, her body was exhumed and found to be incorrupt. An eyewitness reported that neither decay nor bad odour could be detected.[7] Incorruptibility is regarded, theoretically, at least, as a prerequisite for canonization, and exhumation was carried out a further four times. Each time her body was seen to be incorrupt, and she was beatified in 1925. Her body is now on display in a glass coffin in Nevers, visited by thousands of pilgrims every year; 'incorruptible flesh' is certainly a dramatic image of transiting Uranus being exactly conjunct her natal Chiron in Virgo on the day of her death. Despite the commercialization (another Virgoan theme) that has grown to Disneyland proportions, the spirit of this remarkable series of events lives on at Lourdes to this day, with an impressive record of medically documented miracle healings having taken place.[8]

•

IO · Chiron in Context: A Life Story

In looking at the life of a woman whom I shall call 'Sara', and in examining the astrological reflection of it, I will focus on the Chiron configuration, following the themes that are expressed by it, and showing how they have actually unfolded in her inner and outer life. The Chiron configuration in Sara's horoscope is as follows: Chiron is in the 6th house in Scorpio; it opposes Moon in Taurus in the 12th house, is semisquare Mercury in Virgo in the 5th house and square Pluto and Saturn in Leo in the 4th (Saturn is included because it is conjunct Pluto). Furthermore, the Moon is exactly opposite the midpoint of Chiron/Jupiter, both in the same sign and house, so Jupiterian themes are drawn in, as we shall see. In addition to the houses in which these planets fall, the 8th, 9th and 10th houses are implicated in the Chiron configuration, as their respective 'natural' rulers are all aspected by Chiron.

Sara was born into a family of active Christian missionaries. When she was four months old, with transiting Chiron exactly conjunct her natal Jupiter, the family moved from England to a mission in West Africa. The wild beauty, natural environment and rich emotional ambiance of Africa was to play a major role in Sara's inner life; it now symbolizes her true roots, the goal of her inner quest. Chiron squaring both Pluto and Saturn in the 4th house describes very well the feeling of rootlessness that Sara has. Part of her wound, and also her uniqueness, is having been exposed to two irreconcilably different cultures and national archetypes, and feeling unable truly to belong in either. England is a notoriously Saturnian country, and Africa can be very Plutonian, abounding in raw nature and animal life, with tribal societies which at that time were still living in communion with it and closer to both life and death than most European societies.

Since the T-square involving Chiron in Scorpio is opposite the

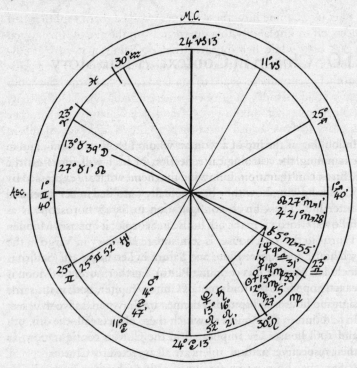

'Sara'

12th-house Moon, and both square 4th-house Pluto, we would expect ancestral and collective as well as personal levels of the feminine to be involved. The ancestral level of Sara's Chiron configuration is reflected in the fact that two generations of her mother's ancestors had also been pioneer missionaries; uncles on both sides of the family had also been involved in this typically Chironian activity, and Jupiter traditionally signifies the uncle. Jupiterian/9th-house issues of foreign travel, religious philosophy and expansion of ideas through teaching and evangelizing are brought into focus as ingredients of the Chiron configuration, as well as profession (10th house) and ancestral themes on her mother's side of the family (Chiron squaring Pluto in the 4th house).

Let us examine how these themes evolved. Sara's mother had been left in England with a guardian from the age of three to ten years old, while her mother (that is, Sara's maternal grand-mother) remained in Africa doing missionary work. The grand-mother eventually returned to England to see Sara's mother, who has a vivid memory of not being recognized by her. Her parents walked past her unknowingly, and subsequently her mother appears to have had a nervous breakdown and was therefore unable to function and take care of the family. Sara's mother took a major role in looking after her brothers and sisters; this is a reflection of the care-taking role which we will see in Sara's own life story. The culture shock of Europe after years of isolation in the African bush, and possibly also the guilt at having betrayed her daughter, all took their toll. This pattern of separation was to be repeated in detail in Sara's life, as we shall see.

With this configuration, we would expect Sara's relationship with her mother likewise to be experienced as one of mutual wounding, fraught with the Plutonian theme of life-and-death struggle. This was indeed the case: Sara nearly did not survive her birth (Chiron/Pluto = trauma concerned with facing death). Her mother developed eclampsia, and during labour began having fits so severe that she was given morphine, and was unconscious during the rest of the birth (Chiron opposite Moon in the 12th house). This drug suppresses the baby's respiration, and is there-fore potentially lethal. The medical decision made upon her entry into the world was that if the worst came to the worst, her life was to be sacrificed so that her mother could live. Although this was normal medical policy, the feeling of always having to fight to survive has accompanied Sara throughout her life, and it is a measure of the depth of conflict which she felt in her relationship with her mother: a life-and-death struggle, amply described by Chiron/Pluto/Moon. (Note that Sara later became a nurse, con-gruent with Chiron in the 6th house.) She was eventually pulled out with forceps, and did not breathe for half an hour. After the birth, her mother was so ill that she could not be with her for a week. Chiron/Moon here is the wounded and absent mother, the wound of premature separation and lack of primary bonding.

The birth also wounded her mother, who was told that, if she wanted another child, she would have to spend the entire pregnancy in England. Perhaps feeling her mission work to be more important, she decided against having another child. This was a further source of anger and guilt for Sara. She felt angry and cheated because she longed for a playmate. Note that the Moon rules Cancer; in her horoscope it is on the cusp of the 3rd house, which is concerned with siblings: here the pain concerns a sibling that never was. She may well have also felt guilty and somehow responsible for wounding her mother, another expression of Chiron opposite the Moon. The patterns around this severe birth trauma have recapitulated several times in Sara's life, as we shall see; the physical and emotional pain connected with it have lain in the background and come powerfully forward from time to time, surfacing whenever separation of any kind threatens and, astrologically, whenever the T-square involving Chiron, Moon, Saturn and Pluto is set off. We all 'lose' mother at birth, but in Sara's case, her first loss was nearly her own life, and this is a measure of the desperation invoked by any impending separation.

Sara's major relationships have tended to follow the pattern of her birth; with Chiron as probable ruler of her Sagittarian Descendant, relationships open up the wounds suggested by the Chiron configuration. Sara has tended to concern herself with other people's feelings and needs rather than her own, and has had to learn to be aware of and assert her own feelings (Chiron opposite Moon in the 12th). This contributes to a relationship beginning to feel stale and toxic (analogous to the morphine used during her birth); she feels suffocated and unable to be herself (Chiron/Saturn). She becomes attracted to someone else, feels reconnected to her sexuality (Chiron/Pluto) and to her vital self, and then a life-and-death struggle follows (Chiron/Pluto, the second stage of labour), to get out of the situation in order to be with the other man (out into life, to be born). Once 'out', however, much pain follows, intensified by the original separation from her mother. She describes herself as 'splitting' from the situation: the image is reminiscent of the forceps which pulled her out of the womb and saved her life.

When Chiron squared its own natal place Sara was seven, and had an experience that was to affect her deeply. She remembers being led into a missionary's bedroom by a young black man. She lay on the bed, and, although he did not penetrate her, he masturbated on her. She remembers vividly the details of the experience; she also remembers agreeing to meet him again, although eventually she told him never to come near her again. Afterwards she suffered a long period of agonizing guilt. She had a recurring image of standing before God in the halls of judgement at the end of time; her name was being called out; her sin was to be exposed to the whole world, and she would be publicly shamed and accused. Remember she was only seven years old, and privately enduring this torment of imminent exposure and punishment. She prayed earnestly to God for forgiveness.

Transiting Chiron was trine her natal Neptune; throughout this period her feeling life was coloured by these characteristically Neptunian experiences of feeling sinful and guilty, of longing for redemption and atonement and asking for forgiveness.

Eventually, she felt indeed forgiven, as though God had lifted her burden of guilt from her. Although on one level she felt relieved, it seems the issue may have sunk from consciousness, merged with other contents, to surface later on. She had 'confessed' to her mother over and over in fantasy, but it was not until the age of fifteen that she realized that she had not in real life told her, and did so. Transiting Chiron had moved into quincunx with Neptune, and transiting Neptune was exactly conjunct her natal Chiron. By this time, in her mind, the unforgivable crime was that she had enjoyed it and gone back for more. The experience was not one of physical rape, although that was the word she used when talking about it, for lack of any other.

At the age of ten, shortly after her inner experience of forgiveness, she was sent to a school in Wales; thus her own mother's life-pattern was repeated. Chiron was exactly opposite her Pluto and squaring her Moon at the time, shortly to square natal Jupiter; the family had moved to Africa when Chiron was exactly conjunct this Jupiter. She hated Britain, and resented being sent away; she remembers feeling cast out and pining for her beloved Africa. It seems possible that she had unconsciously felt she was being punished for enjoying the encounter with the young man, and feared that she had been banished because of her sin and transgression. Archetypally, this pattern is described by her Chiron position: although through this encounter, and the later embellishments of memory and fantasy, she had experienced and expressed her natural sexual curiosity – the physical and instinctual side of her budding womanhood (Chiron in Scorpio squaring Pluto) – everything in her upbringing could only give her permission, as a woman, to be pure, chaste, asexual and dedicated to Christian ideals of service to humanity (Chiron in the 6th house), as expressed within her family. Later on, she was often to subordinate the wild, sexual and passionate side of her in order to serve others (Chiron in the 6th house in Scorpio), and had to bring considerable consciousness to the issue in order not to become merely servile and self-sacrificing with it.

When she arrived in Britain Sara was put in the care of a guardian aunt, who died of cancer the following year, although Sara was not told about the illness until her death. During the preceding period Sara became increasingly 'difficult'; Chiron was transiting her 10th house in Aquarius, and made an exact T-square with her natal 12th-house Moon and 4th-house Pluto, and later, at the time of her aunt's death, opposed Saturn; transiting Saturn was also making its final conjunction with her natal Chiron, amply describing a situation of further loss, separation and also the concretization of the original Chiron-in-Scorpio wound of trauma concerned with death. Thus the emotional ingredients surrounding her birth reconstellated, but this time, the 'life-and-death struggle' culminated in her aunt's death. Transiting Chiron also made a yod formation, quincunx both her natal Mars and the Sun/Venus conjunction in Virgo, and this suggests her emotional reactivity and the fact that she was there against her will. With Chiron in Scorpio, she may well have been acting as a medium for the negative emotion in the environment, sensing the dying woman's feelings, expressing them, and also reacting angrily to them (transiting Chiron = Mars/Venus), responding truthfully but unconsciously to the emotional ambiance of disintegration and death, which was also of course a reminder of her own birth. Equally, the emotional voltage of what she was feeling may have been increased by the ancestral element of repetition of her own mother's life, carrying forward an inheritance of

Plutonic emotion. After her aunt died, Sara felt on some deep level that it was her fault, that her being 'difficult' had killed her aunt. This further ingredient of her aunt's death deepened Sara's guilt, echoing the original guilt at having 'wounded her mother' during birth.

Later in her life, when Sara met her future husband, Chiron was exactly squaring her natal Uranus by transit. She became pregnant before they were married, and, incredibly, before he had penetrated her; she decided to have a termination, which took place during a week when both Chiron and Uranus changed signs, into Aries and Libra respectively, thus opposing each other. The midpoint picture was as follows: Chiron and Uranus = Moon/Saturn, Moon/Pluto, Saturn/Pluto, setting off all three planets involved in the Chiron configuration, and also graphically describing abortion. Not only does this 'immaculate conception' theme, which is medically possible, but extremely rare, express the placement of Chiron in the 6th house (and her three planets in Virgo), but it underscores the polarity of Virgin and Whore which Sara finds within herself as a woman. Chiron was retrograde, and conjuncted exactly the midpoint of Mercury in Virgo and Neptune in Libra during the fortnight after the abortion, when her father discovered, and was shocked by, the news; this describes the way in which the pregnancy wounded forever his image of her as being pure, innocent and sensible. The experience also echoes in an uncanny way her much earlier encounter with the black man, where penetration was not involved; I would speculate that the 'unwanted child' may have unconsciously been seen by Sara as the product of fantasized union with him, the expression of her 'Whore' side, therefore guilt-producing and not allowed. Significantly, however, her mother supported her a great deal during this time, and much healing occurred in their relationship; Sara was also able to express some of her anger for the first time. This is typical of themes threaded together by Chiron: although their ingredients may be reflected elsewhere in the chart, we find the Chiron configuration pin-pointing the main archetypal themes in a person's life, indicating times when there is a true bridging of levels, and areas where the world of duality melts and archetypal patterns take form in events and experiences, often in repeating cycles which can progress towards healing and integration if we pay attention to them.

Chiron was opposite Neptune by transit when at the age of twenty-three Sara finally married. Significantly, she and her husband went to Africa, the scene of the crime, as it were; Chiron was exactly opposite Neptune at the time. In her marriage, which was a happy one for about seven years, she felt the comfort of finally doing something which brought her securely within the fold of family approval. It is interesting how often Chiron/Neptune contacts feature in this major thread of Sara's life. I would see this as connecting with her Chiron being opposite Moon in the 12th house, ruled by Neptune and Pisces. Also, as described in Chapter 9, the Chiron position in a chart often tends to include echoes of the opposite sign and/or house.

If in a horoscope deep ancestral themes are suggested by the Chiron placement, as is the case here with Sara's Chiron in Scorpio and aspecting planets in the 4th and 12th houses, it can be useful to look at the Chiron position of the parents and grandparents; here we may find suggested the kind of wounds which the parents had, and which may be carried forward into the next generation, unless some healing occurs. With Sara and her African background, in terms of collective unconscious influences while she was a child, it is the Plutonian, sexual and instinctual energies which periodically erupt, and which were, no doubt, partly responsible for the breakdown suffered by her grandmother on her return to Europe. Sara, however, has been able to include this aspect of herself and express it in a way that her ancestors were not able to. If we also consider Chiron as suggesting the nature of one's innate and individual connection with the realm of the transpersonal, it clarifies this: Sara's natural means of interface with the divine is through her body and her sexuality. Her powerful emotionality, which she earlier sought to subjugate and felt guilty about, she now increasingly sees as a form of worship of a god other than the rarefied gentle Jesus who featured in her earlier life; the feeling of being out of control, often greatly feared by those with Chiron in the 6th house or in Virgo, has become more of a friend and less of an enemy.

After she had been married for seven years and had had two

children, Chiron opposed its natal place, therefore again beginning to set off the fixed natal T-square. On the last exact opposition Sara went to a party, met a man and later began a disastrous affair with him. Although having very much enjoyed being a wife and mother, she describes herself at this time as having become 'hooked on service' (Chiron in the 6th house) – she was also working as a nurse. She rediscovered her sexuality and her wildness with a vengeance. The marriage began to disintegrate under the strain and, although Sara was eventually discarded by this man, she and her husband decided to separate.

It was at this point that Sara commenced psychotherapy, when Chiron was exactly trine her natal Mercury, ruler of both her Sun and Ascendant, and therefore an important planet in the chart. She started keeping a psychological journal, which has been important to her ever since. With Chiron in the 6th house, and also semisquare her natal Mercury, this is an example of how the Chiron position tends to symbolize things which bring healing for those concerned. Writing is a Mercurial activity; in a psychological journal we can express our deepest private feelings (Scorpio), record our inner journey and reflect upon our life (a 6th-house activity). With Chiron in Scorpio, opposite Moon and square Pluto, a major theme in her therapy was her early relationship with her mother; she felt and expressed a great deal of raw emotion that had been stored for a long time, and had new insights about her life. Another major theme, congruent with Chiron transiting in square to her natal 4th-house Saturn, was her learning to recognize and let go of the paralysing inner voices of self-judgement, self-criticism and punishment, thus slowly building up a solid sense of self-esteem. Also, Chiron in the 6th house or Virgo often accompanies a punishing demand that people be perfect according to standards which actually violate them and do not serve their sense of wholeness.

During the ensuing months, Chiron was to conjunct her North Node in Taurus in the 12th house, square Saturn, and prepare to cross the Ascendant. After the difficult period of separation from her husband, moving into a new house and finding herself responsible for her two children, Sara emerged from the crisis

with a somewhat tentative but growing measure of independence; Chiron squaring Saturn by transit brought challenges in
the typically Saturnian areas of parental, emotional and financial
responsibility, enforced self-reliance and independence. With
Chiron transiting the North Node in Taurus, she was obliged to
deal with a great many practical and financial issues, in the midst
of her deep emotional turmoil (12th house).

At this time, feeling material was released that not only concerned her current situation, but also echoed back to her early life
and her relationship with both parents; working with the patterns
established through her birth trauma became increasingly important. This is certainly congruent with transiting Chiron conjunct her 12th-house Moon, therefore also squaring natal Pluto in
the 4th house. When Chiron transits through the 12th house
people often seek therapy, as the barriers that may be keeping a
potential flood of unconscious material at bay are especially thin at
that time; wounds may become painfully obvious when Chiron
crosses the Ascendant, and thus much healing can also occur.

Shortly before Chiron transited her Ascendant, Sara decided to
train to become a health visitor; she felt able to take on the
challenge of her new life alone and the new self she was getting to
know. The end of this phase of therapy was marked by a great
deal of material concerning her birth (typical of Chiron conjunct
the Ascendant by transit), including a dream of her giving birth to
a half-caste child which everyone said would not survive,
although she knew it would. This dream can be seen to weave
together many threads of her life. It echoes her own physical
birth, when she encountered the Underworld, being born half
dead and half alive; it echoes her African past, as well as her
encounter with the young black man; it also symbolizes a union
between the two halves of herself, the birth of a new sense of
herself, and her conviction that it would live, no matter what
others said.

When Chiron crossed her Ascendant for the second time, she
began her training as a health visitor – a profession symbolized by
her Chiron, a practical form of service (6th house) to the community at large (Moon), often caring for people who are bed-
ridden or isolated at home (12th house). When Chiron made its

last exact transit across her Ascendant – shortly before her birth-day – her father died. In terms of the birth/rebirth sequence evoked by this transit, this is again congruent with the pattern, and the concretization indicates the depth at which the process was in fact taking place. I have frequently observed that, if there is some physical trauma concerned with breathing at birth (stran-gulation, delayed breathing, premature cutting of the cord, and so on), it seems to parallel, on a deep archetypal level, later issues concerned with the father. Jung points out the archetypal and etymological connections (through the Greek word *pneuma*) be-tween spirit, the breath ('air in motion') and the father or wise-old-man figures. At birth Sara had no breath: it was sacrificed in order to save her mother's life. Towards the end of her psycholo-gical rebirth, when she was 'born' out of therapy, her father died. Thus after his death, the wound of her deep grief over her early separation from her mother was also reopened. Once more she met death as she entered life, and was very much alone with her suffering.

Three days after her father's death, she met a man whom I shall call Joel; Joel has several planets in Gemini, including Sun, Mercury, Venus, Saturn, and Uranus; Chiron was about to begin its transit through Gemini. In fact, Sara later discovered that Joel's father died the day after her birthday, in the same year as her father died; this is typical of the web of synchronicities that accompanies any major recapitulation of unconscious material – particularly if birth trauma is involved – and which is commonplace with transits of Chiron. Some time later, when they met again, they began a stormy relationship which lasted until transiting Chiron conjuncted Sara's Uranus. The same pattern occurred again: the situation had become increasingly suffocating for her and helped to precipitate an eventual separation.

Reflecting later on this relationship, Sara realized that part of what had attracted her to Joel was that he reminded her of her own father, whom she had just lost. Because she had not finished mourning for her father she was vulnerable to fulfilling others' images of how she was supposed to be for him. With his planets in Gemini being conjuncted by transiting Chiron, he may be seen as an agent of Chiron in both his wounding and healing capacity.

The healing emerged retrospectively; as Chiron conjuncted her Uranus, Sara realized the unconscious ingredients of her early relationship with her father that were recapitulating during the relationship with Joel, and understood some of the pain she felt within that relationship. Note that Chiron transiting in Gemini squared her Sun, Venus and Mercury in Virgo during the period of the relationship. The depth of Sara's grief about the death of her father was such that, given her primal wounds concerned with loss, she was not able to complete the mourning process at that time; life drew to her someone to fill that gap, but there was a price attached.

Joel has a Moon square Pluto, as does Sara; it was eventually this quality, manifesting itself as jealousy, possessiveness and manipulativeness, that made Sara feel strangled and unable to be herself. She began to see the light, playful and joyful side of her father reflected in one side of this man, while the dark side of him reminded her of her mother. She said: 'It's as if, in order to have my father, I have to do battle with the dark side of my mother.' Her words underline the Oedipal components of the situation, which in this case have deep roots in the birth trauma. During their relationship, Pluto was conjunct her natal Chiron for a period of about eighteen months; Sara decided to be sterilized, as she already had two children and he had four. Chiron in the 6th house or Virgo is sometimes associated with physical sterility, and Chiron in Scorpio is frequently self-destructive; being sterilized is a statement strongly symbolic of the desire to 'kill the mother', as detailed above. By the time the operation was possible, they were no longer living together, and Sara had changed her mind about sterilization; however, pre-malignant cells were discovered growing on her cervix. Although they were detected in time to prevent cancer, Sara was shocked into a definite decision to end the relationship as it was, realizing that these potentially cancerous cells had been growing within her along with her feeling of being wounded within the relationship. She almost literalized her desire to 'kill her mother in order to get to her father', a desire which included reaching the feelings of mourning over her father's death.

However, Joel and Sara had become involved in a mutual

struggle for power, and Sara realized that she had to give up her end of it in order to be released; she could exert considerable power over him because of his strong sexual feelings for her, and his dependence on her as 'the Provider' of many of his needs. This is certainly a very Plutonian theme, congruent with transiting Pluto conjunct her natal Chiron. Note that this was the only manifestation of this typically Plutonian emotional theme in terms of the transits current at the time. The relationship was sexually very fulfilling and powerful, but this made Sara vulnerable to her previous pattern of subordinating herself, becoming 'the Provider' at the service of Joel and ready to become whoever he wanted her to be; again, this is well expressed by her Chiron in the 6th house in Scorpio. Note also that she became 'supermother' in this situation, looking after four children – a typical Chiron/Moon/Pluto theme, further reflected in her profession of health visitor. Also typical of Chiron in Scorpio is the fact that this recapitulation could have actually cost her her own life. Chiron/Pluto contacts by transit, especially the conjunction, often bring experiences which force us to stare death in the face; and often it is our own death and the acceptance of our own mortality that is really the issue.

While I was writing this chapter, Chiron made a series of conjunctions with Sara's Uranus. During the week of the second exact conjunction, she read the first draft, and wrote me a letter.

It seems fitting to allow Sara herself to describe her response to reading her own story. Her first reaction was one of horror and panic. She felt exposed – 'that everyone would instantly recognize who I was and judge me for it'. She mentioned the recurrent dream or fantasy that she had had following the rape experience: 'I believed that when the end of time came, we would all be crowded into the great judgement hall in heaven where God would call my name out among the thousands of people there and expose my "sin" to all and sundry, and then I would be cast out.' Reading the draft had reactivated this fantasy and brought it to the surface. She was thus able to re-embrace this fearful child with all the feelings of vulnerability and guilt that had been cast out before. The experience also brought with it the relief of having survived her worst nightmare coming true. We see here an illustration of Chiron in Gemini at work, where the healing process was facilitated through words written, spoken and read, congruent also with her natal Chiron/Mercury semisquare.

Note that in terms of the birth/rebirth sequence, the re-emergence of the fantasy signals more than the surfacing of a memory of a feeling experience from childhood. Its archetypal magnitude and all-consuming nature are typical of the mental and emotional component of the experience of finally being born. The last step towards liberation from the womb is felt to be an impending disaster of cosmic magnitude, with fantasies of ultimate humiliation, moral defeat and 'damnation of transcendental proportions'.[1] That this experience occurred after Sara's sexual encounter with the black man suggests that birth trauma was reactivated at that time, given that the final stage of labour is often characterized by a strong sexual component. A few weeks later, on the third and last conjunction of transiting Chiron to her natal Uranus, she finally separated from Joel, the intense emotional entanglement having disintegrated, congruent with the recapitulation of birth described above.

As Pluto prepares to oppose her Moon and square its own place, another turn of the spiral represented by Sara's Chiron configuration is forthcoming. She now has considerable insight about the patterns at work within her life, and feels more self-acceptance; she realizes she is about to undergo a cycle of psychological rebirth, and has enough experience to be able to place its ingredients within the larger pattern of her life. She is a woman of great courage, perseverance and optimism, which has enabled her to proceed through these painful trials and rise like a Phoenix out of the ashes – a suitable image indeed for Chiron in Scorpio.

11 · Spirit of the Age

We both create and are created by the times we live in; we are all 'children of our times' in one way or another. As Chiron has but recently been discovered, its themes are now much in evidence, and describe a kind of *Zeitgeist* – Spirit of the Age – which characterizes the collective and psycho-historical context in which we live. By being aware of the archetypal patterns at work, we may perhaps experience more consciously this process of mutual creation. In the following sections some of the themes associated with Chiron are explored by looking at significant trends and events, and by examining the horoscopes of some outstanding individuals whose destiny expresses Chiron's mythic themes in a manner larger than their own personal lives.

Healing and Health

The last twenty years have seen a surge of interest in healing methods that address the whole person rather than merely suppressing symptoms. Many of these techniques originate in other cultures, or in ancient shamanic techniques: healing through flower essences, gem elixirs, art- and music-therapy are examples. The mechanistic view of the body which prevails amongst allopathic medical practitioners is now being juxtaposed with other maps of the body that include the currents of subtle energy linking the body with the rest of the cosmos, and thus are congruent with Chiron's theme of healing the split between body and spirit.

However, such a proliferation of new healing techniques brings with it the danger that we may be enticed into seeing normal human limits and frailties as wounds to be cured or problems to be solved. When the heroic mode enters the field of healing, this too may become a futile struggle which has to be relinquished. Equally, the wounding side of medical orthodoxy has become apparent – for example, in the horrific side-effects of supposed wonder-drugs such as Thalidomide and Opren. The miracles wrought by medical science once dazzled people, but now more and more people are questioning and wanting to take personal responsibility for their health. Like Chiron's pupil Asclepius, who was eventually struck down by Hades for daring to raise the dead, medical orthodoxy is up against its own limits in many areas.

During early 1988, much media attention in Britain was focused on the National Health Service, the ideals upon which it was founded, and the degree to which it seemed to have failed. The Chiron configuration in the chart for the founding of the NHS has Chiron retrograde at 18°34' Scorpio; it is square Saturn and Pluto in Leo in the 11th house, trine Sun in Cancer in the 10th house, widely semisquare Neptune in the 1st house in Libra, and conjunct the South Node in Scorpio. The NHS represented an idealistic plan (Chiron/Neptune/Saturn) that was supposed to transform the health (Chiron in Scorpio, square Pluto) of the whole country (Chiron trine Sun in Cancer, representing the nation). It was to provide good medical services for everyone regardless of economic status – a caring ideal also suggested by Chiron trining the Sun in Cancer in the 10th house: its public image was that of a good mother. The structure of society was to be transformed (Chiron square Saturn and Pluto in the 11th house) as the divisiveness of the class system was bridged; note there are four planets in Gemini in the 9th house, ruled by Chiron and here suggesting the hope of synthesis (9th house). The NHS was to be the envy of Europe, and a model of systematized compassion (Chiron/Sun in the 10th).

In mid January 1988 Chiron was conjunct the Moon, the Sun sign ruler of the NHS chart; thus began a series of conjunctions to the stellium of Geminian planets and the MC, lasting several months. This was intensified by the transiting Saturn/Uranus conjunction lying opposite, exactly on the IC, the foundation, and throwing the entire issue into high profile (MC). The

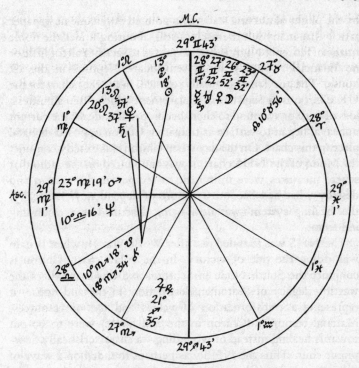

National Health Service (UK)

Saturn/Uranus midpoint, natally and by transit, is a Chiron-sensitive point, as previously mentioned: the established system (Saturn) was challenged (Uranus), and public awareness (Moon) focused on health issues in general (Chiron) as well as the NHS system itself. Several controversial events stand out from the background of turmoil that prevailed: threats to disband the NHS (Chiron/Uranus); drastic strike action by nursing staff prevented by last-minute wage deals (Chiron/Mercury); doctors taking voluntary pay cuts in order to subsidize hospital wards that would otherwise close.

Overall, a high degree of public dissatisfaction was voiced (Chiron in Gemini) and, congruent with transiting Chiron conjunct the Moon of the chart, much public sympathy was elicited by the plight of nursing staff, who pointed out in one newspaper article that many felt themselves still labouring under the noble image of Florence Nightingale, expected to sacrifice all for little or no financial reward (Chiron semisquare Neptune in the 1st house). The good mother finally rebelled. In the 1801 chart for the UK Chiron is in Sagittarius, a placement which often signifies a loss of faith or a wound to cherished hopes and ideals: the current upheaval began to surface as transiting Chiron opposed its natal place in this chart. On the day when Chiron was exactly conjunct the Moon of the NHS chart, it was announced on the radio that severe measures were imminent to reorganize the system and destroy what had become a culture of dependency. Ironically, the 'healing system' was now being described as a wounding influence!

The NHS was founded just after World War II, when Britain was riding the tide of victory. In the NHS chart, Chiron is conjunct the South Node in Scorpio, and this symbolizes the wartime legacy of Plutonian destruction; in the 2nd house, it represents a transformation of values and use of resources. Material resources (Chiron in the 2nd house) were to be put towards healing instead of wounding – a characteristically Scorpionic shift. Thus the NHS was perhaps founded on a wave of collective desire (Chiron/Neptune) to make reparation to the nation for the emotional, mental and physical devastation caused by a war in which the British played a heroic role and inevitably got wounded in the process. This has an echo in the story of Chiron, where the hero Hercules inadvertently causes Chiron's unhealable wound.

Mortality Returns

One feature of recent Western culture has been the suppression of the awareness of death: our 'cult' concerning death has rather been one of denial and minimization, of trying to conquer it in typical heroic mode, aided and abetted by medical science and technology. In rural and so-called primitive cultures children grow up knowing death as part of life; by contrast, many of us will never see a dead human or animal body except on television. In addition, the lack of appropriate mourning rituals in our culture means that the suppressed grief of many people will turn into serious illness, for, if they cannot separate from the dead, they may unconsciously try and follow them. Recently, the work of Elisabeth Kubler Ross and others has increased public awareness of the needs of the dying and the bereaved.[1] The phenomenon of AIDS also means that the experience of death and dying is confronting an increasingly larger number of people. Given that the acceptance of mortality eventually brought an end to Chiron's suffering, it is not surprising that this theme is now much in evidence.

The last two decades have seen increasing public protest against war, nuclear and other. War is often portrayed by governments in an archetypally heroic mode: 'Your country needs you', says the familiar US enrolment poster. As death is removed from reality to a shadow-play of images, human vulnerability goes unnoticed in the fanfare of glory; belief in principles or noble purposes shields us from the full horror of the shattering individual experiences caused by participation in a violent collective insanity. In the years prior to World War II, Jung noticed many of his analysands' dreams were hinting at the devastation about to erupt in Europe. Our individual lives are rooted in the collective, its emotions, beliefs, hopes and fears, and also in its tendency to enact powerful archetypal patterns through historical movements such as wars and revolutions, fashions, fads, cultural and religious trends. In the following story, collective issues are like the loom on which the fabric of individual lives are woven, as wounds are passed from one generation to the next and an accumulation of anguish looks for an outlet.

A year after Chiron's discovery, the world was shocked by a mass suicide in Guyana. Over 900 followers of the Reverend Jim Jones took cyanide, playing for real an act rehearsed several times before as a macabre test of his followers' loyalty. A look at Jones's natal chart and the transits for the evening of this tragic event is revealing, especially in the light of his Chiron. In his natal chart, the Chiron configuration is as follows: Chiron is in Taurus in the

4th house, conjunct Sun in Taurus in the 5th house. It is sextile Jupiter conjunct Pluto in Cancer in the 7th house, square Mars in Leo in the 8th house, biseptile Neptune in Virgo in the 8th house, sesquiquadrate his Capricorn Ascendant, and trine Saturn in Capricorn in the 1st house. With Chiron aspecting the Sun, two 8th-house planets and also both ends of this Saturn/Pluto opposition, we would expect Jones's nature as a 'messiah' to have dark and destructive tones. Also, Mars rules the stellium of planets in Aries in the 3rd house, and this testifies to his powers of persuasion; Mars in the 8th as part of his Chiron configuration adds the likelihood of Jones becoming 'possessed' or taken over by the destructive and irrational qualities of Mars.

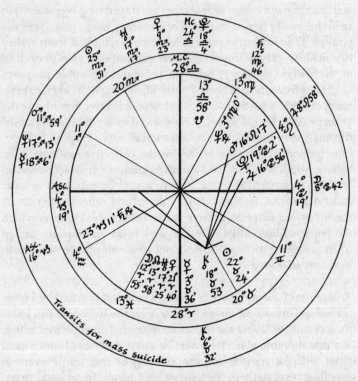

Rev. Jim Jones

Jones's natal Neptune is biseptile Chiron; Meyer describes this aspect as the 'exteriorization of destiny';[2] Jones was indeed at the centre of a Neptunian system of collective delusion, which he manipulated by tactics amply described by the rest of his Chiron configuration. Sexual and economic blackmail were common (Chiron in Taurus sextile Pluto), as were public humiliations and beatings (Chiron/Mars/Pluto); individual personalities were worn down by a punishing regime of work, inadequate diet and frequent mass rituals involving haranguing and violence (here Chiron/Saturn = wounding through discipline and deprivation). Jones's paranoia increased to the point where armed guards patrolled the perimeter of his Guyana settlement, creating a situation of imprisonment. His destiny was indeed to exteriorize the phenomenon of mass self-sacrifice: he informed his followers that the only course of action open to them was mass suicide.[3] Transiting Neptune was in Sagittarius at the time of the mass suicide, here symbolizing the sacrifice (Neptune) of human life for the sake of religious beliefs (Sagittarius).

Continuing the Chiron/Neptune theme, we find that Jones's father was an invalid, having been gassed during World War I, when Chiron was in Pisces. Traditionally, Neptune rules gaseous substances, and thus represents the immediate cause of his father's wound; it was with liquid cyanide (a Mercury/Neptune substance) that Jones lured over 900 people to their apparently willing deaths, like a Neptunian Pied Piper. Here is the Chiron/Saturn theme of an inheritance from the father which presses strongly for resolution or compensation. Chiron in the 4th house implicates father, family, and nation or fatherland: roots.

One cannot but wonder at the unconscious inheritance Jones may have received from his father who was wounded by the collective madness of war. He lacked a strong father to emulate, compete with and be guided by. This is his wound, and one frequently found when Chiron aspects both Sun and Saturn; here the father is literally wounded. Having neither a secure sense of personal individuality (Sun) nor an appropriate sense of limits (Saturn) left Jones's psyche wide open to 'possession' by these two planetary energies, as well as by the other energies of his Chiron configuration. Jones was 'superfather' to his congregation; he had a son of his own and also adopted several children. However, his role escalated out of control as there were no containing limits: tragedy became inevitable as Jones's personality disintegrated and his positive inflation (Chiron/Sun) turned to negative (Chiron/Saturn).

Jones joined a fundamentalist sect in 1950 and, when transiting Chiron was conjunct his Ascendant in Capricorn, he began preaching. He founded his own church in 1953, with Chiron approaching conjunction to his natal Saturn in Capricorn. In 1965, when Chiron was in Pisces, he had a vision of a nuclear holocaust which would supposedly occur on 15 July 1967. His father was incapacitated by gas when Chiron made its previous transit through Pisces, and this vision is perhaps an eruption from the ancestral unconscious, which started the inexorable process of the externalization of Jones's fate. I would speculate that this vision actually comprised undigested elements of his own father's war experience, handed down to him intact and waiting to emerge into consciousness: this phenomenon is a familiar one in depth psychotherapy. The holocaust in question was not to occur in 1967, but had in fact already occurred, wounding his father, and eventually Jones himself in the process. On 15 July 1967 Chiron was in the last degree of Pisces: in this context it symbolizes a holocaust, a final disintegration of life. Tragically, it was probably the demise of his own sanity and ego-boundaries that Jones was foreseeing. On this day, transiting Saturn was exactly conjunct Jones's Moon in Aries, perhaps occluding any sense of personal feeling or containment and contributing to a sense of impotence and frustration (lack of Mars energy) which would later erupt destructively. Transiting Neptune also opposed his natal Chiron/Sun conjunction, 1°2' from their midpoint, echoing yet again the Neptunian theme which gathered increasing momentum and culminated in catastrophe.

When Chiron transited through Jones's Aries stellium, conjuncting each planet in turn, he soared into public view, championing causes in a typically Arian way. With gospel music, social welfare programmes and support for radical political groups, he attracted a sizeable following in San Francisco. During this period, transiting Uranus in the 9th house opposed transiting

Chiron and the natal Aries stellium, emphasizing the sense of mission, purpose and religious destiny (9th house) with which Jones was imbued. His church bought property, amassed considerable wealth (Chiron in Taurus) and acquired land near Georgetown, Guyana. Jones was obsessed with gaining his rightful place in history – a common Chiron/Saturn preoccupation; when we consider that his father had been made an invalid by the machinations of history, it is not surprising. As Chiron opposed Jones's MC in 1975–7, he received public acclaim and numerous honours including, ironically, the Martin Luther King Jr Humanitarian Award.

However, the tide was turning. Reports of brutality and blackmail in unsparing detail began to be filed by former supporters who had managed to extricate themselves; warnings of the possibility of mass suicide were given to the US Government in a written affidavit. All this stood in stark contrast to the sentiments that Jones espoused: 'When you are without ideals, you live alone and die rejected . . . We came here to avoid contributing to the destruction which the country of our birth continues to inflict on less prosperous nations . . . We have found security and fulfilment in collectivism, and we can help build an agricultural nation.'[4] His noble vision – persuasively idealistic but rooted in delusion – soared above the reality of conditions that were reminiscent of a concentration camp: it was a vision of naturalness, simplicity and rural innocence within a caring community, described with macabre irony by his Chiron in Taurus in the 4th house; but Jones's rhetoric took no account of Chiron's aspects to Mars, Saturn and Pluto.

The Sabian Symbol for Jones's Chiron is interesting: 'A new continent rising out of the ocean.' In Rudhyar's interpretation we read:

When the mind has been emptied and light has been called upon to purify the consciousness freed from its attachment and contaminations, a new release of life can emerge out of the infinite Ocean of potentiality, the Virgin SPACE. What will it be used for? . . . The 'technique' is simply to allow the infinite Potential to operate in unconstrained SPONTANEITY. This means to have reached a state in which the conscious, rational ego is no longer a controlling factor.[5]

Jones certainly believed that he and his followers were creating a new nation; his rational ego was certainly no longer in control, and his mind indeed seems to have been emptied – at least of concern for human life. So what was it used for, we might wonder?

The day before the mass suicide, transiting Neptune in Sagittarius was triggered by an exact conjunction from transiting Mercury, falling in Jones's 12th house. As this pair completes no less than three planetary patterns in Jones's natal chart, it is an important one. Neptune is traditionally associated with poisonous liquids, hysteria, deception, victimization and mass delusion; Mercury rules the lungs, bronchials and the nervous system, which are paralysed by cyanide, with death caused by suffocation. Therefore this conjunction accurately symbolizes the means by which the mass suicide was enacted. Mercury also signifies the prominent involvement of the press and media in the affair. Jones and his followers perpetrated an elaborate public-relations deception (Mercury/Neptune) from their Guyanese community base; journalists who pried too deeply found themselves attacked or threatened on their return to the United States; on the day of the suicide, one journalist on his way to Jonestown was killed by Jones's militia.

On the evening of the mass suicide,[6] this Mercury/Neptune conjunction completed a fiery grand trine in Jones's natal chart, with Uranus in Aries in the 3rd house, and Mars in Leo in the 8th. It also completed two yod or 'finger of God' patterns: the first is with natal Chiron sextile both Jupiter and Pluto in Cancer in the 7th, and the second involves transiting Pluto sextile this Mercury/Neptune conjunction, both of which are quincunx natal Chiron in the 4th house. Jones certainly played God, as messiah of the 'good news' of death. Transiting Chiron conjuncts natal Mercury, setting off yet another grand trine in earth signs: Ascendant in Capricorn, trine both Neptune in Virgo in the 8th and Mercury in Taurus in the 4th. Four major configurations thus completed certainly describe something coming to completion. Collective emotion is implicated by the 8th and 12th houses: Mars in the 8th, and also Pluto conjunct Jupiter in the 7th, as part of Jones's natal Chiron configuration, suggest the theme of retribution. It is clear that Jones's personal and ancestral history may have made him the unwitting channel through which collective retribution flowed. Retribution for what and against whom is less clear.

In many primitive societies, premature death or severe illness may cause tremendous fear, as death is not always considered natural but often due to the activity of witchcraft, evil spirits and the like. Suspicious deaths will be followed by a hunt for a scapegoat – one who can be determined to have caused it, directly or indirectly. Once that person is dealt with, often through extreme cruelty, the threat of more unnatural deaths is temporarily removed. Such punishment perhaps mitigates the extreme vulnerability we feel in the face of sudden death or disaster. It comforts us to take control and pursue a victim with righteous indignation.

Here the question is: what happens to the invisible but powerful feelings of desire for retribution within the collective following major disasters, wars and catastrophes where there has been massive loss of life? Who do we blame for the loss of loved ones, health, livelihood, youth or sanity? The Government? The 'enemy'? The monarchy? God? Fate? A journalist's report underlines the helplessness that we seek to avoid with orgies of blame:

Relatives of the dead who had flown desperately to Georgetown, Guyana, ask with helpless grief what point there is in being an American if we had no power to stop such a thing. The implication was that there was *something* the government should have done. These were after all more than 900 American citizens . . . Today it simply haunts us, as *Newsweek* columnist Meg Greenfield observed, with its reminder that 'the jungle is only a few yards away'.[7]

One 'finger of God' completed by transiting Mercury/Neptune points into the 12th house, and thus to the themes of ego-dissolution and sacrifice through collective emotion; the other points to natal Chiron in the 4th house, the place of the father, our ancestry and roots, and also our nation. The 12th house is the deep past, the timeless archetypal world, the raw material of accumulated human experience which underpins individual life. It is perhaps partly because his father could neither re-member his own past nor integrate his experiences and thus passed them on, that Jones's own personality and individual life was dismembered in a wave of desire for retribution that began out in the sea of the collective and finally broke on the shore of Jones's individual life.

Jones's Chiron/Saturn trine is interesting in the light of his relationship with the establishment, as it would typically represent something of his relationship with his father. It is difficult for a man whose father is an invalid to experience many of the feelings of admiration and competition which are normally present in development. He resists emulating an invalid – he cannot compete with him; he feels sorry, resentful, guilty, perhaps longing to do something for the sick father to make him better. At its zenith, Jones's career unfolded in full public view, approved by the establishment (establishment = Saturn = father). As he was an ordained priest who had received accolades and honours for his good works, Jones's débâcle in Guyana was all the more incomprehensible: he 'wounded' the establishment. Was he unconsciously seeking to punish the system that wounded his father, or perhaps to punish his father for his unfortunate inadequacies? During a storm òf public outrage the laws concerning religious freedom were questioned. His track record meant that Jones could not merely be dismissed like Manson as a crank. Something more sinister was at work: Jones's violence was that of the ogre father whose shadowy presence lurks within any Saturnian institution – the negative image of Saturn devouring his children for fear that one would eventually dethrone him. As Jones's desire to 'slay the Terrible Father' grew, it possessed him from within.

Chiron/Mars people are often fated to confront others with their own aggression, and Jones did this on a grand scale. With his Chiron/Jupiter, he wounded the idealism and optimism of many people in his nation: his Jupiter/Pluto conjuncts the Sun/Mercury in Cancer in the US chart. With his Chiron/Sun Jones crushed people's sense of individuality, and replaced it with devotion to him: he became the Sun around which others made their orbit, the shadow of which swallowed them up in death. A sign above Jones's makeshift throne bore silent witness to a sea of bloated bodies: 'Those who do not remember the past are condemned to repeat it' – a gruesome image of Chiron in the 4th house, suggestive of personal, ancestral and national themes. Perhaps this horrific spectacle was a counterpart to, and culmination of, the unbridled religious enthusiasm and Utopian communitarianism current in America at the time. Indeed, it revealed the dark side of the desire for freedom from religious persecution upon which America itself was founded in 1776 in the so-called Age of Enlightenment.[8] Note that Uranus opposed Jones's natal Chiron on the day of the mass suicide.

Racism, the Noble Savage and Black is Beautiful

'At some future time period, not very distant as measured by centuries, the civilized races of men will almost certainly exterminate, and replace, the savage races throughout the world.'[9] These words of Charles Darwin epitomize the attitude towards non-European cultures which has prevailed during the last few centuries. His Chiron is at 11°43' of Aquarius, unaspected except for a square to the Moon's Nodes; thus Darwin was serving as the mouthpiece for ideas within the collective which were ripe for expression – a typical Aquarian theme. He wrote The Origin of Species during his Chiron return. The Sabian Symbol for his Chiron position (12° Aquarius) is ironically appropriate: 'On a vast staircase stand people of different types, graduated upwards.' Rudhyar offers this interpretation.

'The ideal of equalitarianism has to be balanced by a realization that hierarchy of levels is a fact of nature . . . Every human being is *potentially* divine as an individual person, but the natural progression of states of consciousness is an unavoidable reality to accept at the socio-mental level.'[10]

This image, and Rudhyar's interpretation of it, both have their biological precedent in the philosophy of the Chain of Being, which was an attempt to classify the whole of Creation along hierarchical lines, a popular preoccupation amongst European intellectuals during the fifteenth and sixteenth centuries. This in turn was based upon classical beliefs, for example, in Aristotle's famous notion that the world was divided into Greeks and Barbarians. Throughout history, so-called developed cultures have been steeped in this attitude, where what is different, alien and incomprehensible is seen as inferior and even dangerous. It is then feared, judged, reviled, and, if possible, eliminated in the name of preserving one's own clan, tribe or nation and its structures.

When we examine the criteria upon which such hierarchical thinking is in fact based, however, its absurdities and dangers quickly become obvious. In Rudhyar's interpretation, the hierarchy is based on 'consciousness', although he does not specify exactly what that means. However, for anyone living within a Judaeo-Christian framework the obvious danger is that 'spiritual progress' means in practice a progressive divorce from the instincts towards a rarefied and Olympian definition of superiority. In further developments of the Chain of Being, facial and anatomical features, such as width of skull and skin colour, were used by scientists in the late 1700s to create a hierarchy of humanity. The European was placed at the top, and the Negro at the bottom with the apes. This pseudo-scientific model not only served to rationalize prejudices which already existed, but also legitimized slavery and genocide. Racism was even enshrined in language: as late as 1899 the Oxford English Dictionary defined 'hottentot' (a now extinct South African tribe) as 'a person of inferior intellect or culture'.[11]

Before the discovery of the outer planets, when Saturn represented the outer boundary of the cosmos, the myth of the lost Golden Age and its counterpart, the Noble Savage, was a widespread fantasy within the collective European psyche. In Roman mythology the Golden Age was associated with Saturn, and this remote Garden of Eden was at first placed in the past, long ago and far away. However, by the time Uranus was discovered in 1781, a conviction had developed that this paradise literally existed somewhere on earth. The French social philosopher Jean Jacques Rousseau depicted the Noble Savage as a 'good-natured brute', free from suffering and erotic inhibitions, existing in Utopian innocence; his sentimentalizing was to influence the ardent Romanticism of nineteenth-century French and English literature and art. Rousseau has Chiron in Pisces, sesquiquadrate Saturn in Leo, which describes this longing to return to the lost

Golden Age; Chiron in Pisces symbolizes his ability to express and in turn influence the imagination of his time.

In psychological terms, the image of the Noble Savage was projected and concretized, and the drive to find him represents the archetypal backdrop to the voyages of discovery undertaken by explorers such as Vasco da Gama and Captain Cook. From an astrological point of view, we can observe that as Uranian consciousness entered the collective in the late eighteenth century, ideas became literalized and projected in a typically Saturnian way. Perhaps the discovery of Chiron, ruler of Sagittarius and orbiting between Saturn and Uranus, heralds the deconcretizing of such images and the possibility to re-examine some of the beliefs which form the substructure of our collective thinking, and which therefore contribute to our irrational prejudices.

What these explorers found, of course, was not the archetypal Noble Savage, but mortal beings whose appearance and customs were totally alien. Often dismissed with disgust[12] or even slaughtered wholesale,[13] these 'savages' became the representatives of the shadow side of the projected image, the epitome of all that was bestial, sordid and subhuman, the lurid stuff of Victorian nightmare – the 'return of the repressed'. This collective phenomenon has a clear parallel in individual psychology: when we search externally for something which is really an archetypal image, and which we will therefore never find, we often react with destructive rage when our partner, lover, teacher or friend turns out not only to be human and fallible, but also decidedly other and unknown. Although the theme of the quest is central to the meaning of Chiron, this *externalization* is doomed to fail to the extent that it represents a misplaced literalization of inner qualities needed for our own wholeness.

What was Europe really questing for, we might wonder? In the image of the Noble Savage is contained man's longing to return to innocence and his need for reconnection with his natural instinctual self. Symbolically, it is a desire to return to the womb of the Mother, and it is just this return which does eventually provide healing for Chiron's unhealable wound, the ground for which was laid when his mother rejected him, causing his primary wound. The Noble Savage also represents the counterpart to the typical nineteenth-century picture of humanity 'marching forward inexorably . . . towards the ultimate pinnacle, the glorious industrial zenith of Western civilization',[14] an ideal cast in true Herculean and heroic mode, reflecting Chiron's second wound.

All this becomes even more sinister when linked with religion. The image of 'Christian soldiers marching on to war, with the cross of Jesus going on before' is not far removed from the above description of the ideal of Western supremacy. During the mid nineteenth century theological debate raged as to whether or not all races could have been created by God through Adam and Eve. Collective consensus was deeply influenced by philosophers such as Comte de Saint-Simon, whose attitude was that, even if all humanity had common parents in the Garden of Eden, civilization was the exclusive province of the white European; Darwin's *The Origin of Species* provided ammunition for this line of thinking. This period also saw the re-emergence of the idea of the Aryan super-race, which was the mythical inspiration for Hitler and his 'Final Solution'. In another form, it provides the basis of the *Broederbond* (brotherhood), a secret society formed in South Africa in 1918 by a few religious zealots; this *Broederbond* now has thousands of members who control almost every aspect of the establishment, and who are dedicated to ideals of racial purity entrenched in a fundamentalist interpretation of the Bible, as mentioned in the section on Chiron/Pluto aspects (p. 257). The apartheid system is an institutionalization of these beliefs.

Missionary fervour reached a peak in many parts of the world during the nineteenth century, with the belief that God created nature to be subdued and conquered by man so he could eventually master the entire earth. There are now few areas of the world which have not been irrevocably influenced by Western culture and/or religion. I believe that the soul-impulse, so to speak, of this collective movement may have been the urgent need to reconnect with the 'primitive', as described above. This being unconscious, however, it functioned in reverse. Instead of being able to allow religious and cultural cross-fertilization, it became a phenomenon of superiority which resulted in enslavement, domination and exploitation, the repercussions of which are still with us.

However, synchronous with the discovery of Chiron, we have

seen a revival of interest in primitive cultures; with the benefit of hindsight some exchange is now occurring. During the 1960s, just as in the late 1700s, a common collective attitude was to reject Western society, its values and traditions, in the search for something better. However, the outer trappings of another culture may be adopted without any deep change of inner attitude. The image of the Noble Savage lives on, but in a form modified to compensate for the materialism of our times, whose high standards of living have often been made possible by cheap labour of non-Western ethnic origin. Following the recent 'sexual revolution' which reacted against the repressiveness of Victorian attitudes, the Noble Savage has returned in the form of the shaman, and this perhaps describes the need for *spiritual* revitalization as well as the reconnecting of body and spirit.

Reflecting on the above network of associations, we can see how strongly Chiron is connected with the phenomenon of racism, which represents the collective parallel to a process which can also be seen at work within our individual psyches. For apartheid describes an archetypal pattern, a cultural and religious heritage of unrelated opposites split apart and set against each other. At an individual level it symbolizes the inner warfare provoked by social adaptation and ego-development where our instinctual wounds or religious needs are ignored, and the destructiveness invoked through our attempts to conform by endorsing this denial. In Jungian terms, it represents the split between the ego and the unconscious, which may result in self-righteousness, denial, splitting and projection, leading to paranoia, defensive retaliation and persecution. Whether or not we are consciously aware of it, the collective mind, the root-system of our individual thinking, contains the belief structures I have tried to describe. Just as the collective development of Western man occurred through the progressive divorce from the instinctual and earthy side of his nature, so we have individually been educated over many centuries. Thus our collective, as well as our individual shadows, contain chaotic elements of unconscious and unintegrated instinctual energy, collectively projected on to the black races who have historically been reviled accordingly.

The Republic of South Africa currently represents for the

world the ultimate symbol of this divided self: apartheid evokes intense emotion even in people who have no personal connection with the situation. Perhaps it is safer to campaign to free Nelson Mandela than to face the pain of the maltreated and imprisoned natural man within one's own soul. Steve Biko, a poet and revolutionary leader, died in jail in September 1977, a few weeks before the discovery of Chiron. Many consider his death as a turning-point: it provoked millions into an open commitment to violence, having given up hope of a negotiated dismantling of apartheid. Examining the chart for the Republic of South Africa will serve to demonstrate how the Chiron configuration in mundane astrology tells us something about the 'national

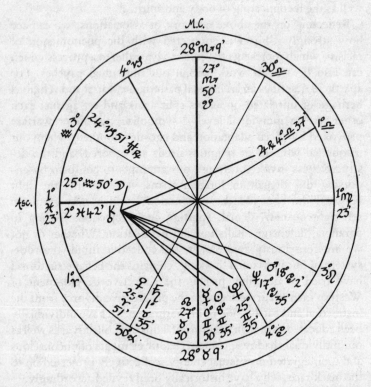

South Africa (Union)

individuality' of a country, to use a paradoxical expression. It certainly shows the dominant archetypal patterns at work, their themes unfolding through the twists and turns of history.

Before exploring the chart for the Republic of South Africa, let us look at a previous chart, for when South Africa became a self-governing British Dominion on 31 May 1910. Both charts have Chiron conjunct the Ascendant in Pisces: it is in the 1st house of the Union chart, and in the 12th house of the Republic chart. Many of the laws which cumulatively became the policy of apartheid were passed during previous transits of Chiron through Pisces, a literal expression of a wound frequently found with Chiron in Pisces: the inability to intuit, much less honour any sense of the unity of all life and humanity within it. Instead of the compassion, acceptance and ability to tolerate and include differences – which can be the gift of Pisces – here we surely have the discriminating Virgoan underside of Pisces at its worst, for Virgo defines itself by what it is not. The identity of South Africa as a Dominion was hard-won, in a manner typical of Chiron in the 1st house, through the two Boer wars. The fight for the right to exist, another theme typical of Chiron in the 1st house, is strong in all racial groups in South Africa. Among the Afrikaners the idea was spread of their being a Chosen People, similar to the mythic image prevalent amongst Jews; they feel persecuted by both blacks and foreigners (English-speaking white South Africans). This conferred upon the Afrikaners a sense of destiny which demanded adherence to ideals of Christian purity and self-discipline that neither group of their persecutors was considered capable of. This inflated sense of identity, fight for existence, self-righteousness and arrogance are all common expressions of Chiron in the 1st house. On the Chiron return of the Union chart, South Africa became a Republic, and a new cycle of its destiny began to unfold.

The Chiron configuration in the Republic chart is as follows: Chiron is in the 12th house, conjunct both Ascendant and South Node in the 12th house, all in Pisces. It forms a mutable grand cross involving all angles of the chart; it forms a T-square by opposing Pluto and North Node in Virgo in the 6th house and squaring the Sun in Gemini in the 4th house, which is conjunct the

IC. The Sagittarius Moon in the 10th house is widely conjunct the MC of this chart and, while not directly part of the grand cross itself, is opposite the Sun, and therefore frequently drawn into the configuration by transiting planets. Chiron also completes a grand trine in water, with Neptune in Scorpio in the 9th house and Mercury in Cancer in the 4th house. Chiron in the 12th house here symbolizes isolationism and the role of exile and scapegoat, currently being literalized by international pressure to ostracize South Africa. Chiron in Pisces represents the level of collective anguish and guilt evoked by the situation, both within South Africa and elsewhere. Perhaps during this present Chiron cycle, the structure of the present system will be eroded altogether, the final dissolution suggested by the 12th house.

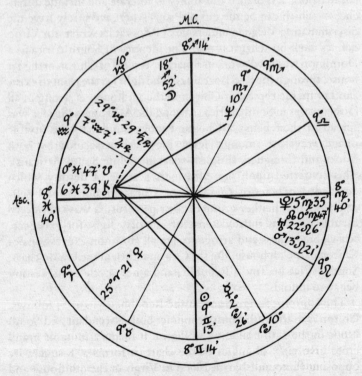

South Africa (Republic)

In mundane astrology the Sun represents the ruling class.[15] Here it is in Gemini, conjunct the IC; it squares Chiron and symbolizes clearly the clashing of opposites and the policy of 'divide and rule' which forms the basis (4th house) of South African society. Chiron's 12th-house position suggests a deeply embedded historical wound or conflict, which is indeed reflected in the longer history of the region: in addition to the divisive and damaging colonial policies, internecine tribal warfare raged and many tribal groups were slaughtered; some were absorbed into the Zulu empire of Shaka while others proceeded northwards with the rebel Mzilikazi. This Chiron/Sun square and the trine to Mercury also symbolize the strict censorship of publications and media; the information system (Mercury) is wounded, and maintaining political ignorance is a major weapon of the state (Chiron/Mercury in the 4th house). These 4th-house planets signify the passionate nationalism, the love of the motherland or fatherland that abounds in the people of South Africa, of whatever race. Chiron aspecting both symbolizes the wound of forced 'resettlement' of black people and, through this, destruction of family and clan groups (4th house).

In mundane astrology Pluto and Neptune represent the dispossessed classes, here meaning everyone except the whites. Chiron is opposite Pluto in Virgo in the 6th house, conjuncting the Moon's Nodes; this describes a distinctive combination of exploitive and brutal practicality (Pluto/North Node in the 6th house) and other worldliness (Chiron/South Node in the 12th house). Fear of being overrun (12th house) by the 'Black Peril' has prompted the Government to take 'draconian measures' (Pluto/North Node, sometimes called 'draco') including interrogation (Chiron aspecting Sun in Gemini and Mercury) and torture (Chiron/Pluto). The ideals of Christian and racial purity and self-discipline are described by the sixth/twelfth axis. Pluto in the 6th house here represents the workers, increasingly committed to the goal of armed revolution, setting the dispossessed (Pluto) firmly against the ruling class (Chiron square Sun, opposite Pluto). Revolutionary activities, on the part of blacks or whites, brew underground in typically Plutonian danger and secrecy, exacting a high toll on personal relationships (Pluto is conjunct the Descendant), and affecting every aspect of daily life (6th house).

The grand trine in water signs suggests an emotional closed circuit; Chiron trining Neptune in Scorpio in the 9th and Mercury in the 4th in Cancer here signifies emotionally biased (Mercury in Cancer) and dogmatic religious beliefs (9th house), defended with Scorpionic zeal. The religious justification for apartheid was challenged by Bishop Desmond Tutu, via the World Council of Churches, which formally declared that there could be no such biblical justification. This caused a massive crisis of religious faith (Chiron trine Neptune in the 9th house) among rank-and-file Afrikaners, but was followed by a resurgence of militant national-ism at grass-roots level, still continuing·at the time of writing.

During Chiron's recent transit through Gemini, it was con-junct the Sun of South Africa's chart in mid 1985, activating the mutable cross; the situation escalated and began increasingly to impinge on the consciousness of the world at large. A state of emergency was declared and an information blackout enforced (transiting Chiron in Gemini); a number of minor and largely cosmetic reforms took place during this period. Education, another Geminian concern, was severely disrupted in several black townships, and for a time ground to a halt altogether. The final transit of Chiron over the Sun in South Africa's chart saw the publication of the still highly controversial Kairos document. Written by black Christian theologians, it has an apocalyptic focus, drawing upon the Gospels and the Revelations of St John, and invoking biblical support for the use of force against oppres-sion. Doing violent battle with the Devil of apartheid is seen as performing a Christian duty: apartheid might yet be hoist on its own petard of religious justification. The nature of this *kairos* is poignantly expressive of Chiron in Gemini: the apocalypse is here the mythic image of the ultimate war of opposites.

The week of the final transit of Chiron in Gemini opposite the 10th-house Moon in Sagittarius saw a cover article in *Time* magazine, entitled 'Hints of Hope – Afrikaners Begin to Unbend' (Chiron was also almost exactly opposite Saturn!). It reported the resignation of twenty-seven senior academicians from an exclus-ive Afrikaans-speaking university, who issued a manifesto 'demanding abolition of all residuals of apartheid'. In the words of a former member of the *Broederbond*, 'the government is the captive of its own meaningless rhetoric'.[16] However, although the transit of Chiron through Gemini did perhaps weaken the stranglehold of the ideas which form its basis, it has also brought increased polarization (Chiron in Gemini) within the Government. Afrikanerdom is split between those committed to the neo-fascist path of total separation, and those who are beginning to accept that reform of the apartheid system is necessary and inevitable.

The planets in the Chiron configuration of the horoscope of the United States are strikingly similar to those in the Republic chart of South Africa: in the United States' chart Chiron is also square both Sun and Pluto, and also aspects Moon and Mercury. In their treatment of their indigenous people, these two countries share a similar collective karmic burden, and time will tell whether the United States will seek vicariously to expiate its own genocidal crimes by future direct or indirect involvement in the affairs of South Africa. Given the archetypal themes which these two nations share, it would not be surprising.

The racism which exists in many countries mirrors the same sickness within the individual psyche. However, over the last few decades, and especially since the discovery of Chiron, many elements of black culture have influenced the music, dress style and aspirations of the collective. Given the phenomenon of collective projection I have described, 'Black is Beautiful' perhaps symbolizes at a collective level the recognition that to face and integrate the shadow of our own denied selves brings the possibility of renewal and redemption to both individual and society.

Ecology

The earth today is wounded and sore . . . The reason we exploit, damage and savage the earth is because we are out of balance. We have lost our sense of proportion. And we cannot be proportionate unless we honour the wilderness and the natural person within ourselves.

Laurens van der Post[17]

As man's intellectual understanding and physical mastery over the outer world has increased, he has lost sight of the wholeness of nature. In the chart for the time of Chiron's discovery, Chiron is focal in Taurus in the 4th house, pointing to this wound, lying at the foundation (4th house) of this period of history. The recent science of ecology seeks to redress this imbalance, being concerned with the interrelatedness of different biological species, including man, and with the intimate network of interdependency which is necessary for survival. The word 'ecology' comes from the Greek *oikos*, meaning 'house' or 'home'. Lack of appreciation of the interconnectedness of all life inevitably brings alienation, a feeling of being not 'at home' either within oneself or, indeed, on the earth. We can then value neither, as 'excessive interference with *outer* nature creates of necessity disorder of the *inner* nature, for the two are intimately connected'.[18]

An ecological attitude to life could be seen as the contemporary and scientific counterpart to the shamanic world-view (see Chapter 1). Wilderness man lived with an instinctive awareness of his place within the totality; the visionary and *conscious* awareness of this was earned by the shaman through his suffering, initiation and submission to his vocation. For 'the wilderness is the original biotype of the soul'.[19] Laurens van der Post points out that as the few remaining areas of wilderness on earth are rapidly being encroached upon, wilderness man is also disappearing.

In a way that is the greatest loss of all, because this person could have been our real bridge to knowing wilderness and nature in the way in which it is known by the Creator, and in which it should really be known . . . we have (also) destroyed the wilderness person in ourselves. And because of (his) absence . . . we are left with a kind of loneliness, an inadequate comprehension of what life can be.[20]

Taking a psychological perspective, C. A. Meier suggests that as man has tamed and subjugated the dangerous aspects of nature, those same aspects which used once to keep our forebears watchful and humble have reappeared from within,

so that the whole of Western society rapidly approaches the physical and mental cracking point from the inner dangers alone. This is no joking matter for should the outer wilderness disappear altogether, it would inevitably resurrect powerfully from within, whereupon it would immediately be projected. Enemies would be created, and its terrifying aspects would take revenge for our neglect, our lack of reverence, our ruthless interference with that beautiful order of things.[21]

We can discern behind these eloquent quotations the archetypal figure whom we met in Chapter 4: here indeed is Artemis, the *potnia theron*, Lady of the Wild Things. She represents nature in the raw, unspoilt and untamed; she demands respect and even human sacrifice; she supports all life, she is the Mother of mothers, and woe betide those who ignore her. The inner search for the wilderness man will inevitably connect us to the child within, with its joy and perhaps also its indescribable suffering, its capacity for play as well as its grief at being wrenched from primordial innocence in the interests of 'socialization', 'education' and other processes designed to make it fit into a system which no longer pays its dues to the primordial origins of life. Living in urban Western society, far from the healing benefits of an unspoilt geographical wilderness, it is perhaps by reconnecting with this wound that we may finally be able to appreciate our own 'wilderness within', the psychological habitat which supports our true individual natures. Like an ignorant traveller amongst the undisturbed life of the wild, we must go quietly and carefully to learn the laws of this inner terrain. For if we should transgress these natural laws, the wilderness within may arise in all its primordial power and perhaps even demand a bloody sacrifice from us.

Just eight days before the discovery of Chiron, the first World Wilderness Congress began, and the story of how this important international forum was conceived and born clearly illustrates Chiron at work. The impetus behind it came from the friendship between two South African men, Dr Ian Player and Qumbu Magqubu Ntombela, who had long worked together in a huge conservation area and game reserve. During the transits of Chiron opposite his natal Moon and Neptune (1958–62), Dr Player had an idea that developed into the Wilderness Leadership School, which provides an opportunity for people to experience the healing powers of the wilderness. He and Magqubu would lead wilderness trails, taking small groups of people to encounter the spirit of Africa and to meet nature and themselves in the raw. In this way, both individual growth and awareness of the importance of conservation are fostered and, to date, over 12,000 people have had life-changing experiences on these trails. This project is also multi-racial, a truly Chironian bridging of the political divide, and an attempt to reintroduce and reconnect both black and white people with the healing powers of their wilderness heritage.

The Chiron configuration in Dr Player's horoscope is as follows: Chiron is at 29°26' Aries, conjunct Venus in Aries in the 1st

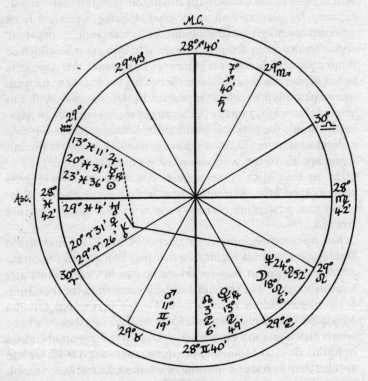

Ian Player

house. It is trine Neptune in the 5th house, biseptile Saturn in Capricorn in the 9th house, and semisquare Jupiter in the 12th house. Here Chiron/Venus indicates the capacity for relationships that bridge cultural divides and collective prejudices, and bring healing to others. The School emphasizes the three relationships of man to God, man to man, and man to earth – an eloquent statement of Chiron conjunct Venus with its expanded vision of relationship. Dr Player's chart also has a stellium of planets in Pisces including Jupiter, Mercury, Sun, Ascendant and Uranus, all in the 12th house except Uranus. This suggests a subliminal sensitivity to the collective with its suffering and longing for redemption and unity, and further emphasizes an already strong Neptune, the overall dispositor of the chart and trine Chiron. Uranus in Pisces conjunct the Ascendant shows the capacity to be an innovator, a medium of change in the realm of ideas, while Chiron in the 1st house in Aries gives the urge to take action and to do something positive. The School was started in 1962, as transiting Chiron began to conjunct Jupiter, the first planet of his 12th-house Pisces stellium, suggesting the expansion and actualization of a Neptunian vision. Dr Player's Jupiter in Pisces conjuncts Chiron in the chart of South Africa, describing his role in addressing the wounds of his country; his natal Mars, ruler of Chiron in Aries, is conjunct the Sun in the chart of South Africa, symbolizing action taken to reconcile opposites.

In 1940, Dr Player's mentor Magqubu was bitten by a poisonous snake and went into a coma for three days, during which time he experienced an inner visionary journey. Two years of serious illness followed and precipitated a quest for healing, as neither his traditional medicine nor the white man's medicine seemed to help. Magqubu was eventually led to the Zulu prophet Shembe, through which connection he was eventually healed; he embraced Christianity, although also maintaining his traditional Zulu way of life. Birth data is unfortunately not available for Magqubu; he was born between 1900 and 1902, with Chiron somewhere between mid-Sagittarius and mid-Capricorn. However, even from this scant information we can see some interesting Chironian patterns in terms of Magqubu's role in the evolution of the World Wilderness Congress (WWC).

From November 1900 until December 1901, Chiron was continuously conjunct either Jupiter or Saturn or both, in late Sagittarius and/or early Capricorn; hence it is likely that Magqubu's
Chiron is conjunct Jupiter and/or Saturn. Note also that Dr
Player's MC is at 28°40′ Sagittarius, conjunct the Ascendant of
the WWC chart (28°7′ Sagittarius); all three horoscopes therefore
align in a significant way with the Galactic Centre, as discussed in
Chapter 6, which underlines the breadth of vision involved in this
project. Magqubu's full name means 'Bloated Grudge', as he was
born during a serious family dispute over cattle, involving his
father and his uncle.[22] Jupiter rules Sagittarius and is the traditional significator for uncle, while Saturn rules Capricorn and is
associated with the father. Given names often reflect our fate:
parents may unwittingly bestow a gift or curse with a name
symbolizing issues that need resolution, unfinished business that
will be carried forward into the next generation. The 'Bloated
Grudge' was literalized in Magqubu's initiatory sickness: he
swelled up so large that he was immobilized, no longer able to get
around without help. Jupiter is associated with swellings, and
Saturn with being immobilized and helpless. In the course of his
quest (Chiron), Magqubu departed radically from the traditional
religious customs of his father (Saturn). His healing finally came
through his own unique synthesis (Jupiter) of African and European cosmologies, and thus is clearly symbolized by Chiron,
Jupiter and Saturn.

In early 1975, just before Dr Player's first exact Chiron return,
he and Magqubu conceived the idea of a forum, modelled on the
indaba, a Zulu word meaning a gathering to debate important
matters – a get-together or powwow: people from all over the
world would gather to create awareness of the importance of the
wilderness, and to promote action to conserve it. Plans were set in
motion, and, two and a half years later, vision became reality a
few days before Chiron was discovered. Vance Martin also joined
the project; his Chiron is in Sagittarius in the 7th house, focal by
virtue of its numerous aspects. He played a key role in organizing
subsequent congresses (his Chiron squares Saturn in Virgo),
helping synthesize the various scientific disciplines involved
(Chiron in Sagittarius), and articulating the importance of the

spiritual and inner aspects of wilderness conservation (his Chiron trines a Sun/Mercury conjunction in Leo).

The first countries to participate were South Africa, Australia, the United States and Canada, all of whom have on their national consciences abuse of their indigenous people, whose customs and religion were not appreciated, and whose land was appropriated. Like all conquering nations, they have incurred a collective karmic debt. The activities of WWC work towards paying this debt, healing these rifts and thus expiating the 'sins of the fathers'. The theme of ancestral issues connected with the father immediately suggests Chiron/Saturn at work, so let us explore that.

The chart for the WWC has Chiron trine Saturn, and, as we have seen, Magqubu probably has either Chiron conjunct Saturn, or Chiron in Capricorn, or indeed both. Vance Martin has Chiron squaring Saturn, and Dr Player's natal Saturn is in Sagittarius in the 9th house, biquintile Chiron: the quintile represents creative transformation and thus the biquintile represents its externalization,[23] which can be clearly seen in Dr Player's life. His Chiron in Aries symbolizes action taken to resolve issues involving both ancestral themes connected with the father (Saturn), and also religious and philosophical issues (9th house); the 12th-house Jupiter in Pisces squaring Saturn widens the scope of this task to include the collective at large. As Dr Player is South African, the nature of these collective issues will already be clear from the above analysis of the chart of South Africa. In addition, at the age of twelve, one of Dr Player's knees (ruled by Saturn) was punctured by a stone, leaving the joint permanently deformed and frequently very painful; at the time transiting Chiron was opposing his natal Pluto in the 4th house while transiting Saturn was conjunct his Chiron. This disability made him more introverted than he would otherwise have been, but did not stop him from pioneering the sport of canoe-racing in South Africa, true to Chiron in the 1st house in Aries.

The WWC chart has Chiron in Taurus in the 5th house trine Saturn in Leo in the 9th, symbolizing the expression of healing intent (Chiron in the 5th house), a reconciliation of past issues (Saturn) as well as visions and ideals (9th house) and a formulation of something tangible that works in the world. The WWC encourages practical idealism, supports the pursuit of personal meaning within the framework of its preoccupations, and also serves to educate across national and racial barriers: all this is described by the Chiron/Saturn aspect. Chiron also opposes a stellium of Scorpio planets in the 11th house: Sun, Mercury and Uranus. This same combination appears in Dr Player's horoscope: through the vehicle of the WWC, his Piscean empathy and responsiveness to collective issues have achieved focus and directed power within Scorpio. In the WWC chart Chiron symbolizes the expression (5th house) of powerful ideas (Chiron/Mercury) which can transform collective attitudes (Chiron/

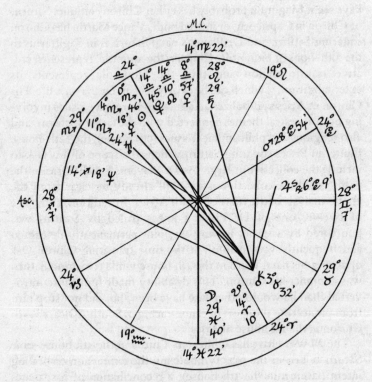

World Wilderness Congress

Uranus in the 11th). The linking of inner and outer is typically Chironian, as well as the bridging of cultural, racial and national divides. Chiron also squares Mars in Cancer in the 8th house, suggesting healing (Chiron) the wounds of aggression (Mars) against Mother Earth (Cancer), and promoting awareness (Chiron) of the exploitation of natural resources (8th house = others' resources). Chiron is sextile Jupiter stationary-direct in its exaltation in Cancer, symbolizing the vision (Jupiter), and also the ecological necessity, of finding ourselves again at home (Cancer) on the earth, and through this to renew our capacity to connect with the numinous dimension of life (Jupiter). Dr Player's MC conjunct the Ascendant of the WWC chart, both in Sagittarius and therefore ruled by Chiron, shows the progression whereby one man's aspirations (MC) gave birth (Ascendant) to a project benefiting the world at large. All this occurred during Dr Player's Chiron return, and serves as an example of individuality being fulfilled by its consecration to larger collective concerns.

Drug Abuse and the Quest for Consciousness

During the decade or so preceding the discovery of Chiron, millions of people travelled to the East to meet the cultural 'other', in search of enlightenment, peace and an alternative to materialistic Western values. When gurus of the drug culture began to adopt Eastern religions, the world of drugs and the quest for consciousness became inextricably linked. After indigestible experiences of expanded consciousness (negative Uranus), some eventually abandoned their quest and retreated into a guilty materialism and cynicism (negative Saturn) as the discrepancy between their actual life and their visions became intolerable. In an attempt to 'stay high', others obsessively pursued psychological-growth techniques or followed gurus of various kinds. More recently, abuse of prescribed drugs such as amphetamines and hard drugs such as heroin is becoming widespread – the pronunciation of the word *hero-in* underlines the mythic context of this: one is reminded of Chiron, accidentally wounded by the hero Hercules, his friend and pupil. The cult of the hero lives on in our craving for the bright, the beautiful and the heroic within ourselves and others, and our need for mind-altering substances to sustain it.

For many people, however, drugs began or accompanied a serious quest for understanding of the strange other world of perception that was thus opened. Ritual use of hallucinogenic plant substances is an intrinsic part of many shamanic cultures; knowledge and use of plants to alter one's state of mind are an ancient accessory to mankind's cultural and religious development, perhaps as old as consciousness itself. Robert Graves suggests that the Centaurs became wild and unruly through eating *amanita muscaria* mushrooms.[24] These mushrooms are a common hallucinogenic substance of great antiquity, eaten for stamina against the cold and to facilitate ecstatic experience and shamanic trance; in some cultures the plant itself is regarded as a symbol of primary cosmological significance.[25] The goddess Artemis bestowed upon Chiron an intimate knowledge of the healing properties of plants, which he passed on to his students, notably the famous hero-physician Asclepius; we have no reason to suppose this excluded their psychotropic properties. Indeed, in one version of Chiron's story, he eventually discovered a plant which healed his wound, and was named 'Centaury' after him.[26]

However, the use of hallucinogenic substances within shamanic cultural forms is usually surrounded with ritual, taboo and strict observances, or at least approached with an attitude of awe and reverence, being regarded as the means directly to experience the god thus invoked. In contrast, the recent explosion of drug use has perhaps been characterized rather by ego-gratification and escapism, which have collectively outweighed transcendental or devotional intentions.

The Centaurs were part of the retinue of Dionysus, the Greek god of wine, who is connected with Chiron's half-brothers, Zeus and Hades. Dios is another name for Zeus, and Nysa was where Persephone was abducted by Hades into the Underworld. Thus the name 'Dionysus' means 'Zeus of the Underworld': the Dionysian ecstasy spans both the celestial heights of Zeus and the chthonic depths and potential terrors of Pluto's realm. Mare-headed Demeter, whose ancient cult we have met before, is sometimes called 'Melania': 'The Black One'. It was she who roamed in anguish and rage, mourning the loss of her daughter Persephone and threatening to lay waste the earth and everything on it if she was not returned; it was also she who featured in the Eleusinian mysteries.

It has been suggested by Gordon Wasson et al. that the abduction of Persephone symbolizes the onset of a hallucinogenic seizure,[27] and that the Eleusinian mysteries involved the ritual drinking of a special potion, the *kykeon*, containing the psychotropic alkaloid of ergot, a fungal parasite hosted by cereal crops such as barley, of which the *kykeon* was known to be made. Lysergic acid, from which LSD is synthesized, is the nucleus common to most ergot alkaloids.[28] Thus, it is likely that the substance which facilitated the transcendent experiences at Eleusis was similar in effect to LSD. These mysteries were considered so sacred that to speak of them was an offence punishable by death; indeed, there remains not one existing account of exactly what happened there, although scholars have pieced together oblique allusions, hints and fragments of evidence to recreate a description of some of the rituals. Candidates for initiation underwent extensive preparation, and to witness the mysteries was considered the highest spiritual blessing. They were celebrated for about 2000 years, until the sanctuary of Demeter was destroyed in AD 396 by the invading Goth king Alarich and the Christian monks who accompanied him.

Almost 1500 years later, LSD was synthesized by Dr Albert Hofmann, who realized its psychotropic effects when he took it himself in 1943. LSD was distributed by Sandoz laboratories as a psychochemical agent to psychiatric-research units in England and America. But by the mid 1960s LSD hysteria was rife; its use had reached epidemic proportions, promoted by influential figures such as Ken Kesey, Richard Alpert and Timothy Leary, by now the high priest of the drug subculture whose credo was: 'Turn on, tune in, drop out.'

Let us look at Chiron in the horoscopes of Albert Hofmann, the creator of LSD, and Timothy Leary, its apostle. The Chiron configuration in the chart of Albert Hofmann is as follows: Chiron is in Aquarius in the 8th house, opposite Moon in Leo in the 2nd house, and sesquiquadrate Pluto in Gemini in the 12th house, conjunct the Ascendant. These ingredients aptly symbolize the creation which earned Hofmann a place in history; the era of sexual liberation (8th house) and social revolution (Aquarius) followed in the wake of LSD; it was synthesized from an organic substance (Chiron/Moon in the 2nd). Pluto here alludes to the mass transformation of consciousness through the dissolving (12th house) of duality and ordinary perceptions (Gemini). In the light of the above reference to the Eleusinian mysteries, the Sabian Symbol for Hofmann's Chiron is extraordinarily specific: 'A masked figure performs ritualistic acts in a mystery play.' The interpretation speaks of the 'great Mysteries of the past' having been created to transform instinctual energies to a mentally conscious level.

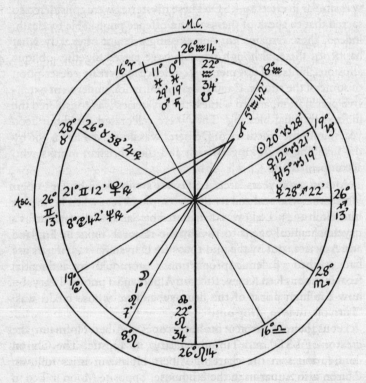

Albert Hofmann

'Biological and cosmic energies can thus be used to ensure that social processes do not lose touch with the deeper realities of planetary and universal life. The individual is seen as having assumed a transpersonal responsibility.'[29]

As a child, before he had any knowledge of Greek culture, Hofmann was fascinated by pictures of antique Greek sculptures.[30] The obvious metaphor suggested by this intriguing network of symbolic connections is a past-life connection, where Dr Hofmann in this life was 'doing what he had done before', but in a manner congruent with the culture of present-day Europe, facilitating the mass expansion of consciousness through his creation of LSD.

On the day of Hofmann's self-experiment, the first ever consciously induced LSD trip, transiting Pluto was about to make its final opposition to his natal Chiron, exact within 46', and transiting Chiron was three days from its station, conjunct within 24' his natal North Node in Leo: this describes the fulfilling of a Plutonian destiny. In Hofmann's own words,

I see the importance of LSD in the possibility of providing material aid to meditation aimed at the mystical experience of a deeper, comprehensive reality. Such a use accords entirely with the essence and working character of LSD as a sacred drug.[31]

Hofmann's natal Saturn in the 10th house in Pisces gives him a sense of reserve and caution as regards other dimensions of experience; he recognized the profanation involved in 'stealing the fire' of substances sacred to other people's religions. He participated in such ceremonies himself with Mexican shamans, when transiting Chiron was conjunct his natal Saturn and Mars, and transiting Saturn was conjunct his natal Chiron; this double combination here suggests the bridging of the personal world of ego-boundaries (Saturn) and the eternal realm (Chiron). Unlike Leary, however, Hofmann was never caught up in messianic fervour; he maintained a strong sense of rational discrimination (Gemini Ascendant, opposite Mercury in Sagittarius in the 7th house) and social responsibility (Chiron in Aquarius opposite Moon, also Saturn in the 10th house).

By way of contrast, in Timothy Leary's horoscope we see the

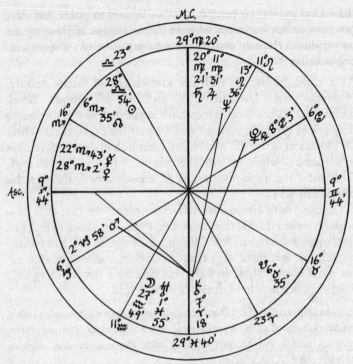

Timothy Leary

Chiron configuration as follows: Chiron is in Aries in the 4th house, forming a grand cross, opposite the MC in Virgo, and square both Mars in Capricorn in the 1st house and Pluto in Cancer in the 8th house. It is also sesquiquadrate Mercury in the 12th house, and completes a grand trine in fire, with his Sagittarian Ascendant and Neptune in the 9th house in Leo. When transiting Chiron was moving from Aquarius into Pisces, conjunct his natal Moon and Uranus in the 3rd house, Leary had his first experience of sacred mushrooms. This transit here symbolizes expansion of consciousness through ordinary perceptions (Moon in the 3rd) being opened to the mind-world beyond (Uranus in Pisces). After this, Leary dedicated himself to researching the effects of psychedelic drugs in a project which he carried out while teaching at Harvard University. He was dismissed from Harvard when transiting Chiron was exactly opposite his 9th-house Jupiter and transiting Pluto exactly conjunct it, symbolizing the end of his formal career in higher education (9th house) and the inauguration of himself as psychedelic guru (Chiron/Jupiter). Here is also illustrated the danger of hubris typical of the 9th house, where gaining higher knowledge for personal power can reach obsessional proportions, especially when Jupiter, Neptune and Pluto are involved.

When transiting Chiron was exactly opposite his natal Saturn in Virgo, Leary went to India and converted to Hinduism. Leary's translation of Hindu philosophy shows the Chiron/Saturn tendency to make things inappropriately and externally concrete. Ironically, his all-or-nothing message to reject society and turn inward stems from the same dualism as expressed in the materialism from which he and countless others were trying to escape. As Chiron approached his IC, Leary founded the League for Spiritual Discovery (LSD): establishing something in the outer world was a 10th-house response to this transit, and perhaps represented an escape from his own inner world. With Chiron in the 4th house, this would be a likely line of least resistance: conflicts (Chiron in Aries) with his father are indicated (Chiron in the 4th house) – here extended to society (echo of the opposite 10th house) – as well as the deep-seated insecurity typical of Chiron in Aries, for which the Mars/Pluto opposition would compensate with an enormous and potentially destructive power drive. Leary spent most of his Chiron return in prison, scapegoated (a Neptune/Chiron theme) and made an example of.

When the retrograde conjunction of transiting Chiron to natal Chiron was approaching, Leary managed to escape and went into exile (Neptune/Chiron). The midpoint configuration for the night of his escape (13/14 September 1970) is interesting: transiting Chiron was 48' from exactly opposite transiting Uranus, and semisquare transiting Saturn, so we have the Chiron = Saturn/Uranus combination again! The Chiron/Uranus midpoint also activates the following pairs of natal planets: Chiron/Pluto, Sun/Saturn, Jupiter/Neptune; these describe a sudden (Uranus) release (Jupiter/Neptune) which transgressed the law (Sun/Saturn), and involved personal risk (Chiron/Pluto). Leary was imprisoned again shortly after his Chiron return, when Saturn squared the midpoint of his natal Saturn/Jupiter; he was finally freed when transiting Neptune in Sagittarius had just crossed his Ascendant and was square his natal Jupiter. During this second period of imprisonment, transiting Pluto in the 10th house continuously opposed his Chiron, thus setting off the entire Chiron configuration. This transit could have represented an opportunity for deepening an individual through a confrontation with inner pain and the results of the abuse of power, a breaking down and transformation of his role in the world.

Saturn as natural ruler of the MC is loosely associated with Leary's Chiron configuration, and the Saturnian principle indeed appears wounded in Leary's life, especially as, during the mid 1960s, at the height of Leary's activity, transiting Chiron made a series of exact oppositions to his natal Saturn. Saturn in the 9th house may ask that we honour Saturn and his principles as a divine image deserving of respect, but also suggests that it might darkly colour our view of reality – in which case it may be projected and we then 'fight the Devil' somewhere in the outer world. Those with Saturn in Virgo fulfil themselves through duty and service to others. Leary perhaps had literally to 'serve (Virgo) time (Saturn)' in order for this to happen, as in his previous manifesto Saturn was the enemy, projected outside and reviled. Those with Saturn in Virgo often struggle with a deep feeling of inner restriction, mental and emotional retentiveness, narrow-mindedness, and a fear of anything which they cannot control. One can imagine the terror that they might feel in the midst of an uncontrollable psychedelic experience: Leary in turn controlled others' minds and influenced the attitudes of millions, and this is also reflected by his Chiron/Mercury aspect.

Natal Chiron completing the fiery grand trine with Neptune and the Ascendant here exacerbated the messianic touch commonly found with Chiron, and Neptune is traditionally associated with drugs. Leary's 'trip', as described by his Chiron configuration, included rejection of Saturnian structures and values. He encouraged the pursuit of chemical enlightenment, without apparent consideration of human limits or reverence for the archetypal world into which he was intruding. There was rather an ego-inflation and perhaps even an exaltation in the destruction involved (Chiron/Mars/Pluto in a T-square). On the other hand, Leary's influence upon the collective was profound: he boldly explored (Chiron in Aries) regions of inner space (Chiron/Mercury in the 12th) and exhorted others to do likewise (Chiron/Mercury in Scorpio). Millions were subsequently forced, true Mars/Pluto style, to explore the content of their own minds in order to digest their experiences, and this in turn contributed to the revolution in consciousness synchronous with the discovery of Chiron. Finally, a look at the Sabian Symbol for Leary's Chiron position: 'A large woman's hat with streamers blown by an east wind.' The interpretation specifically mentions Eastern philosophies and speaks of largely undeveloped mental processes, still needing protection. 'A too great openness to the sky-energies on the "spiritual level" could lead to obsessions of various kinds.'[32]

To return to the mythic background of the drug phenomenon, Wasson further suggests that the fire which Prometheus stole was in fact a hallucinogenic substance: it is described by Aeschylus as 'the flowery splendour of all-fashioning fire',[33] as flower, drug and promoter of all human science.[34] Herb-gatherers in ancient Greece used fennel stalks for collecting herbs, and we are told that Prometheus concealed the 'glowing ember' within a fennel stalk when he stole it from Olympus. Prometheus' stealing fire from the gods and returning it to humanity is perhaps also a metaphor for the gathering of psychotropic plants, man's lost connection with the gods thus being restored through ritual participation in ecstatic hallucinatory experience.

We have already seen how the stories of Chiron and Prometheus interconnect and, in the light of the above network of associations, the mass use of drugs could be seen as symbolizing 'stealing fire' – in the sense of consciousness – and the drive to re-establish a personal connection with the world of the numinous. However, when the essentially religious nature of this need is ignored and not honoured, taboos and rituals are not observed, and, without appropriate preparations, we risk over-exposure to the archetypal world which then unleashes regressive tendencies and self-destructiveness: we become chained and tormented like Prometheus.

In our time, however, such has been the hunger to reconnect with the source of spiritual renewal within our own soul, that greed for power in the form of knowledge of inner dimensions now represents the dark underside of psychological-growth techniques, spiritual quests and also our own discipline, astrology. A new world is opening up, but we take to it our old attitudes of exploitation and arrogance: this Promethean conquest of inner space is paralleled by the conquest of outer space for political power. However, perhaps the discovery of Chiron symbolizes the rekindling within the collective psyche of an attitude of awe and reverence towards the immensity of which we are but a small part, and the respect for life which follows this realization. Laurens van der Post made these comments on the Sermon on the Mount:

Recognition of what it lacks is one of the most dynamic forces in the human spirit. Realization of our greater selves comes first through the recognition of what we are not . . . Only the spirit that recognizes itself to be poor, through what it is not, has any promise of increase. We are beggars always to what we were meant to be.[35]

Epilogue

I would like to end with a personal story. While writing this book, I had the unexpected pleasure of a visit from Christina La Barre, a dear friend whom I had not seen for many years. When I told her I was writing an astrology book about Chiron, she asked me what Chiron was. I replied: 'He was that wounded Centaur in Greek mythology.' Her eyes widened and she said: 'Really? I must tell you a dream I had.' Christina is a gifted story-teller, and I sat listening for what seemed to be an eternity, entranced and drawn into the dream with her, feeling it was no accident that she had arrived out of the blue to tell it to me.

Christina is a nurse, midwife and mother of two daughters. She has the Sun in Capricorn, and her Chiron configuration is as follows: Chiron is in Virgo in the 2nd house, trine a Taurus MC and also Mercury in Capricorn, square Saturn and Mars in Gemini and sextile Venus in Scorpio. She had this dream about six weeks after Chiron was discovered, and although she had never told it to anyone before, every detail remained crystal-clear, still reverberating within her nine years later. Transiting Chiron was conjunct her Saturn in Gemini when she related it to me, symbolizing a healing experience (Chiron) formulated into words (Saturn in Gemini). On a personal level, Christina relates the dream to a stage of her personal life which was then culminating. She was experiencing the profound psychological and physical upheavals of hormonal shifts that were occurring as she emerged from a seven-year period of intensive mothering. However, I felt that this dream also portrayed an archetypal sequence of wider significance, and that she had dreamed her dream for all of us – congruent with natal Saturn in the 11th house Saturn squaring

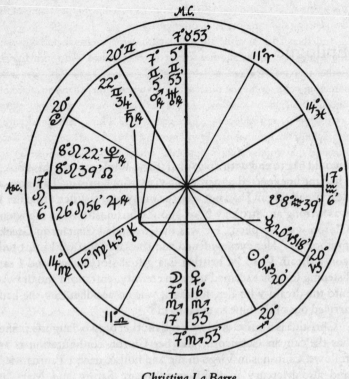

Christina La Barre

$$\chi = \hbar / \text{\#}$$

Chiron. Here follows a transcript of what she told: I will let the dream speak for itself . . .

In the dream I knew that there were two parts that had to come together: each image was very contained, wholly complete within itself before they met . . .

In the beginning was a Centaur, young, beautiful, muscles rippling and full of energy. It was a glistening reddish colour like a roan horse, leaping and playing in a meadow rich with flowers and green grass. It was rolling about and playing, just feeling the air and the greenness and the fertility.

Very young, like spring and early summer – revelling in the feeling of its own energy shooting out and coming back.

And then after a while the Centaur became aware that there was something else: it had another search to make, it had to do something. Rather than go back and look for more Centaurs, it knew it must seek something else, someone different, somewhere other than this place of beautiful valleys and meadows, fertility and lush youth. And the Centaur started searching and looking, eyes open, just looking. It had to go up, up, up into the mountains, slowly moving away from the fertile plains, through the woods, always upwards, where it's harder and harder to live. And the Centaur became more and more ascetic, searching and searching, eyes always open, very clear and masculine: a straightforward searching energy that was pure and alert, yet still unaware.

It was not afraid in its search: searching through the trees, along the pathways, up and up into a far more rarefied atmosphere, way, way up into the mountains, until it came to a high place, not barren but windswept and spare, rarefied and brilliantly clear. It was all of life at the same time.

And then the searching gaze of the Centaur was absolutely clear. It looked and looked and there it was! It saw a vast lake and started towards it . . . a high lake, absolutely vast, not wide or reaching from horizon to horizon, but vast in the sense of being so utterly deep. Utterly, utterly deep. Not a shallow mountain stream, or a little pool, but very, very deep.

Immediately jumping in, down to the bottom of this deep mountain lake that reaches to the core of the earth where there's heat and generation and the nest of the beginnings. Now there's swirling warmth and utter encompassment, until there emerges the consciousness of a fish, slowly separating from being simply the warmth and the sway. A beautiful, glistening thing, all muscle, swimming and rolling about, so much part of everything that consciousness comes slowly: the muscle is part of the water, which is part of the warmth that is part of the earth that is part of everything. Swimming and playing, slowly developing the consciousness that it exists playing within the environment, feeling encompassed by the nestling, cradling warmth of generation.

Then the muscles start working and swimming up and up. At one point the eyes look upwards and see the surface of the water. Seeing that, desire springs forth, knowing it's got to get there, wants to get there, the desire is to go up, straight up. Once the nose breaks through the surface of the water, the top part of this fish-being becomes a goat, an air-breathing creature, a creature of the land, with a nose that cannot go underwater again, but for a second, trying to swim with these perfectly ridiculous hooves. Its only saving is the fish-tail that brought it up out of the depths. Breaking surface will be the death of the tail, the death of its whole being, because the goat can't breathe down in its previous watery environment. It's impossible, no matter what. It's going to die. And therefore the head tells the tail: 'I've got to get to the bank, I've got to get to the shore', even though the tail knows nothing of the shore.

And so the head of this struggling hoofed beast is telling the tail to impel it, and they work together towards the shore. And the hooves clamber up over rocks not soft and worn, but sharp with the newness of life, cracked by the opening of things. At long last the goat pulls itself up: 'Oooh, I'll be able to breathe up here.' It clambers up on to the rocky shore, while the tail that impelled it there still thrashes with the energy of the attempt to save it. Now it's beating itself raw and ragged and bleeding on these rocks. The goat turns around and looks at the nether half of its being. It's been ripped to shreds and hurts like hell – it can't separate. The tail has to go back into the water – it's hurting too much. The feet have to go forward – although it's utter agony this creature can't go back. If it dives back into the water to save the tail it will die. Knowing that the head is what will keep it alive to breathe and to eat, what must it do? Drag this bleeding tail through the woods and over the rocks for the rest of its life? Is that what must be? Is that the only way forward? To go back means to die, to go forward means shredding itself up and eventually bleeding to death. My God, now what?

At this point, the Centaur sees the goat-fish. First there is utter fascination and amazement, and then just pity because this creature is an absolute mess. As an archer the Centaur knows what it has to do. Out of pity, because there's nothing left to save, it lifts up its bow, fits the arrow and aims. The agonized goat-fish is thrashing wildly and looking at this beautiful Centaur. When it realizes the Centaur is going to kill it, at first there's more desperate thrashing: 'My God! Is this it? Is this what life is about? I'm here just to get shot?' Then the goat-fish looks and knows: 'This is it. This is the path. There's no way back.' And so, with courage and straightness, the goat turns his head to face the Centaur, for of course to wound the tail would have meant nothing. The Centaur shoots, and the goat puts its brow forward to meet the arrow, which kills it, going straight in between the eyes and disappearing.

Then the Centaur must weep, mourning the loss of its innocence. 'Is this what I came here for? Is my job to kill? That's what it is. That's who I am and that's what I do well, and so I had to kill.' But such sorrow! 'This was such a beautiful beast that went through this beautiful world, and I had to kill it, knowing somehow there was no choice.' And so it weeps and mourns. Because that too is part of it: to weep for this thing that was hurting so much, knowing that it's over.

When the Centaur looks up, he sees that from the body of the dead goat with the fish's tail has emerged a glistening, pure white female unicorn. It is fully mature, delicate, but not fragile. And the two beings eye each other, male and female, aware that mating is a bit ridiculous because they're two such different beasts. Yet their gift from the gods is that they can each be what they were made to be: the Centaur will for ever hunt and search with its own sheer pointed masculine energy, and the unicorn can also be for ever itself – hunted, yes, but elusive, playful and transformatively aware that this is the game. The Centaur has to keep on searching, so that the unicorn will gladly play the game of leaping and hiding.

Thus the unicorn can then give its gift of death and transformation back to the Centaur, who suffered so innocently and unknowingly, having to carry out the killing. Thus she can say: 'That's fine, we go beyond.'

That was the end of the dream: the feeling of delight in the chase of consciousness.

Appendix 1

Astronomical Information

Discovery

1 November 1977, 10.00 am, Pasadena, California. Astrologer Al Morrison suggests a rectification of four minutes earlier.

Discoverer

Charles T. Kowal, b. 8 November 1940, Buffalo, New York. He also discovered the thirteenth and fourteenth moons of Jupiter, a comet, and eighty supernovae, which is the second largest number of astronomical discoveries ever made by one person. Of the asteroids he discovered, one was named after his daughter Loretta, and one after the town of Naples where he met his wife in 1968. He graduated from Buffalo High School in 1957; he won a scholarship to USC and majored in astronomy; he graduated with a BA in 1961. He began working for Hale Observatories in the same year.[1]

Diameter

Unknown; estimated at 100–400 kilometres, although one source gives 100–400 miles!

Orbit Time

49–51 years. Its movement is erratic, affected by perturbations from its neighbours, Saturn and Uranus.

Orbital Eccentricity

Chiron has the greatest orbital eccentricity of any planet. Where 0.0000 is a circle, and 1.0000 is a line, Chiron's eccentricity is

0.3786. Formerly, Pluto's orbit was the most eccentric, at 0.2482; before its discovery, Mercury's orbit showed the greatest eccentricity, at 0.2056.[2]

Orbital Inclination
6.9° to the ecliptic.

Positions of North Node

8 September 1856	0° Scorpio
16 November 1881	29° Libra 45'
25 January 1907	29° Libra
3 April 1932	29° Libra
11 June 1957	28° Libra 30'
19 August 1962	28° Libra 45'

Chiron's North Node will remain around this degree throughout the rest of this century. It will conjunct its own Nodal Position in December 1996.[3]

Perihelion and Aphelion
At perihelion, Chiron is 1.27 billion kilometres (8.5 AU) distant from the Sun, and situated between Saturn and Jupiter, having crossed Saturn's orbit on its way. At aphelion, Chiron is 2.8 billion kilometres from the Sun (18.9 AU).[4]

Dates for This Century[5]

2 June 1920	aphelion
29 August 1945	perihelion
7 December 1970	aphelion
14 February 1996	perihelion

Appendix 2

Details and Sources of Astrological Data Used

The Rodden ratings of data accuracy are included in brackets. Koch house cusps are used throughout, rounded up to the next degree.

Abbreviations for Sources

AA – The Data Bank of the Astrological Association, UK
Am. Bk. – Rodden, Lois M., *The American Book of Charts*
BWH – Campion, Nicholas, *The Book of World Horoscopes*
MR – my own files
SS – Jones, Marc Edmund, *Sabian Symbols*

ATKINS, Susan Denise (A) (p. 190)
    7.5.1948; 1.03 am PDT; San Gabriel, California.
    Source: AA.

BERNADETTE OF LOURDES (Marie-Bernarde Soubirous)
(A) (p. 281)
    7.1.1844; 2.00 pm LMT; Lourdes, France.
    Vision: 11.2.1858; time unknown, noon used.
    Death: 16.4.1879; time unknown, noon used.
    Canonized 1933.
    Source: AA.

FREUD, Sigmund (A) (p. 255)
    6.5.1856; 6.30 pm LMT; Freiberg, Moravia (now Pribor, Czechoslovakia).
    Source: Am. Bk.

HEISENBERG, Werner (C) (p. 115)
5.12.1901; 4.45 am MET; Würzburg, Germany.
Source: AA.

HOFMANN, Albert (A) (p. 336)
11.1.1906; 3.00 pm CET; Baden, Switzerland.
Source: MR (letter from Hofmann to myself). Chart used with permission.

JONES, Jim (A) (p. 308)
13.5.1931; 10.00 pm CST; Lynn, Indiana.
Source: AA.

KING, Martin Luther (DD) (p. 247)
15.1.1929; 11.21 am CST; Atlanta, Georgia.
Source: AA. Of the alternative charts listed I have used the one rectified by Jim Lewis (Astrocartography). My thanks to Chester Kemp who helped me check it.

LA BARRE, Christina (A) (p. 344)
22.12.1943; 8.15 pm EDT; New York City.
Source: MR. Chart used with permission.

LAWRENCE, David Herbert (A) (p. 63)
11.9.1885; 9.45 am GMT; Eastwood, Nottingham.
Source: AA.

LEARY, Timothy (A) (p. 338)
22.10.1920; 10.45 am EDT; Springfield, Massachusetts.
Source: AA.

MANSON, Charles (A) (p. 197)
12.11.1934; 4.40 pm EST; Cincinnati, Ohio.
Source: AA.

PLAYER, Ian (A) (p. 328)
15.3.1927; 6.35 am EET (rectified); Johannesburg, South Africa.
Source: MR. Chart used with permission.

NATIONAL HEALTH SERVICE (p. 305)
5.7.48; 12.00 pm BST; London.
Source: AA.

RHODES, Cecil John (DD) (p. 216)
5.7.1853; 7.00 pm LMT; Bishops Stortford, Hertfordshire.
Source: AA.

RHODESIA (Unilateral Declaration of Independence) (A) (p. 180)
11.11.1965; 11.00 am EET; Salisbury (now Harare).
Source: MR (noted down from radio broadcast 11.11.1965).

'SARA' (A) (p. 290)
5.9.1947; 10.05 pm BST; Glasgow, Scotland.
Source: MR (from client herself). Chart used with permission.

SOUTH AFRICA (Republic) (p. 322)
31.5.1961; midnight EET; Pretoria.
Source: BWH.

SOUTH AFRICA (Union) (p. 320)
31.5.1961; midnight EET; Cape Town.
Source: BWH. Union was instituted at midnight, although the oath was signed at noon on the same day.

VAN DER POST, Laurens (A) (p. 165)
13.12.1906; 2.00 am EET; Philippolis, South Africa.
Source: AA.

WORLD WILDERNESS CONGRESS (beginning of inaugural lecture) (A) (p. 332)
24.10.77; 9.00 am EET; Johannesburg, South Africa.
Source: MR (letter from Ian Player to myself).

Appendix 3 · Ephemeris of Chiron
1900—2030

The ephemeris for the years 1900–2000 was computed by James Neely and Eric Tarkington utilizing a set of orbital elements published by Brian Marsden of the Smithsonian Astrophysical Laboratory, Cambridge, Massachusetts. The information was originally published in 1978 in the Monograph Series of Phenomena Publications, Toronto, Canada.

The ephemeris listing for the years 2001–2030 was calculated by the Solar Fire™ astrological program (further information available from Esoteric Technologies Pty Ltd, Adelaide, Australia, via the Internet at: http://www.esotech.com.au/).

Notes
  i) Astrological longitude only is listed. For any other information, you will need to consult a more detailed ephemeris.
 ii) Stations are listed at the end of each year.
iii) All positions are for midnight.

1900

Date		Long.
Jan	1	18SA55
	11	20SA00
	21	21SA02
	31	21SA58
Feb	10	22SA49
	20	23SA32
Mar	2	24SA07
	12	24SA34
	22	24SA52
Apr	1	25SA00
	11	24SA58
	21	24SA48
May	1	24SA28
	11	24SA02
	21	23SA28
	31	22SA51
Jun	10	22SA11
	20	21SA30
	30	20SA51
Jul	10	20SA15
	20	19SA44
	30	19SA20
Aug	9	19SA04
	19	18SA56
	29	18SA57
Sep	8	19SA08
	18	19SA27
	28	19SA54
Oct	8	20SA30
	18	21SA13
	28	22SA01
Nov	7	22SA56
	17	23SA54
	27	24SA56
Dec	7	26SA01
	17	27SA06
	27	28SA12

Stations	Date	
Retrograde	Apr	4
Direct	Aug	22

1901

Date		Long.
Jan	6	29SA17
	16	00CP19
	26	01CP18
Feb	5	02CP14
	15	03CP03
	25	03CP47
Mar	7	04CP24
	17	04CP53
	27	05CP13
Apr	6	05CP25
	16	05CP28
	26	05CP22
May	6	05CP08
	16	04CP46
	26	04CP17
Jun	5	03CP44
	15	03CP06
	25	02CP27
Jul	5	01CP48
	15	01CP12
	25	00CP39
Aug	4	00CP11
	14	29SA50
	24	29SA37
Sep	3	29SA32
	13	29SA35
	23	29SA47
Oct	3	00CP08
	13	00CP36
	23	01CP11
Nov	2	01CP53
	12	02CP41
	22	03CP33
Dec	2	04CP29
	12	05CP28
	22	06CP29

Stations	Date	
Retrograde	Apr	14
Direct	Sep	3

1902

Date		Long.
Jan	1	07CP30
	11	08CP31
	21	09CP30
	31	10CP27
Feb	10	11CP20
	20	12CP09
Mar	2	12CP52
	12	13CP29
	22	13CP58
Apr	1	14CP21
	11	14CP35
	21	14CP40
May	1	14CP38
	11	14CP27
	21	14CP09
	31	13CP44
Jun	10	13CP14
	20	12CP39
	30	12CP02
Jul	10	11CP25
	20	10CP48
	30	10CP15
Aug	9	09CP45
	19	09CP21
	29	09CP04
Sep	8	08CP55
	18	08CP53
	28	09CP00
Oct	8	09CP15
	18	09CP37
	28	10CP06
Nov	7	10CP43
	17	11CP25
	27	12CP12
Dec	7	13CP03
	17	13CP57
	27	14CP53

Stations	Date	
Retrograde	Apr	22
Direct	Sep	14

1903

Date		Long.
Jan	6	15CP50
	16	16CP47
	26	17CP43
Feb	5	18CP37
	15	19CP28
	25	20CP15
Mar	7	20CP57
	17	21CP34
	27	22CP04
Apr	6	22CP26
	16	22CP42
	26	22CP49
May	6	22CP49
	16	22CP41
	26	22CP25
Jun	5	22CP03
	15	21CP36
	25	21CP04
Jul	5	20CP29
	15	19CP53
	25	19CP17
Aug	4	18CP44
	14	18CP14
	24	17CP48
Sep	3	17CP29
	13	17CP16
	23	17CP11
Oct	3	17CP14
	13	17CP24
	23	17CP42
Nov	2	18CP07
	12	18CP39
	22	19CP16
Dec	2	19CP59
	12	20CP45
	22	21CP35

Stations	Date	
Retrograde	Apr	30
Direct	Sep	24

1904		1905	
Date	**Long.**	**Date**	**Long.**
Jan 1	22CP27	Jan 5	29CP20
11	23CP21	15	00AQ11
21	24CP15	25	01AQ02
31	25CP08	Feb 4	01AQ52
Feb 10	25CP59	14	02AQ41
20	26CP48	24	03AQ28
Mar 1	27CP33	Mar 6	04AQ11
11	28CP14	16	04AQ50
21	28CP49	26	05AQ25
31	29CP19	Apr 5	05AQ53
Apr 10	29CP42	15	06AQ16
20	29CP58	25	06AQ32
30	00AQ06	May 5	06AQ41
May 10	00AQ07	15	06AQ43
20	00AQ01	25	06AQ38
30	29CP48	Jun 4	06AQ26
Jun 9	29CP28	14	06AQ08
19	29CP03	24	05AQ45
29	28CP33	Jul 4	05AQ17
Jul 9	28CP00	14	04AQ45
19	27CP26	24	04AQ12
29	26CP51	Aug 3	03AQ39
Aug 8	26CP18	13	03AQ06
18	25CP47	23	02AQ36
28	25CP21	Sep 2	02AQ09
Sep 7	25CP00	12	01AQ48
17	24CP46	22	01AQ32
27	24CP38	Oct 2	01AQ23
Oct 7	24CP38	12	01AQ21
17	24CP45	22	01AQ26
27	25CP00	Nov 1	01AQ38
Nov 6	25CP21	11	01AQ56
16	25CP49	21	02AQ21
26	26CP23	Dec 1	02AQ52
Dec 6	27CP02	11	03AQ28
16	27CP45	21	04AQ08
26	28CP31	31	04AQ52

Stations	Date	Stations	Date
Retrograde	May 6	Retrograde	May 12
Direct	Oct 2	Direct	Oct 10

1906

Date		Long.
Jan	10	05AQ38
	20	06AQ26
	30	07AQ14
Feb	9	08AQ02
	19	08AQ49
Mar	1	09AQ34
	11	10AQ15
	21	10AQ53
	31	11AQ26
Apr	10	11AQ54
	20	12AQ16
	30	12AQ32
May	10	12AQ41
	20	12AQ44
	30	12AQ39
Jun	9	12AQ29
	19	12AQ12
	29	11AQ50
Jul	9	11AQ23
	19	10AQ53
	29	10AQ21
Aug	8	09AQ48
	18	09AQ17
	28	08AQ47
Sep	7	08AQ20
	17	07AQ59
	27	07AQ42
Oct	7	07AQ32
	17	07AQ28
	27	07AQ32
Nov	6	07AQ42
	16	07AQ59
	26	08AQ21
Dec	6	08AQ50
	16	09AQ24
	26	10AQ01

Stations	Date
Retrograde	May 18
Direct	Oct 17

1907

Date		Long.
Jan	5	10AQ43
	15	11AQ26
	25	12AQ12
Feb	4	12AQ58
	14	13AQ44
	24	14AQ29
Mar	6	15AQ12
	16	15AQ52
	26	16AQ28
Apr	5	17AQ00
	15	17AQ27
	25	17AQ48
May	5	18AQ04
	15	18AQ13
	25	18AQ16
Jun	4	18AQ12
	14	18AQ02
	24	17AQ46
Jul	4	17AQ24
	14	16AQ59
	24	16AQ30
Aug	3	15AQ59
	13	15AQ27
	23	14AQ56
Sep	2	14AQ27
	12	14AQ01
	22	13AQ39
Oct	2	13AQ22
	12	13AQ11
	22	13AQ07
Nov	1	13AQ09
	11	13AQ18
	21	13AQ33
Dec	1	13AQ54
	11	14AQ21
	21	14AQ53
	31	15AQ29

Stations	Date
Retrograde	May 24
Direct	Oct 23

1908		1909	
Date	**Long.**	**Date**	**Long.**
Jan 10	16AQ08	Jan 4	20AQ35
20	16AQ50	14	21AQ13
30	17AQ33	24	21AQ53
Feb 9	18AQ18	Feb 3	22AQ35
19	19AQ02	13	23AQ17
29	19AQ45	23	24AQ00
Mar 10	20AQ26	Mar 5	24AQ41
20	21AQ05	15	25AQ21
30	21AQ40	25	25AQ58
Apr 9	22AQ10	Apr 4	26AQ32
19	22AQ36	14	27AQ02
29	22AQ57	24	27AQ27
May 9	23AQ12	May 4	27AQ47
19	23AQ21	14	28AQ01
29	23AQ24	24	28AQ09
Jun 8	23AQ20	Jun 3	28AQ12
18	23AQ10	13	28AQ08
28	22AQ55	23	27AQ59
Jul 8	22AQ34	Jul 3	27AQ44
18	22AQ10	13	27AQ24
28	21AQ42	23	27AQ00
Aug 7	21AQ12	Aug 2	26AQ32
17	20AQ41	12	26AQ03
27	20AQ10	22	25AQ33
Sep 6	19AQ41	Sep 1	25AQ03
16	19AQ16	11	24AQ35
26	18AQ54	21	24AQ10
Oct 6	18AQ37	Oct 1	23AQ48
16	18AQ26	11	23AQ32
26	18AQ21	21	23AQ20
Nov 5	18AQ23	31	23AQ15
15	18AQ31	Nov 10	23AQ16
25	18AQ45	20	23AQ24
Dec 5	19AQ05	30	23AQ37
15	19AQ30	Dec 10	23AQ56
25	20AQ01	20	24AQ21
		30	24AQ50

Stations	**Date**	**Stations**	**Date**
Retrograde	May 28	Retrograde	Jun 1
Direct	Oct 28	Direct	Nov 3

1910

Date		Long.
Jan	9	25AQ23
	19	26AQ00
	29	26AQ38
Feb	8	27AQ19
	18	28AQ00
	28	28AQ41
Mar	10	29AQ21
	20	00PI00
	30	00PI35
Apr	9	01PI08
	19	01PI37
	29	02PI01
May	9	02PI20
	19	02PI34
	29	02PI42
Jun	8	02PI44
	18	02PI40
	28	02PI30
Jul	8	02PI16
	18	01PI56
	28	01PI32
Aug	7	01PI06
	17	00PI37
	27	00PI07
Sep	6	29AQ38
	16	29AQ11
	26	28AQ46
Oct	6	28AQ25
	16	28AQ09
	26	27AQ58
Nov	5	27AQ52
	15	27AQ53
	25	28AQ00
Dec	5	28AQ13
	15	28AQ32
	25	28AQ55

Stations	Date
Retrograde	Jun 6
Direct	Nov 8

1911

Date		Long.
Jan	4	29AQ24
	14	29AQ56
	24	00PI31
Feb	3	01PI09
	13	01PI48
	23	02PI28
Mar	5	03PI08
	15	03PI47
	25	04PI24
Apr	4	04PI59
	14	05PI31
	24	05PI58
May	4	06PI22
	14	06PI40
	24	06PI53
Jun	3	07PI00
	13	07PI02
	23	06PI58
Jul	3	06PI48
	13	06PI34
	23	06PI14
Aug	2	05PI51
	12	05PI25
	22	04PI56
Sep	1	04PI27
	11	03PI59
	21	03PI32
Oct	1	03PI08
	11	02PI47
	21	02PI31
	31	02PI20
Nov	10	02PI15
	20	02PI16
	30	02PI23
Dec	10	02PI36
	20	02PI54
	30	03PI17

Stations	Date
Retrograde	Jun 10
Direct	Nov 13

1912

Date		Long.
Jan	9	03PI45
	19	04PI16
	29	04PI51
Feb	8	05PI28
	18	06PI06
	28	06PI45
Mar	9	07PI24
	19	08PI02
	29	08PI38
Apr	8	09PI12
	18	09PI42
	28	10PI09
May	8	10PI31
	18	10PI49
	28	11PI01
Jun	7	11PI08
	17	11PI09
	27	11PI05
Jul	7	10PI55
	17	10PI40
	27	10PI21
Aug	6	09PI58
	16	09PI32
	26	09PI04
Sep	5	08PI35
	15	08PI07
	25	07PI41
Oct	5	07PI17
	15	06PI57
	25	06PI41
Nov	4	06PI31
	14	06PI26
	24	06PI27
Dec	4	06PI34
	14	06PI47
	24	07PI05

Stations	Date	
Retrograde	Jun	14
Direct	Nov	17

1913

Date		Long.
Jan	3	07PI28
	13	07PI55
	23	08PI26
Feb	2	09PI00
	12	09PI36
	22	10PI14
Mar	4	10PI52
	14	11PI30
	24	12PI07
Apr	3	12PI42
	13	13PI15
	23	13PI44
May	3	14PI10
	13	14PI32
	23	14PI48
Jun	2	15PI00
	12	15PI06
	22	15PI07
Jul	2	15PI02
	12	14PI52
	22	14PI37
Aug	1	14PI18
	11	13PI55
	21	13PI29
	31	13PI02
Sep	10	12PI33
	20	12PI06
	30	11PI40
Oct	10	11PI17
	20	10PI57
	30	10PI42
Nov	9	10PI32
	19	10PI27
	29	10PI29
Dec	9	10PI36
	19	10PI49
	29	11PI07

Stations	Date	
Retrograde	Jun	18
Direct	Nov	21

1914

Date		Long.
Jan	8	11Pl29
	18	11Pl56
	28	12Pl27
Feb	7	13Pl01
	17	13Pl36
	27	14Pl13
Mar	9	14Pl50
	19	15Pl28
	29	16Pl04
Apr	8	16Pl38
	18	17Pl10
	28	17Pl39
May	8	18Pl03
	18	18Pl24
	28	18Pl40
Jun	7	18Pl51
	17	18Pl57
	27	18Pl57
Jul	7	18Pl52
	17	18Pl41
	27	18Pl26
Aug	6	18Pl07
	16	17Pl44
	26	17Pl18
Sep	5	16Pl51
	15	16Pl23
	25	15Pl56
Oct	5	15Pl30
	15	15Pl08
	25	14Pl49
Nov	4	14Pl34
	14	14Pl25
	24	14Pl21
Dec	4	14Pl22
	14	14Pl30
	24	14Pl43

Stations	Date
Retrograde	Jun 22
Direct	Nov 26

1915

Date		Long.
Jan	3	15Pl01
	13	15Pl23
	23	15Pl50
Feb	2	16Pl21
	12	16Pl54
	22	17Pl29
Mar	4	18Pl05
	14	18Pl42
	24	19Pl19
Apr	3	19Pl54
	13	20Pl28
	23	20Pl59
May	3	21Pl26
	13	21Pl51
	23	22Pl11
Jun	2	22Pl26
	12	22Pl36
	22	22Pl41
Jul	2	22Pl41
	12	22Pl35
	22	22Pl24
Aug	1	22Pl09
	11	21Pl49
	21	21Pl26
	31	21Pl01
Sep	10	20Pl34
	20	20Pl06
	30	19Pl39
Oct	10	19Pl14
	20	18Pl52
	30	18Pl33
Nov	9	18Pl19
	19	18Pl10
	29	18Pl07
Dec	9	18Pl09
	19	18Pl17
	29	18Pl30

Stations	Date
Retrograde	Jun 26
Direct	Nov 30

1916

Date	Long.
Jan 8	18PI48
18	19PI11
28	19PI38
Feb 7	20PI08
17	20PI41
27	21PI16
Mar 8	21PI52
18	22PI28
28	23PI04
Apr 7	23PI39
17	24PI12
27	24PI42
May 7	25PI09
17	25PI33
27	25PI52
Jun 6	26PI07
16	26PI16
26	26PI21
Jul 6	26PI20
16	26PI14
26	26PI02
Aug 5	25PI47
15	25PI27
25	25PI04
Sep 4	24PI38
14	24PI11
24	23PI44
Oct 4	23PI17
14	22PI52
24	22PI31
Nov 3	22PI13
13	21PI59
23	21PI51
Dec 3	21PI48
13	21PI50
23	21PI59

Stations	Date
Retrograde	Jun 29
Direct	Dec 3

1917

Date	Long.
Jan 2	22PI12
12	22PI31
22	22PI54
Feb 1	23PI21
11	23PI51
21	24PI24
Mar 3	24PI58
13	25PI34
23	26PI10
Apr 2	26PI45
12	27PI20
22	27PI52
May 2	28PI22
12	28PI48
22	29PI11
Jun 1	29PI29
11	29PI43
21	29PI52
Jul 1	29PI56
11	29PI55
21	29PI48
31	29PI36
Aug 10	29PI20
20	29PI00
30	28PI37
Sep 9	28PI11
19	27PI44
29	27PI17
Oct 9	26PI51
19	26PI26
29	26PI05
Nov 8	25PI47
18	25PI35
28	25PI27
Dec 8	25PI24
18	25PI28
28	25PI36

Stations	Date
Retrograde	Jul 3
Direct	Dec 7

1918			1919		
Date		**Long.**	**Date**		**Long.**
Jan	7	25PI50	Jan	2	29PI11
	17	26PI09		12	29PI25
	27	26PI33		22	29PI45
Feb	6	27PI00	Feb	1	00AR08
	16	27PI30		11	00AR36
	26	28PI03		21	01AR06
Mar	8	28PI37	Mar	3	01AR39
	18	29PI13		13	02AR13
	28	29PI48		23	02AR49
Apr	7	00AR23	Apr	2	03AR24
	17	00AR57		12	03AR59
	27	01AR29		22	04AR32
May	7	01AR58	May	2	05AR03
	17	02AR24		12	05AR32
	27	02AR46		22	05AR57
Jun	6	03AR04	Jun	1	06AR19
	16	03AR17		11	06AR36
	26	03AR25		21	06AR49
Jul	6	03AR29	Jul	1	06AR57
	16	03AR26		11	06AR59
	26	03AR19		21	06AR56
Aug	5	03AR07		31	06AR49
	15	02AR50	Aug	10	06AR36
	25	02AR30		20	06AR19
Sep	4	02AR07		30	05AR58
	14	01AR41	Sep	9	05AR34
	24	01AR14		19	05AR08
Oct	4	00AR47		29	04AR41
	14	00AR21	Oct	9	04AR14
	24	29PI57		19	03AR49
Nov	3	29PI36		29	03AR25
	13	29PI19	Nov	8	03AR05
	23	29PI07		18	02AR48
Dec	3	28PI59		28	02AR36
	13	28PI58	Dec	8	02AR30
	23	29PI02		18	02AR29
				28	02AR33

Stations	**Date**		**Stations**	**Date**	
Retrograde	Jul	6	Retrograde	Jul	10
Direct	Dec	11	Direct	Dec	14

1920			1921		
Date		**Long.**	**Date**		**Long.**
Jan	7	02AR43	Jan	1	06AR04
	17	02AR58		11	06AR14
	27	03AR18		21	06AR30
Feb	6	03AR42		31	06AR51
	16	04AR10	Feb	10	07AR15
	26	04AR41		20	07AR43
Mar	7	05AR13	Mar	2	08AR14
	17	05AR48		12	08AR47
	27	06AR23		22	09AR22
Apr	6	06AR58	Apr	1	09AR57
	16	07AR33		11	10AR32
	26	08AR06		21	11AR07
May	6	08AR37	May	1	11AR39
	16	09AR05		11	12AR10
	26	09AR30		21	12AR38
Jun	5	09AR51		31	13AR02
	15	10AR08	Jun	10	13AR23
	25	10AR20		20	13AR39
Jul	5	10AR27		30	13AR51
	15	10AR29	Jul	10	13AR57
	25	10AR25		20	13AR59
Aug	4	10AR17		30	13AR55
	14	10AR04	Aug	9	13AR46
	24	09AR46		19	13AR32
Sep	3	09AR25		29	13AR14
	13	09AR01	Sep	8	12AR52
	23	08AR35		18	12AR28
Oct	3	08AR08		28	12AR02
	13	07AR41	Oct	8	11AR34
	23	07AR15		18	11AR08
Nov	2	06AR52		28	10AR42
	12	06AR32	Nov	7	10AR19
	22	06AR16		17	09AR59
Dec	2	06AR05		27	09AR44
	12	05AR59	Dec	7	09AR34
	22	05AR59		17	09AR28
				27	09AR29

Stations	Date		Stations	Date	
Retrograde	Jul	13	Retrograde	Jul	17
Direct	Dec	17	Direct	Dec	21

1922   1923

Date	Long.		Date	Long.
Jan 6	09AR35		Jan 1	13AR00
16	09AR46		11	13AR06
26	10AR02		21	13AR18
Feb 5	10AR23		31	13AR35
15	10AR48		Feb 10	13AR57
25	11AR17		20	14AR23
Mar 7	11AR48		Mar 2	14AR52
17	12AR21		12	15AR23
27	12AR56		22	15AR57
Apr 6	13AR32		Apr 1	16AR32
16	14AR07		11	17AR08
26	14AR41		21	17AR43
May 6	15AR14		May 1	18AR17
16	15AR44		11	18AR50
26	16AR12		21	19AR20
Jun 5	16AR36		31	19AR48
15	16AR56		Jun 10	20AR12
25	17AR12		20	20AR31
Jul 5	17AR23		30	20AR47
15	17AR29		Jul 10	20AR57
25	17AR30		20	21AR03
Aug 4	17AR25		30	21AR03
14	17AR16		Aug 09	20AR58
24	17AR01		19	20AR48
Sep 3	16AR43		29	20AR33
13	16AR21		Sep 08	20AR14
23	15AR56		18	19AR52
Oct 3	15AR29		28	19AR26
13	15AR02		Oct 08	18AR59
23	14AR35		18	18AR32
Nov 2	14AR10		28	18AR05
12	13AR47		Nov 07	17AR40
22	13AR28		17	17AR17
Dec 2	13AR13		27	16AR58
12	13AR03		Dec 07	16AR44
22	12AR59		17	16AR35
			27	16AR31

Stations	Date		Stations	Date
Retrograde	Jul 21		Retrograde	Jul 25
Direct	Dec 25		Direct	Dec 28

1924

Date		Long.
Jan	6	16AR33
	16	16AR40
	26	16AR53
Feb	5	17AR10
	15	17AR33
	25	17AR59
Mar	6	18AR29
	16	19AR01
	26	19AR35
Apr	5	20AR11
	15	20AR46
	25	21AR22
May	5	21AR56
	15	22AR29
	25	22AR59
Jun	4	23AR27
	14	23AR50
	24	24AR10
Jul	4	24AR25
	14	24AR35
	24	24AR40
Aug	3	24AR40
	13	24AR35
	23	24AR24
Sep	2	24AR09
	12	23AR49
	22	23AR26
Oct	2	23AR00
	12	22AR33
	22	22AR05
Nov	1	21AR38
	11	21AR13
	21	20AR51
Dec	1	20AR32
	11	20AR18
	21	20AR10
	31	20AR06

Stations	Date
Retrograde	Jul 28
Direct	Dec 31

1925

Date		Long.
Jan	10	20AR09
	20	20AR17
	30	20AR31
Feb	9	20AR49
	19	21AR12
Mar	1	21AR39
	11	22AR09
	21	22AR42
	31	23AR17
Apr	10	23AR53
	20	24AR29
	30	25AR05
May	10	25AR39
	20	26AR12
	30	26AR42
Jun	9	27AR10
	19	27AR33
	29	27AR53
Jul	9	28AR08
	19	28AR18
	29	28AR22
Aug	8	28AR22
	18	28AR16
	28	28AR05
Sep	7	27AR49
	17	27AR29
	27	27AR05
Oct	7	26AR39
	17	26AR11
	27	25AR43
Nov	6	25AR16
	16	24AR51
	26	24AR29
Dec	6	24AR10
	16	23AR57
	26	23AR49

Stations	Date
Retrograde	Aug 1

1926			1927	

Date		Long.	Date		Long.
Jan	5	23AR46	Jan	10	27AR32
	15	23AR50		20	27AR36
	25	23AR58		30	27AR46
Feb	4	24AR13	Feb	9	28AR01
	14	24AR32		19	28AR21
	24	24AR56	Mar	1	28AR46
Mar	6	25AR24		11	29AR14
	16	25AR55		21	29AR46
	26	26AR28		31	00TA20
Apr	5	27AR03	Apr	10	00TA56
	15	27AR40		20	01TA33
	25	28AR16		30	02TA10
May	5	28AR52	May	10	02TA47
	15	29AR27		20	03TA22
	25	00TA01		30	03TA56
Jun	4	00TA31	Jun	9	04TA27
	14	00TA59		19	04TA54
	24	01TA22		29	05TA18
Jul	4	01TA42	Jul	9	05TA38
	14	01TA57		19	05TA52
	24	02TA06		29	06TA02
Aug	3	02TA11	Aug	8	06TA06
	13	02TA10		18	06TA05
	23	02TA03		28	05TA58
Sep	2	01TA51	Sep	7	05TA46
	12	01TA35		17	05TA29
	22	01TA14		27	05TA08
Oct	2	00TA50	Oct	7	04TA43
	12	00TA24		17	04TA16
	22	29AR55		27	03TA47
Nov	1	29AR27	Nov	6	03TA19
	11	29AR00		16	02TA51
	21	28AR35		26	02TA26
Dec	1	28AR13	Dec	6	02TA04
	11	27AR55		16	01TA46
	21	27AR42		26	01TA33
	31	27AR34			

Stations	Date		Stations	Date	
Direct	Jan	4	Direct	Jan	8
Retrograde	Aug	6	Retrograde	Aug	10

1928

Date		Long.
Jan	5	01TA26
	15	01TA25
	25	01TA29
Feb	4	01TA40
	14	01TA56
	24	02TA17
Mar	5	02TA42
	15	03TA12
	25	03TA44
Apr	4	04TA19
	14	04TA56
	24	05TA34
May	4	06TA12
	14	06TA49
	24	07TA25
Jun	3	07TA59
	13	08TA30
	23	08TA58
Jul	3	09TA23
	13	09TA42
	23	09TA57
Aug	2	10TA07
	12	10TA11
	22	10TA09
Sep	1	10TA02
	11	09TA50
	21	09TA32
Oct	1	09TA10
	11	08TA45
	21	08TA17
	31	07TA48
Nov	10	07TA19
	20	06TA51
	30	06TA26
Dec	10	06TA03
	20	05TA46
	30	05TA33

Stations	Date
Direct	Jan 12
Retrograde	Aug 14

1929

Date		Long.
Jan	9	05TA27
	19	05TA26
	29	05TA31
Feb	8	05TA42
	18	05TA59
	28	06TA21
Mar	10	06TA47
	20	07TA18
	30	07TA51
Apr	9	08TA27
	19	09TA05
	29	09TA43
May	9	10TA22
	19	11TA00
	29	11TA37
Jun	8	12TA12
	18	12TA44
	28	13TA13
Jul	8	13TA37
	18	13TA57
	28	14TA13
Aug	7	14TA22
	17	14TA26
	27	14TA25
Sep	6	14TA17
	16	14TA04
	26	13TA47
Oct	6	13TA24
	16	12TA58
	26	12TA30
Nov	5	12TA00
	15	11TA30
	25	11TA02
Dec	5	10TA36
	15	10TA14
	25	09TA56

Stations	Date
Direct	Jan 15
Retrograde	Aug 19

1930

Date		Long.
Jan	4	09TA44
	14	09TA38
	24	09TA37
Feb	3	09TA43
	13	09TA55
	23	10TA13
Mar	5	10TA36
	15	11TA03
	25	11TA34
Apr	4	12TA09
	14	12TA46
	24	13TA24
May	4	14TA04
	14	14TA44
	24	15TA23
Jun	3	16TA01
	13	16TA36
	23	17TA09
Jul	3	17TA39
	13	18TA04
	23	18TA25
Aug	2	18TA40
	12	18TA50
	22	18TA55
Sep	1	18TA53
	11	18TA46
	21	18TA33
Oct	1	18TA14
	11	17TA51
	21	17TA25
	31	16TA56
Nov	10	16TA25
	20	15TA55
	30	15TA26
Dec	10	15TA00
	20	14TA37
	30	14TA19

Stations	Date	
Direct	Jan	19
Retrograde	Aug	24

1931

Date		Long.
Jan	9	14TA07
	19	14TA01
	29	14TA01
Feb	8	14TA08
	18	14TA20
	28	14TA39
Mar	10	15TA02
	20	15TA31
	30	16TA03
Apr	9	16TA38
	19	17TA17
	29	17TA56
May	9	18TA37
	19	19TA18
	29	19TA58
Jun	8	20TA37
	18	21TA14
	28	21TA48
Jul	8	22TA19
	18	22TA45
	28	23TA07
Aug	7	23TA23
	17	23TA34
	27	23TA38
Sep	6	23TA37
	16	23TA30
	26	23TA16
Oct	6	22TA58
	16	22TA34
	26	22TA07
Nov	5	21TA37
	15	21TA06
	25	20TA35
Dec	5	20TA05
	15	19TA38
	25	19TA15

Stations	Date	
Direct	Jan	23
Retrograde	Aug	29

1932

Date		Long.
Jan	4	18TA57
	14	18TA45
	24	18TA39
Feb	3	18TA39
	13	18TA46
	23	19TA00
Mar	4	19TA19
	14	19TA43
	24	20TA13
Apr	3	20TA46
	13	21TA23
	23	22TA02
May	3	22TA44
	13	23TA26
	23	24TA08
Jun	2	24TA50
	12	25TA30
	22	26TA09
Jul	2	26TA44
	12	27TA16
	22	27TA43
Aug	1	28TA06
	11	28TA23
	21	28TA35
	31	28TA40
Sep	10	28TA40
	20	28TA32
	30	28TA19
Oct	10	28TA00
	20	27TA36
	30	27TA08
Nov	9	26TA38
	19	26TA06
	29	25TA34
Dec	9	25TA03
	19	24TA36
	29	24TA12

Stations	Date	
Direct	Jan	28
Retrograde	Sep	3

1933

Date		Long.
Jan	8	23TA53
	18	23TA41
	28	23TA35
Feb	7	23TA35
	17	23TA43
	27	23TA56
Mar	9	24TA16
	19	24TA42
	29	25TA12
Apr	8	25TA47
	18	26TA25
	28	27TA06
May	8	27TA49
	18	28TA33
	28	29TA17
Jun	7	00GE00
	17	00GE42
	27	01GE22
Jul	7	01GE59
	17	02GE33
	27	03GE02
Aug	6	03GE26
	16	03GE45
	26	03GE58
Sep	5	04GE04
	15	04GE04
	25	03GE58
Oct	5	03GE44
	15	03GE26
	25	03GE01
Nov	4	02GE33
	14	02GE02
	24	01GE29
Dec	4	00GE56
	14	00GE24
	24	29TA55

Stations	Date	
Direct	Feb	1
Retrograde	Sep	9

1934

Date		Long.
Jan	3	29TA31
	13	29TA11
	23	28TA58
Feb	2	28TA52
	12	28TA53
	22	29TA00
Mar	4	29TA14
	14	29TA35
	24	00GE01
Apr	3	00GE33
	13	01GE09
	23	01GE49
May	3	02GE31
	13	03GE15
	23	04GE01
Jun	2	04GE47
	12	05GE33
	22	06GE17
Jul	2	06GE59
	12	07GE38
	22	08GE14
Aug	1	08GE45
	11	09GE12
	21	09GE32
	31	09GE47
Sep	10	09GE55
	20	09GE56
	30	09GE50
Oct	10	09GE37
	20	09GE19
	30	08GE54
Nov	9	08GE26
	19	07GE53
	29	07GE19
Dec	9	06GE45
	19	06GE12
	29	05GE42

Stations	Date	
Direct	Feb	6
Retrograde	Sep	16

1935

Date		Long.
Jan	8	05GE17
	18	04GE56
	28	04GE42
Feb	7	04GE35
	17	04GE36
	27	04GE43
Mar	9	04GE58
	19	05GE19
	29	05GE46
Apr	8	06GE19
	18	06GE56
	28	07GE37
May	8	08GE22
	18	09GE08
	28	09GE56
Jun	7	10GE44
	17	11GE32
	27	12GE19
Jul	7	13GE03
	17	13GE45
	27	14GE24
Aug	6	14GE58
	16	15GE27
	26	15GE50
Sep	5	16GE06
	15	16GE16
	25	16GE19
Oct	5	16GE15
	15	16GE04
	25	15GE46
Nov	4	15GE21
	14	14GE52
	24	14GE19
Dec	4	13GE44
	14	13GE09
	24	12GE34

Stations	Date	
Direct	Feb	11
Retrograde	Sep	24

1936

Date	Long.
Jan 3	12GE03
13	11GE35
23	11GE14
Feb 2	10GE59
12	10GE51
22	10GE50
Mar 3	10GE58
13	11GE12
23	11GE34
Apr 2	12GE02
12	12GE35
22	13GE14
May 2	13GE57
12	14GE43
22	15GE32
Jun 1	16GE22
11	17GE13
21	18GE03
Jul 1	18GE53
11	19GE41
21	20GE26
31	21GE08
Aug 10	21GE45
20	22GE17
30	22GE44
Sep 9	23GE04
19	23GE17
29	23GE22
Oct 9	23GE20
19	23GE10
29	22GE53
Nov 8	22GE30
18	22GE01
28	21GE27
Dec 8	20GE51
18	20GE14
28	19GE38

Stations	Date
Direct	Feb 17
Retrograde	Oct 1

1937

Date	Long.
Jan 7	19GE04
17	18GE35
27	18GE12
Feb 6	17GE55
16	17GE45
26	17GE44
Mar 8	17GE50
18	18GE04
28	18GE26
Apr 7	18GE55
17	19GE29
27	20GE09
May 7	20GE54
17	21GE42
27	22GE33
Jun 6	23GE26
16	24GE20
26	25GE14
Jul 6	26GE07
16	26GE58
26	27GE48
Aug 5	28GE33
15	29GE15
25	29GE51
Sep 4	00CN22
14	00CN46
24	01CN02
Oct 4	01CN12
14	01CN13
24	01CN05
Nov 3	00CN51
13	00CN28
23	00CN00
Dec 3	29GE27
13	28GE50
23	28GE11

Stations	Date
Direct	Feb 22
Retrograde	Oct 10

1938

Date		Long.
Jan	2	27GE33
	12	26GE57
	22	26GE25
Feb	1	25GE59
	11	25GE40
	21	25GE28
Mar	3	25GE25
	13	25GE30
	23	25GE43
Apr	2	26GE05
	12	26GE33
	22	27GE08
May	2	27GE49
	12	28GE36
	22	29GE26
Jun	1	00CN19
	11	01CN15
	21	02CN12
Jul	1	03CN10
	11	04CN07
	21	05CN03
	31	05CN57
Aug	10	06CN48
	20	07CN35
	30	08CN16
Sep	9	08CN52
	19	09CN21
	29	09CN43
Oct	9	09CN57
	19	10CN03
	29	10CN00
Nov	8	09CN48
	18	09CN28
	28	09CN02
Dec	8	08CN29
	18	07CN52
	28	07CN12

Stations	Date	
Direct	Mar	2
Retrograde	Oct	20

1939

Date		Long.
Jan	7	06CN32
	17	05CN53
	27	05CN18
Feb	6	04CN49
	16	04CN26
	26	04CN11
Mar	8	04CN05
	18	04CN08
	28	04CN20
Apr	7	04CN40
	17	05CN08
	27	05CN43
May	7	06CN25
	17	07CN12
	27	08CN04
Jun	6	09CN00
	16	09CN59
	26	11CN00
Jul	6	12CN02
	16	13CN04
	26	14CN05
Aug	5	15CN04
	15	16CN01
	25	16CN54
Sep	4	17CN42
	14	18CN24
	24	19CN00
Oct	4	19CN29
	14	19CN49
	24	20CN01
Nov	3	20CN04
	13	19CN57
	23	19CN42
Dec	3	19CN18
	13	18CN47
	23	18CN10

Stations	Date	
Direct	Mar	9
Retrograde	Oct	31

1940

Date	Long.
Jan 2	17CN30
12	16CN48
22	16CN07
Feb 1	15CN28
11	14CN55
21	14CN28
Mar 2	14CN09
12	13CN59
22	13CN58
Apr 1	14CN06
11	14CN24
21	14CN51
May 1	15CN25
11	16CN07
21	16CN55
31	17CN49
Jun 10	18CN47
20	19CN49
30	20CN53
Jul 10	21CN59
20	23CN06
30	24CN13
Aug 9	25CN18
19	26CN21
29	27CN21
Sep 8	28CN17
18	29CN08
28	29CN52
Oct 8	00LE29
18	00LE58
28	01LE18
Nov 7	01LE28
17	01LE29
27	01LE20
Dec 7	01LE02
17	00LE35
27	00LE01

Stations	Date
Direct	Mar 17
Retrograde	Nov 12

1941

Date	Long.
Jan 6	29CN21
16	28CN38
26	27CN55
Feb 5	27CN13
15	26CN34
25	26CN02
Mar 7	25CN37
17	25CN22
27	25CN15
Apr 6	25CN19
16	25CN33
26	25CN56
May 6	26CN28
16	27CN08
26	27CN56
Jun 5	28CN50
15	29CN50
25	00LE54
Jul 5	02LE01
15	03LE11
25	04LE23
Aug 4	05LE35
14	06LE47
24	07LE58
Sep 3	09LE05
13	10LE10
23	11LE09
Oct 3	12LE03
13	12LE51
23	13LE30
Nov 2	14LE01
12	14LE22
22	14LE33
Dec 2	14LE33
12	14LE23
22	14LE03

Stations	Date
Direct	Mar 28
Retrograde	Nov 27

1942

Date		Long.
Jan	1	13LE34
	11	12LE58
	21	12LE16
	31	11LE31
Feb	10	10LE46
	20	10LE03
Mar	2	09LE25
	12	08LE53
	22	08LE30
Apr	1	08LE16
	11	08LE13
	21	08LE20
May	1	08LE38
	11	09LE05
	21	09LE42
	31	10LE27
Jun	10	11LE20
	20	12LE19
	30	13LE24
Jul	10	14LE33
	20	15LE46
	30	17LE02
Aug	9	18LE19
	19	19LE37
	29	20LE54
Sep	8	22LE10
	18	23LE23
	28	24LE33
Oct	8	25LE37
	18	26LE36
	28	27LE27
Nov	7	28LE10
	17	28LE44
	27	29LE08
Dec	7	29LE21
	17	29LE22
	27	29LE13

Stations	Date	
Direct	Apr	9
Retrograde	Dec	13

1943

Date		Long.
Jan	6	28LE53
	16	28LE24
	26	27LE47
Feb	5	27LE04
	15	26LE18
	25	25LE31
Mar	7	24LE47
	17	24LE08
	27	23LE36
Apr	6	23LE13
	16	23LE00
	26	22LE58
May	6	23LE07
	16	23LE26
	26	23LE56
Jun	5	24LE36
	15	25LE24
	25	26LE20
Jul	5	27LE23
	15	28LE32
	25	29LE46
Aug	4	01VI04
	14	02VI24
	24	03VI46
Sep	3	05VI09
	13	06VI31
	23	07VI52
Oct	3	09VI10
	13	10VI25
	23	11VI35
Nov	2	12VI38
	12	13VI34
	22	14VI22
Dec	2	15VI00
	12	15VI28
	22	15VI44

Stations	Date	
Direct	Apr	22
Retrograde	Dec	31

1944

Date		Long.
Jan	1	15VI49
	11	15VI42
	21	15VI24
	31	14VI56
Feb	10	14VI20
	20	13VI37
Mar	1	12VI50
	11	12VI03
	21	11VI18
	31	10VI37
Apr	10	10VI04
	20	09VI40
	30	09VI26
May	10	09VI23
	20	09VI31
	30	09VI50
Jun	9	10VI20
	19	11VI00
	29	11VI49
Jul	9	12VI46
	19	13VI51
	29	15VI02
Aug	8	16VI18
	18	17VI38
	28	19VI02
Sep	7	20VI27
	17	21VI53
	27	23VI19
Oct	7	24VI44
	17	26VI06
	27	27VI25
Nov	6	28VI39
	16	29VI47
	26	00LI48
Dec	6	01LI40
	16	02LI23
	26	02LI55

Stations	Date	
Direct	May	7

1945

Date		Long.
Jan	5	03LI15
	15	03LI24
	25	03LI21
Feb	4	03LI06
	14	02LI41
	24	02LI06
Mar	6	01LI25
	16	00LI39
	26	29VI51
Apr	5	29VI05
	15	28VI23
	25	27VI48
May	5	27VI21
	15	27VI04
	25	26VI58
Jun	4	27VI03
	14	27VI20
	24	27VI47
Jul	4	28VI25
	14	29VI13
	24	00LI09
Aug	3	01LI12
	13	02LI22
	23	03LI38
Sep	2	04LI59
	12	06LI22
	22	07LI48
Oct	2	09LI16
	12	10LI43
	22	12LI10
Nov	1	13LI34
	11	14LI55
	21	16LI12
Dec	1	17LI22
	11	18LI26
	21	19LI21
	31	20LI07

Stations	Date	
Retrograde	Jan	17
Direct	May	25

	1946			1947	
Date		**Long.**	**Date**		**Long.**
Jan	10	20LI42	Jan	5	06SC35
	20	21LI06		15	07SC22
	30	21LI19		25	07SC58
Feb	9	21LI19	Feb	4	08SC24
	19	21LI08		14	08SC38
Mar	1	20LI46		24	08SC41
	11	20LI14	Mar	6	08SC32
	21	19LI35		16	08SC13
	31	18LI50		26	07SC43
Apr	10	18LI03	Apr	5	07SC07
	20	17LI17		15	06SC24
	30	16LI34		25	05SC38
May	10	15LI56	May	5	04SC53
	20	15LI26		15	04SC09
	30	15LI06		25	03SC30
Jun	9	14LI56	Jun	4	02SC58
	19	14LI57		14	02SC35
	29	15LI10		24	02SC22
Jul	9	15LI33	Jul	4	02SC19
	19	16LI07		14	02SC27
	29	16LI50		24	02SC45
Aug	8	17LI42	Aug	3	03SC14
	18	18LI43		13	03SC53
	28	19LI50		23	04SC41
Sep	7	21LI03	Sep	2	05SC36
	17	22LI21		12	06SC39
	27	23LI43		22	07SC48
Oct	7	25LI07	Oct	2	09SC02
	17	26LI33		12	10SC19
	27	27LI59		22	11SC40
Nov	6	29LI25	Nov	1	13SC02
	16	00SC48		11	14SC25
	26	02SC09		21	15SC47
Dec	6	03SC25	Dec	1	17SC08
	16	04SC35		11	18SC25
	26	05SC39		21	19SC39
				31	20SC47

Stations	**Date**		**Stations**	**Date**	
Retrograde	Feb	4	Retrograde	Feb	21
Direct	Jun	12	Direct	Jul	1

1948

Date		Long.
Jan	10	21SC48
	20	22SC42
	30	23SC27
Feb	9	24SC02
	19	24SC27
	29	24SC41
Mar	10	24SC44
	20	24SC36
	30	24SC17
Apr	9	23SC50
	19	23SC15
	29	22SC34
May	9	21SC50
	19	21SC05
	29	20SC22
Jun	8	19SC43
	18	19SC11
	28	18SC46
Jul	8	18SC31
	18	18SC25
	28	18SC29
Aug	7	18SC44
	17	19SC09
	27	19SC43
Sep	6	20SC27
	16	21SC18
	26	22SC16
Oct	6	23SC20
	16	24SC29
	26	25SC42
Nov	5	26SC58
	15	28SC15
	25	29SC33
Dec	5	00SA51
	15	02SA06
	25	03SA19

Stations	Date	
Retrograde	Mar	7
Direct	Jul	18

1949

Date		Long.
Jan	4	04SA28
	14	05SA31
	24	06SA28
Feb	3	07SA18
	13	07SA59
	23	08SA31
Mar	5	08SA53
	15	09SA04
	25	09SA05
Apr	4	08SA56
	14	08SA37
	24	08SA10
May	4	07SA36
	14	06SA57
	24	06SA14
Jun	3	05SA31
	13	04SA49
	23	04SA12
Jul	3	03SA40
	13	03SA15
	23	02SA59
Aug	2	02SA52
	12	02SA55
	22	03SA08
Sep	1	03SA30
	11	04SA01
	21	04SA41
Oct	1	05SA28
	11	06SA22
	21	07SA22
	31	08SA27
Nov	10	09SA35
	20	10SA46
	30	11SA59
Dec	10	13SA11
	20	14SA23
	30	15SA34

Stations	Date	
Retrograde	Mar	21
Direct	Aug	4

1950		1951	
Date	**Long.**	**Date**	**Long.**
Jan 9	16SA41	Jan 4	26SA27
19	17SA43	14	27SA31
29	18SA41	24	28SA32
Feb 8	19SA32	Feb 3	29SA29
18	20SA16	13	00CP20
28	20SA52	23	01CP05
Mar 10	21SA19	Mar 5	01CP42
20	21SA36	15	02CP12
30	21SA44	25	02CP33
Apr 9	21SA42	Apr 4	02CP45
19	21SA30	14	02CP48
29	21SA10	24	02CP41
May 9	20SA42	May 4	02CP26
19	20SA08	14	02CP04
29	19SA29	24	01CP34
Jun 8	18SA48	Jun 3	01CP00
18	18SA07	13	00CP22
28	17SA27	23	29SA42
Jul 8	16SA51	Jul 3	29SA03
18	16SA21	13	28SA25
28	15SA58	23	27SA52
Aug 7	15SA43	Aug 2	27SA25
17	15SA37	12	27SA05
27	15SA40	22	26SA52
Sep 6	15SA52	Sep 1	26SA48
16	16SA13	11	26SA52
26	16SA43	21	27SA06
Oct 6	17SA21	Oct 1	27SA27
16	18SA06	11	27SA57
26	18SA57	21	28SA34
Nov 5	19SA54	31	29SA18
15	20SA54	Nov 10	00CP07
25	21SA59	20	01CP01
Dec 5	23SA05	30	01CP59
15	24SA13	Dec 10	03CP00
25	25SA20	20	04CP02
		30	05CP05

Stations	**Date**	**Stations**	**Date**
Retrograde	Apr 1	Retrograde	Apr 12
Direct	Aug 18	Direct	Aug 31

1952			1953		
Date		**Long.**	**Date**		**Long.**
Jan	9	06CP08	Jan	3	13CP48
	19	07CP09		13	14CP47
	29	08CP07		23	15CP45
Feb	8	09CP02	Feb	2	16CP40
	18	09CP52		12	17CP33
	28	10CP37		22	18CP21
Mar	9	11CP14	Mar	4	19CP04
	19	11CP45		14	19CP42
	29	12CP08		24	20CP13
Apr	8	12CP23	Apr	3	20CP37
	18	12CP29		13	20CP53
	28	12CP27		23	21CP01
May	8	12CP16	May	3	21CP01
	18	11CP57		13	20CP54
	28	11CP32		23	20CP38
Jun	7	11CP01	Jun	2	20CP16
	17	10CP26		12	19CP48
	27	09CP48		22	19CP16
Jul	7	09CP10	Jul	2	18CP41
	17	08CP33		12	18CP04
	27	07CP59		22	17CP28
Aug	6	07CP29	Aug	1	16CP53
	16	07CP05		11	16CP23
	26	06CP48		21	15CP57
Sep	5	06CP39		31	15CP37
	15	06CP38	Sep	10	15CP25
	25	06CP45		20	15CP20
Oct	5	07CP01		30	15CP22
	15	07CP24	Oct	10	15CP33
	25	07CP55		20	15CP51
Nov	4	08CP32		30	16CP17
	14	09CP15	Nov	9	16CP49
	24	10CP04		19	17CP28
Dec	4	10CP56		29	18CP11
	14	11CP52	Dec	9	18CP59
	24	12CP49		19	19CP50
				29	20CP43

Stations	**Date**		**Stations**	**Date**	
Retrograde	Apr	20	Retrograde	Apr	28
Direct	Sep	11	Direct	Sep	21

1954

Date		Long.
Jan	8	21CP38
	18	22CP33
	28	23CP28
Feb	7	24CP21
	17	25CP11
	27	25CP57
Mar	9	26CP39
	19	27CP16
	29	27CP47
Apr	8	28CP11
	18	28CP28
	28	28CP37
May	8	28CP39
	18	28CP33
	28	28CP20
Jun	7	28CP01
	17	27CP35
	27	27CP05
Jul	7	26CP32
	17	25CP57
	27	25CP22
Aug	6	24CP48
	16	24CP17
	26	23CP50
Sep	5	23CP29
	15	23CP14
	25	23CP06
Oct	5	23CP06
	15	23CP13
	25	23CP27
Nov	4	23CP49
	14	24CP17
	24	24CP52
Dec	4	25CP31
	14	26CP15
	24	27CP02

Stations	Date	
Retrograde	May	5
Direct	Sep	30

1955

Date		Long.
Jan	3	27CP52
	13	28CP44
	23	29CP36
Feb	2	00AQ27
	12	01AQ18
	22	02AQ06
Mar	4	02AQ50
	14	03AQ31
	24	04AQ07
Apr	3	04AQ37
	13	05AQ00
	23	05AQ17
May	3	05AQ28
	13	05AQ30
	23	05AQ26
Jun	2	05AQ15
	12	04AQ57
	22	04AQ33
Jul	2	04AQ05
	12	03AQ34
	22	03AQ00
Aug	1	02AQ26
	11	01AQ53
	21	01AQ22
	31	00AQ55
Sep	10	00AQ33
	20	00AQ17
	30	00AQ07
Oct	10	00AQ04
	20	00AQ09
	30	00AQ21
Nov	9	00AQ39
	19	01AQ05
	29	01AQ36
Dec	9	02AQ12
	19	02AQ53
	29	03AQ37

Stations	Date	
Retrograde	May	11
Direct	Oct	8

1956

Date		Long.
Jan	8	04AQ24
	18	05AQ12
	28	06AQ02
Feb	7	06AQ51
	17	07AQ39
	27	08AQ24
Mar	8	09AQ07
	18	09AQ46
	28	10AQ21
Apr	7	10AQ50
	17	11AQ13
	27	11AQ30
May	7	11AQ40
	17	11AQ44
	27	11AQ40
Jun	6	11AQ30
	16	11AQ14
	26	10AQ52
Jul	6	10AQ25
	16	09AQ55
	26	09AQ23
Aug	5	08AQ50
	15	08AQ18
	25	07AQ47
Sep	4	07AQ20
	14	06AQ58
	24	06AQ41
Oct	4	06AQ30
	14	06AQ26
	24	06AQ28
Nov	3	06AQ38
	13	06AQ54
	23	07AQ17
Dec	3	07AQ46
	13	08AQ19
	23	08AQ58

Stations	Date
Retrograde	May 16
Direct	Oct 14

1957

Date		Long.
Jan	2	09AQ39
	12	10AQ24
	22	11AQ10
Feb	1	11AQ57
	11	12AQ43
	21	13AQ29
Mar	3	14AQ13
	13	14AQ54
	23	15AQ32
Apr	2	16AQ05
	12	16AQ33
	22	16AQ56
May	2	17AQ13
	12	17AQ23
	22	17AQ26
Jun	1	17AQ23
	11	17AQ14
	21	16AQ59
Jul	1	16AQ38
	11	16AQ12
	21	15AQ44
	31	15AQ13
Aug	10	14AQ41
	20	14AQ09
	30	13AQ39
Sep	9	13AQ12
	19	12AQ50
	29	12AQ32
Oct	9	12AQ21
	19	12AQ15
	29	12AQ17
Nov	8	12AQ25
	18	12AQ40
	28	13AQ01
Dec	8	13AQ28
	18	13AQ59
	28	14AQ35

Stations	Date
Retrograde	May 22
Direct	Oct 21

1958			1959		
Date		**Long.**	**Date**		**Long.**
Jan	7	15AQ15	Jan	2	19AQ50
	17	15AQ57		12	20AQ28
	27	16AQ41		22	21AQ08
Feb	6	17AQ26	Feb	1	21AQ51
	16	18AQ11		11	22AQ34
	26	18AQ55		21	23AQ17
Mar	8	19AQ37	Mar	3	23AQ59
	18	20AQ16		13	24AQ40
	28	20AQ53		23	25AQ18
Apr	7	21AQ25	Apr	2	25AQ53
	17	21AQ52		12	26AQ24
	27	22AQ14		22	26AQ50
May	7	22AQ30	May	2	27AQ11
	17	22AQ40		12	27AQ26
	27	22AQ43		22	27AQ36
Jun	6	22AQ41	Jun	1	27AQ39
	16	22AQ32		11	27AQ37
	26	22AQ17		21	27AQ28
Jul	6	21AQ57	Jul	1	27AQ14
	16	21AQ33		11	26AQ54
	26	21AQ05		21	26AQ31
Aug	5	20AQ35		31	26AQ04
	15	20AQ04	Aug	10	25AQ34
	25	19AQ33		20	25AQ04
Sep	4	19AQ03		30	24AQ34
	14	18AQ37	Sep	9	24AQ05
	24	18AQ15		19	23AQ39
Oct	4	17AQ57		29	23AQ17
	14	17AQ45	Oct	9	23AQ00
	24	17AQ39		19	22AQ48
Nov	3	17AQ40		29	22AQ42
	13	17AQ47	Nov	8	22AQ42
	23	18AQ01		18	22AQ48
Dec	3	18AQ20		28	23AQ01
	13	18AQ46	Dec	8	23AQ20
	23	19AQ16		18	23AQ44
				28	24AQ13

Stations	**Date**		**Stations**	**Date**	
Retrograde	May	27	Retrograde	Jun	1
Direct	Oct	27	Direct	Nov	2

1960

Date		Long.
Jan	7	24AQ46
	17	25AQ22
	27	26AQ01
Feb	6	26AQ42
	16	27AQ23
	26	28AQ05
Mar	7	28AQ46
	17	29AQ25
	27	00PI02
Apr	6	00PI35
	16	01PI05
	26	01PI31
May	6	01PI51
	16	02PI06
	26	02PI15
Jun	5	02PI18
	15	02PI15
	25	02PI07
Jul	5	01PI53
	15	01PI34
	25	01PI10
Aug	4	00PI44
	14	00PI15
	24	29AQ46
Sep	3	29AQ16
	13	28AQ48
	23	28AQ23
Oct	3	28AQ01
	13	27AQ44
	23	27AQ32
Nov	2	27AQ26
	12	27AQ25
	22	27AQ32
Dec	2	27AQ44
	12	28AQ02
	22	28AQ25

Stations	Date
Retrograde	Jun 5
Direct	Nov 7

1961

Date		Long.
Jan	1	28AQ53
	11	29AQ25
	21	00PI00
	31	00PI38
Feb	10	01PI18
	20	01PI58
Mar	2	02PI38
	12	03PI18
	22	03PI56
Apr	1	04PI31
	11	05PI04
	21	05PI33
May	1	05PI57
	11	06PI16
	21	06PI30
	31	06PI39
Jun	10	06PI42
	20	06PI39
	30	06PI30
Jul	10	06PI16
	20	05PI58
	30	05PI35
Aug	9	05PI09
	19	04PI41
	29	04PI12
Sep	8	03PI43
	18	03PI15
	28	02PI50
Oct	8	02PI29
	18	02PI12
	28	02PI00
Nov	7	01PI54
	17	01PI54
	27	02PI00
Dec	7	02PI12
	17	02PI29
	27	02PI52

Stations	Date
Retrograde	Jun 9
Direct	Nov 12

1962

Date		Long.
Jan	6	03Pl19
	16	03Pl50
	26	04Pl25
Feb	5	05Pl02
	15	05Pl40
	25	06Pl19
Mar	7	06Pl59
	17	07Pl37
	27	08Pl14
Apr	6	08Pl49
	16	09Pl20
	26	09Pl48
May	6	10Pl11
	16	10Pl30
	26	10Pl43
Jun	5	10Pl51
	15	10Pl54
	25	10Pl50
Jul	5	10Pl41
	15	10Pl27
	25	10Pl09
Aug	4	09Pl46
	14	09Pl21
	24	08Pl53
Sep	3	08Pl24
	13	07Pl56
	23	07Pl29
Oct	3	07Pl04
	13	06Pl44
	23	06Pl27
Nov	2	06Pl16
	12	06Pl10
	22	06Pl10
Dec	2	06Pl16
	12	06Pl28
	22	06Pl45

Stations	Date	
Retrograde	Jun	14
Direct	Nov	16

1963

Date		Long.
Jan	1	07Pl07
	11	07Pl34
	21	08Pl04
	31	08Pl38
Feb	10	09Pl14
	20	09Pl52
Mar	2	10Pl30
	12	11Pl09
	22	11Pl46
Apr	1	12Pl22
	11	12Pl55
	21	13Pl26
May	1	13Pl53
	11	14Pl15
	21	14Pl33
	31	14Pl46
Jun	10	14Pl53
	20	14Pl55
	30	14Pl51
Jul	10	14Pl42
	20	14Pl28
	30	14Pl09
Aug	9	13Pl47
	19	13Pl22
	29	12Pl54
Sep	8	12Pl26
	18	11Pl58
	28	11Pl32
Oct	8	11Pl08
	18	10Pl47
	28	10Pl31
Nov	7	10Pl20
	17	10Pl15
	27	10Pl15
Dec	7	10Pl21
	17	10Pl33
	27	10Pl50

Stations	Date	
Retrograde	Jun	18
Direct	Nov	21

1964

Date		Long.
Jan	6	11PI12
	16	11PI39
	26	12PI09
Feb	5	12PI42
	15	13PI17
	25	13PI54
Mar	6	14PI32
	16	15PI09
	26	15PI46
Apr	5	16PI21
	15	16PI54
	25	17PI23
May	5	17PI49
	15	18PI11
	25	18PI28
Jun	4	18PI40
	14	18PI47
	24	18PI48
Jul	4	18PI44
	14	18PI34
	24	18PI20
Aug	3	18PI01
	13	17PI39
	23	17PI14
Sep	2	16PI46
	12	16PI19
	22	15PI51
Oct	2	15PI25
	12	15PI01
	22	14PI42
Nov	1	14PI26
	11	14PI16
	21	14PI10
Dec	1	14PI11
	11	14PI17
	21	14PI29
	31	14PI47

Stations	Date	
Retrograde	Jun	21
Direct	Nov	24

1965

Date		Long.
Jan	10	15PI09
	20	15PI35
	30	16PI05
Feb	9	16PI38
	19	17PI13
Mar	1	17PI49
	11	18PI26
	21	19PI03
	31	19PI38
Apr	10	20PI13
	20	20PI44
	30	21PI13
May	10	21PI38
	20	21PI59
	30	22PI15
Jun	9	22PI27
	19	22PI33
	29	22PI34
Jul	9	22PI29
	19	22PI19
	29	22PI05
Aug	8	21PI46
	18	21PI23
	28	20PI58
Sep	7	20PI31
	17	20PI03
	27	19PI36
Oct	7	19PI11
	17	18PI48
	27	18PI28
Nov	6	18PI13
	16	18PI03
	26	17PI59
Dec	6	18PI00
	16	18PI06
	26	18PI19

Stations	Date	
Retrograde	Jun	25
Direct	Nov	29

1966

Date		Long.
Jan	5	18PI36
	15	18PI58
	25	19PI24
Feb	4	19PI54
	14	20PI27
	24	21PI01
Mar	6	21PI37
	16	22PI13
	26	22PI50
Apr	5	23PI25
	15	23PI58
	25	24PI29
May	5	24PI57
	15	25PI22
	25	25PI42
Jun	4	25PI57
	14	26PI08
	24	26PI13
Jul	4	26PI14
	14	26PI08
	24	25PI58
Aug	3	25PI43
	13	25PI24
	23	25PI02
Sep	2	24PI36
	12	24PI09
	22	23PI42
Oct	2	23PI15
	12	22PI50
	22	22PI27
Nov	1	22PI09
	11	21PI54
	21	21PI45
Dec	1	21PI41
	11	21PI42
	21	21PI49
	31	22PI02

Stations	Date	
Retrograde	Jun	29
Direct	Dec	3

1967

Date		Long.
Jan	10	22PI19
	20	22PI42
	30	23PI08
Feb	9	23PI38
	19	24PI10
Mar	1	24PI44
	11	25PI20
	21	25PI56
	31	26PI32
Apr	10	27PI06
	20	27PI39
	30	28PI09
May	10	28PI37
	20	29PI00
	30	29PI20
Jun	9	29PI35
	19	29PI45
	29	29PI49
Jul	9	29PI49
	19	29PI43
	29	29PI33
Aug	8	29PI17
	18	28PI58
	28	28PI35
Sep	7	28PI10
	17	27PI43
	27	27PI16
Oct	7	26PI49
	17	26PI24
	27	26PI02
Nov	6	25PI44
	16	25PI30
	26	25PI21
Dec	6	25PI18
	16	25PI20
	26	25PI27

Stations	Date	
Retrograde	Jul	3
Direct	Dec	7

1968

Date		Long.
Jan	5	25PI40
	15	25PI58
	25	26PI21
Feb	4	26PI47
	14	27PI17
	24	27PI50
Mar	5	28PI24
	15	28PI59
	25	29PI35
Apr	4	00AR10
	14	00AR44
	24	01AR16
May	4	01AR46
	14	02AR13
	24	02AR36
Jun	3	02AR55
	13	03AR09
	23	03AR18
Jul	3	03AR22
	13	03AR21
	23	03AR15
Aug	2	03AR04
	12	02AR48
	22	02AR28
Sep	1	02AR05
	11	01AR40
	21	01AR13
Oct	1	00AR46
	11	00AR19
	21	29PI55
	31	29PI33
Nov	10	29PI16
	20	29PI02
	30	28PI54
Dec	10	28PI51
	20	28PI54
	30	29PI02

1969

Date		Long.
Jan	9	29PI16
	19	29PI34
	29	29PI57
Feb	8	00AR24
	18	00AR53
	28	01AR26
Mar	10	02AR00
	20	02AR35
	30	03AR11
Apr	9	03AR45
	19	04AR19
	29	04AR51
May	9	05AR20
	19	05AR46
	29	06AR09
Jun	8	06AR27
	18	06AR40
	28	06AR49
Jul	8	06AR53
	18	06AR51
	28	06AR44
Aug	7	06AR32
	17	06AR16
	27	05AR56
Sep	6	05AR33
	16	05AR07
	26	04AR40
Oct	6	04AR13
	16	03AR47
	26	03AR23
Nov	5	03AR02
	15	02AR45
	25	02AR32
Dec	5	02AR24
	15	02AR22
	25	02AR26

Stations	Date		Stations	Date	
Retrograde	Jul	5	Retrograde	Jul	9
Direct	Dec	10	Direct	Dec	13

1970		1971	
Date	**Long.**	**Date**	**Long.**
Jan 4	02AR34	Jan 9	06AR06
14	02AR49	19	06AR20
24	03AR07	29	06AR40
Feb 3	03AR31	Feb 8	07AR03
13	03AR58	18	07AR31
23	04AR28	28	08AR01
Mar 5	05AR00	Mar 10	08AR34
15	05AR34	20	09AR08
25	06AR10	30	09AR43
Apr 4	06AR45	Apr 9	10AR18
14	07AR19	19	10AR53
24	07AR53	29	11AR26
May 4	08AR24	May 9	11AR57
14	08AR53	19	12AR25
24	09AR19	29	12AR51
Jun 3	09AR40	Jun 8	13AR12
13	09AR58	18	13AR29
23	10AR11	28	13AR42
Jul 3	10AR19	Jul 8	13AR49
13	10AR22	18	13AR51
23	10AR20	28	13AR48
Aug 2	10AR12	Aug 7	13AR40
12	10AR00	17	13AR28
22	09AR43	27	13AR11
Sep 1	09AR23	Sep 6	12AR50
11	08AR59	16	12AR26
21	08AR34	26	12AR00
Oct 1	08AR07	Oct 6	11AR33
11	07AR40	16	11AR06
21	07AR14	26	10AR40
31	06AR50	Nov 5	10AR17
Nov 10	06AR29	15	09AR56
20	06AR13	25	09AR40
30	06AR00	Dec 5	09AR29
Dec 10	05AR54	15	09AR22
20	05AR52	25	09AR21
30	05AR56		

Stations	**Date**	**Stations**	**Date**
Retrograde	Jul 13	Retrograde	Jul 17
Direct	Dec 17	Direct	Dec 21

1972

Date		Long.
Jan	4	09AR26
	14	09AR36
	24	09AR52
Feb	3	10AR12
	13	10AR36
	23	11AR04
Mar	4	11AR35
	14	12AR07
	24	12AR42
Apr	3	13AR17
	13	13AR52
	23	14AR27
May	3	15AR00
	13	15AR30
	23	15AR59
Jun	2	16AR23
	12	16AR44
	22	17AR01
Jul	2	17AR13
	12	17AR20
	22	17AR22
Aug	1	17AR18
	11	17AR10
	21	16AR56
	31	16AR39
Sep	10	16AR17
	20	15AR53
	30	15AR27
Oct	10	15AR00
	20	14AR33
	30	14AR07
Nov	9	13AR44
	19	13AR24
	29	13AR08
Dec	9	12AR57
	19	12AR52
	29	12AR52

Stations	Date	
Retrograde	Jul	20
Direct	Dec	24

1973

Date		Long.
Jan	8	12AR57
	18	13AR08
	28	13AR24
Feb	7	13AR45
	17	14AR10
	27	14AR38
Mar	9	15AR09
	19	15AR42
	29	16AR17
Apr	8	16AR52
	18	17AR27
	28	18AR02
May	8	18AR35
	18	19AR06
	28	19AR33
Jun	7	19AR58
	17	20AR19
	27	20AR35
Jul	7	20AR46
	17	20AR53
	27	20AR54
Aug	6	20AR50
	16	20AR41
	26	20AR27
Sep	5	20AR09
	15	19AR47
	25	19AR22
Oct	5	18AR56
	15	18AR28
	25	18AR01
Nov	4	17AR36
	14	17AR13
	24	16AR53
Dec	4	16AR38
	14	16AR28
	24	16AR23

Stations	Date	
Retrograde	Jul	24
Direct	Dec	27

1974

Date		Long.
Jan	3	16AR24
	13	16AR30
	23	16AR41
Feb	2	16AR58
	12	17AR20
	22	17AR45
Mar	4	18AR14
	14	18AR46
	24	19AR19
Apr	3	19AR54
	13	20AR30
	23	21AR05
May	3	21AR40
	13	22AR13
	23	22AR43
Jun	2	23AR11
	12	23AR35
	22	23AR56
Jul	2	24AR12
	12	24AR23
	22	24AR29
Aug	1	24AR29
	11	24AR25
	21	24AR15
	31	24AR01
Sep	10	23AR42
	20	23AR20
	30	22AR55
Oct	10	22AR28
	20	22AR00
	30	21AR33
Nov	9	21AR08
	19	20AR45
	29	20AR26
Dec	9	20AR11
	19	20AR01
	29	19AR57

1975

Date		Long.
Jan	8	19AR58
	18	20AR05
	28	20AR18
Feb	7	20AR35
	17	20AR57
	27	21AR23
Mar	9	21AR53
	19	22AR25
	29	22AR59
Apr	8	23AR35
	18	24AR11
	28	24AR46
May	8	25AR21
	18	25AR54
	28	26AR25
Jun	7	26AR52
	17	27AR17
	27	27AR37
Jul	7	27AR52
	17	28AR03
	27	28AR09
Aug	6	28AR09
	16	28AR04
	26	27AR54
Sep	5	27AR39
	15	27AR20
	25	26AR57
Oct	5	26AR31
	15	26AR04
	25	25AR36
Nov	4	25AR09
	14	24AR43
	24	24AR21
Dec	4	24AR02
	14	23AR48
	24	23AR39

Stations	Date		Stations	Date
Retrograde	Jul 28		Retrograde	Aug 1
Direct	Dec 31			

1976		1977	
Date	**Long.**	**Date**	**Long.**
Jan 3	23AR35	Jan 7	27AR18
13	23AR37	17	27AR20
23	23AR45	27	27AR29
Feb 2	23AR58	Feb 6	27AR43
12	24AR16	16	28AR02
22	24AR39	26	28AR25
Mar 3	25AR06	Mar 8	28AR53
13	25AR36	18	29AR24
23	26AR09	28	29AR57
Apr 2	26AR43	Apr 7	00TA33
12	27AR19	17	01TA09
22	27AR56	27	01TA46
May 2	28AR32	May 7	02TA23
12	29AR07	17	02TA58
22	29AR40	27	03TA32
Jun 1	00TA11	Jun 6	04TA03
11	00TA39	16	04TA31
21	01TA03	26	04TA55
Jul 1	01TA23	Jul 6	05TA15
11	01TA38	16	05TA31
21	01TA49	26	05TA41
31	01TA54	Aug 5	05TA46
Aug 10	01TA54	15	05TA46
20	01TA49	25	05TA40
30	01TA38	Sep 4	05TA29
Sep 9	01TA22	14	05TA13
19	01TA03	24	04TA52
29	00TA39	Oct 4	04TA28
Oct 9	00TA13	14	04TA02
19	29AR45	24	03TA33
29	29AR17	Nov 3	03TA05
Nov 8	28AR50	13	02TA37
18	28AR24	23	02TA12
28	28AR02	Dec 3	01TA49
Dec 8	27AR43	13	01TA31
18	27AR29	23	01TA17
28	27AR21		

Stations	**Date**	**Stations**	**Date**
Direct	Jan 4	Direct	Jan 7
Retrograde	Aug 4	Retrograde	Aug 9

1978

Date		Long.
Jan	2	1TA09
	12	1TA06
	22	1TA10
Feb	1	1TA19
	11	1TA34
	21	1TA54
Mar	3	2TA18
	13	2TA47
	23	3TA18
Apr	2	3TA53
	12	4TA29
	22	5TA06
May	2	5TA43
	12	6TA20
	22	6TA56
Jun	1	7TA30
	11	8TA02
	21	8TA30
Jul	1	8TA55
	11	9TA15
	21	9TA31
	31	9TA41
Aug	10	9TA46
	20	9TA45
	30	9TA39
Sep	9	9TA27
	19	9TA11
	29	8TA50
Oct	9	8TA25
	19	7TA58
	29	7TA29
Nov	8	7TA00
	18	6TA32
	28	6TA07
Dec	8	5TA44
	18	5TA26
	28	5TA12

Stations	Date
Direct	Jan 11
Retrograde	Aug 13

1979

Date		Long.
Jan	7	05TA05
	17	05TA03
	27	05TA07
Feb	6	05TA17
	16	05TA32
	26	05TA53
Mar	8	06TA18
	18	06TA48
	28	07TA20
Apr	7	07TA56
	17	08TA32
	27	09TA10
May	7	09TA49
	17	10TA27
	27	11TA03
Jun	6	11TA38
	16	12TA10
	26	12TA39
Jul	6	13TA04
	16	13TA24
	26	13TA40
Aug	5	13TA51
	15	13TA55
	25	13TA55
Sep	4	13TA48
	14	13TA36
	24	13TA19
Oct	4	12TA57
	14	12TA32
	24	12TA04
Nov	3	11TA35
	13	11TA06
	23	10TA37
Dec	3	10TA11
	13	09TA48
	23	09TA30

Stations	Date
Direct	Jan 15
Retrograde	Aug 18

1980

Date		Long.
Jan	2	09TA17
	12	09TA10
	22	09TA08
Feb	1	09TA13
	11	09TA24
	21	09TA40
Mar	2	10TA02
	12	10TA28
	22	10TA58
Apr	1	11TA32
	11	12TA08
	21	12TA46
May	1	13TA25
	11	14TA04
	21	14TA43
	31	15TA20
Jun	10	15TA56
	20	16TA28
	30	16TA58
Jul	10	17TA24
	20	17TA45
	30	18TA01
Aug	9	18TA11
	19	18TA16
	29	18TA16
Sep	8	18TA09
	18	17TA57
	28	17TA39
Oct	8	17TA17
	18	16TA51
	28	16TA23
Nov	7	15TA53
	17	15TA23
	27	14TA54
Dec	7	14TA27
	17	14TA04
	27	13TA46

Stations	Date	
Direct	Jan	19
Retrograde	Aug	22

1981

Date		Long.
Jan	6	13TA33
	16	13TA26
	26	13TA25
Feb	5	13TA30
	15	13TA41
	25	13TA59
Mar	7	14TA21
	17	14TA48
	27	15TA20
Apr	6	15TA54
	16	16TA31
	26	17TA11
May	6	17TA51
	16	18TA31
	26	19TA11
Jun	5	19TA49
	15	20TA26
	25	21TA00
Jul	5	21TA30
	15	21TA57
	25	22TA18
Aug	4	22TA35
	14	22TA46
	24	22TA52
Sep	3	22TA51
	13	22TA44
	23	22TA32
Oct	3	22TA14
	13	21TA51
	23	21TA25
Nov	2	20TA55
	12	20TA25
	22	19TA54
Dec	2	19TA24
	12	18TA57
	22	18TA34

Stations	Date	
Direct	Jan	22
Retrograde	Aug	27

1982

Date		Long.
Jan	1	18TA15
	11	18TA02
	21	17TA55
	31	17TA55
Feb	10	18TA00
	20	18TA13
Mar	2	18TA31
	12	18TA54
	22	19TA22
Apr	1	19TA55
	11	20TA30
	21	21TA09
May	1	21TA49
	11	22TA30
	21	23TA12
	31	23TA53
Jun	10	24TA33
	20	25TA11
	30	25TA46
Jul	10	26TA18
	20	26TA45
	30	27TA08
Aug	9	27TA26
	19	27TA38
	29	27TA43
Sep	8	27TA43
	18	27TA36
	28	27TA24
Oct	8	27TA06
	18	26TA43
	28	26TA16
Nov	7	25TA46
	17	25TA14
	27	24TA42
Dec	7	24TA12
	17	23TA44
	27	23TA20

Stations	Date	
Direct	Jan	26
Retrograde	Sep	2

1983

Date		Long.
Jan	6	23TA01
	16	22TA48
	26	22TA41
Feb	5	22TA41
	15	22TA47
	25	23TA00
Mar	7	23TA19
	17	23TA43
	27	24TA12
Apr	6	24TA46
	16	25TA23
	26	26TA03
May	6	26TA44
	16	27TA27
	26	28TA10
Jun	5	28TA53
	15	29TA34
	25	00GE14
Jul	5	00GE51
	15	01GE24
	25	01GE53
Aug	4	02GE17
	14	02GE36
	24	02GE49
Sep	3	02GE55
	13	02GE56
	23	02GE50
Oct	3	02GE37
	13	02GE19
	23	01GE55
Nov	2	01GE28
	12	00GE57
	22	00GE25
Dec	2	29TA52
	12	29TA21
	22	28TA52

Stations	Date	
Direct	Jan	31
Retrograde	Sep	8

1984

Date	Long.
Jan 1	28TA27
11	28TA08
21	27TA54
31	27TA47
Feb 10	27TA47
20	27TA53
Mar 1	28TA06
11	28TA26
21	28TA51
31	29TA21
Apr 10	29TA56
20	00GE35
30	01GE16
May 10	01GE59
20	02GE44
30	03GE29
Jun 9	04GE13
19	04GE57
29	05GE38
Jul 9	06GE17
19	06GE52
29	07GE23
Aug 8	07GE49
18	08GE09
28	08GE24
Sep 7	08GE32
17	08GE33
27	08GE28
Oct 7	08GE16
17	07GE58
27	07GE34
Nov 6	07GE06
16	06GE34
26	06GE01
Dec 6	05GE27
16	04GE55
26	04GE25

Stations	Date
Direct	Feb 5
Retrograde	Sep 14

1985

Date	Long.
Jan 5	03GE59
15	03GE39
25	03GE24
Feb 4	03GE17
14	03GE16
24	03GE23
Mar 6	03GE36
16	03GE57
26	04GE23
Apr 5	04GE54
15	05GE30
25	06GE10
May 5	06GE53
15	07GE38
25	08GE25
Jun 4	09GE12
14	09GE59
24	10GE44
Jul 4	11GE28
14	12GE09
24	12GE47
Aug 3	13GE20
13	13GE48
23	14GE11
Sep 2	14GE27
12	14GE37
22	14GE40
Oct 2	14GE36
12	14GE25
22	14GE07
Nov 1	13GE44
11	13GE15
21	12GE43
Dec 1	12GE09
11	11GE34
21	11GE00
31	10GE29

Stations	Date
Direct	Feb 9
Retrograde	Sep 21

1986

Date		Long.
Jan	10	10GE01
	20	09GE40
	30	09GE24
Feb	9	09GE16
	19	09GE15
Mar	1	09GE21
	11	09GE35
	21	09GE56
	31	10GE22
Apr	10	10GE55
	20	11GE32
	30	12GE14
May	10	12GE59
	20	13GE46
	30	14GE35
Jun	9	15GE24
	19	16GE14
	29	17GE02
Jul	9	17GE49
	19	18GE33
	29	19GE13
Aug	8	19GE49
	18	20GE21
	28	20GE46
Sep	7	21GE05
	17	21GE18
	27	21GE23
Oct	7	21GE20
	17	21GE11
	27	20GE54
Nov	6	20GE31
	16	20GE02
	26	19GE30
Dec	6	18GE54
	16	18GE18
	26	17GE43

Stations	Date	
Direct	Feb	15
Retrograde	Sep	28

1987

Date		Long.
Jan	5	17GE10
	15	16GE41
	25	16GE17
Feb	4	16GE01
	14	15GE51
	24	15GE49
Mar	6	15GE55
	16	16GE08
	26	16GE29
Apr	5	16GE57
	15	17GE30
	25	18GE09
May	5	18GE52
	15	19GE39
	25	20GE28
Jun	4	21GE19
	14	22GE12
	24	23GE04
Jul	4	23GE56
	14	24GE46
	24	25GE33
Aug	3	26GE18
	13	26GE58
	23	27GE33
Sep	2	28GE02
	12	28GE25
	22	28GE40
Oct	2	28GE48
	12	28GE49
	22	28GE42
Nov	1	28GE27
	11	28GE05
	21	27GE36
Dec	1	27GE04
	11	26GE27
	21	25GE50
	31	25GE12

Stations	Date	
Direct	Feb	21
Retrograde	Oct	7

1988

Date		Long.
Jan	10	24GE37
	20	24GE06
	30	23GE41
Feb	9	23GE22
	19	23GE10
	29	23GE07
Mar	10	23GE11
	20	23GE24
	30	23GE45
Apr	9	24GE12
	19	24GE47
	29	25GE26
May	9	26GE11
	19	27GE00
	29	27GE52
Jun	8	28GE46
	18	29GE41
	28	00CN37
Jul	8	01CN33
	18	02CN27
	28	03CN19
Aug	7	04CN07
	17	04CN52
	27	05CN32
Sep	6	06CN06
	16	06CN33
	26	06CN53
Oct	6	07CN06
	16	07CN10
	26	07CN06
Nov	5	06CN54
	15	06CN34
	25	06CN07
Dec	5	05CN34
	15	04CN58
	25	04CN19

Stations	Date
Direct	Feb 28
Retrograde	Oct 16

1989

Date		Long.
Jan	4	03CN40
	14	03CN02
	24	02CN28
Feb	3	02CN00
	13	01CN38
	23	01CN24
Mar	5	01CN18
	15	01CN21
	25	01CN32
Apr	4	01CN52
	14	02CN19
	24	02CN54
May	4	03CN34
	14	04CN20
	24	05CN11
Jun	3	06CN05
	13	07CN03
	23	08CN01
Jul	3	09CN01
	13	10CN01
	23	11CN00
Aug	2	11CN57
	12	12CN51
	22	13CN41
Sep	1	14CN27
	11	15CN07
	21	15CN40
Oct	1	16CN06
	11	16CN24
	21	16CN34
	31	16CN35
Nov	10	16CN27
	20	16CN10
	30	15CN46
Dec	10	15CN15
	20	14CN38
	30	13CN59

Stations	Date
Direct	Mar 6
Retrograde	Oct 26

1990

Date		Long.
Jan	9	13CN18
	19	12CN37
	29	12CN00
Feb	8	11CN28
	18	11CN02
	28	10CN44
Mar	10	10CN35
	20	10CN35
	30	10CN44
Apr	9	11CN02
	19	11CN28
	29	12CN02
May	9	12CN43
	19	13CN30
	29	14CN22
Jun	8	15CN19
	18	16CN19
	28	17CN22
Jul	8	18CN26
	18	19CN30
	28	20CN34
Aug	7	21CN37
	17	22CN37
	27	23CN34
Sep	6	24CN27
	16	25CN14
	26	25CN55
Oct	6	26CN29
	16	26CN55
	26	27CN12
Nov	5	27CN19
	15	27CN18
	25	27CN06
Dec	5	26CN46
	15	26CN18
	25	25CN43

Stations	Date	
Direct	Mar	15
Retrograde	Nov	8

1991

Date		Long.
Jan	4	25CN04
	14	24CN21
	24	23CN39
Feb	3	22CN58
	13	22CN21
	23	21CN51
Mar	5	21CN28
	15	21CN14
	25	21CN09
Apr	4	21CN14
	14	21CN28
	24	21CN52
May	4	22CN25
	14	23CN05
	24	23CN52
Jun	3	24CN45
	13	25CN44
	23	26CN46
Jul	3	27CN52
	13	29CN00
	23	00LE09
Aug	2	01LE19
	12	02LE28
	22	03LE35
Sep	1	04LE40
	11	05LE40
	21	06LE36
Oct	1	07LE26
	11	08LE10
	21	08LE45
	31	09LE11
Nov	10	09LE29
	20	09LE36
	30	09LE33
Dec	10	09LE19
	20	08LE57
	30	08LE26

Stations	Date	
Direct	Mar	24
Retrograde	Nov	21

1992

Date		Long.
Jan	9	07LE49
	19	07LE06
	29	06LE22
Feb	8	05LE38
	18	04LE57
	28	04LE20
Mar	9	03LE51
	19	03LE30
	29	03LE19
Apr	8	03LE18
	18	03LE28
	28	03LE47
May	8	04LE15
	18	04LE53
	28	05LE39
Jun	7	06LE32
	17	07LE30
	27	08LE35
Jul	7	09LE43
	17	10LE54
	27	12LE08
Aug	6	13LE23
	16	14LE38
	26	15LE52
Sep	5	17LE05
	15	18LE14
	25	19LE20
Oct	5	20LE20
	15	21LE14
	25	22LE01
Nov	4	22LE39
	14	23LE08
	24	23LE26
Dec	4	23LE34
	14	23LE32
	24.	23LE18

1993

Date		Long.
Jan	3	22LE55
	13	22LE22
	23	21LE43
Feb	2	21LE00
	12	20LE14
	22	19LE28
Mar	4	18LE46
	14	18LE10
	24	17LE41
Apr	3	17LE21
	13	17LE12
	23	17LE13
May	3	17LE25
	13	17LE47
	23	18LE20
Jun	2	19LE01
	12	19LE51
	22	20LE48
Jul	2	21LE52
	12	23LE01
	22	24LE14
Aug	1	25LE31
	11	26LE50
	21	28LE10
	31	29LE30
Sep	10	00VI50
	20	02VI08
	30	03VI23
Oct	10	04VI33
	20	05VI39
	30	06VI37
Nov	9	07VI29
	19	08VI11
	29	08VI44
Dec	9	09VI06
	19	09VI16
	29	09VI16

Stations	Date	
Direct	Apr	4
Retrograde	Dec	6

Stations	Date	
Direct	Apr	16
Retrograde	Dec	23

1994

Date		Long.
Jan	8	09VI04
	18	08VI41
	28	08VI09
Feb	7	07VI30
	17	06VI45
	27	05VI58
Mar	9	05VI12
	19	04VI28
	29	03VI51
Apr	8	03VI21
	18	03VI01
	28	02VI52
May	8	02VI53
	18	03VI06
	28	03VI29
Jun	7	04VI03
	17	04VI46
	27	05VI38
Jul	7	06VI38
	17	07VI44
	27	08VI56
Aug	6	10VI13
	16	11VI33
	26	12VI56
Sep	5	14VI21
	15	15VI46
	25	17VI10
Oct	5	18VI33
	15	19VI52
	25	21VI08
Nov	4	22VI18
	14	23VI22
	24	24VI18
Dec	4	25VI05
	14	25VI42
	24	26VI08

Stations	Date	
Direct	May	1

1995

Date		Long.
Jan	3	26VI23
	13	26VI26
	23	26VI17
Feb	2	25VI57
	12	25VI27
	22	24VI49
Mar	4	24VI05
	14	23VI18
	24	22VI30
Apr	3	21VI46
	13	21VI07
	23	20VI35
May	3	20VI13
	13	20VI01
	23	20VI00
Jun	2	20VI11
	12	20VI33
	22	21VI06
Jul	2	21VI48
	12	22VI40
	22	23VI39
Aug	1	24VI46
	11	25VI59
	21	27VI17
	31	28VI39
Sep	10	00LI04
	20	01LI30
	30	02LI58
Oct	10	04LI25
	20	05LI50
	30	07LI13
Nov	9	08LI32
	19	09LI46
	29	10LI53
Dec	9	11LI53
	19	12LI44
	29	13LI25

Stations	Date	
Retrograde	Jan	10
Direct	May	18

1996

Date		Long.
Jan	8	13LI55
	18	14LI14
	28	14LI21
Feb	7	14LI16
	17	13LI59
	27	13LI32
Mar	8	12LI56
	18	12LI14
	28	11LI28
Apr	7	10LI40
	17	09LI55
	27	09LI14
May	7	08LI39
	17	08LI14
	27	07LI59
Jun	6	07LI55
	16	08LI02
	26	08LI20
Jul	6	08LI49
	16	09LI28
	26	10LI17
Aug	5	11LI14
	15	12LI19
	25	13LI30
Sep	4	14LI46
	14	16LI07
	24	17LI31
Oct	4	18LI57
	14	20LI24
	24	21LI51
Nov	3	23LI17
	13	24LI40
	23	26LI00
Dec	3	27LI15
	13	28LI24
	23	29LI25

1997

Date		Long.
Jan	2	00SC18
	12	01SC01
	22	01SC34
Feb	1	01SC55
	11	02SC05
	21	02SC02
Mar	3	01SC49
	13	01SC25
	23	00SC52
Apr	2	00SC12
	12	29LI27
	22	28LI40
May	2	27LI54
	12	27LI12
	22	26LI36
Jun	1	26LI08
	11	25LI49
	21	25LI41
Jul	1	25LI44
	11	25LI57
	21	26LI22
	31	26LI56
Aug	10	27LI40
	20	28LI33
	30	29LI33
Sep	9	00SC40
	19	01SC53
	29	03SC10
Oct	9	04SC31
	19	05SC54
	29	07SC19
Nov	8	08SC43
	18	10SC07
	28	11SC28
Dec	8	12SC46
	18	13SC59
	28	15SC06

Stations	Date	
Retrograde	Jan	28
Direct	Jun	4

Stations	Date	
Retrograde	Feb	14
Direct	Jun	23

1998

Date		Long.
Jan	7	16SC06
	17	16SC58
	27	17SC41
Feb	6	18SC14
	16	18SC35
	26	18SC46
Mar	8	18SC45
	18	18SC33
	28	18SC11
Apr	7	17SC40
	17	17SC02
	27	16SC19
May	7	15SC33
	17	14SC48
	27	14SC06
Jun	6	13SC29
	16	12SC59
	26	12SC38
Jul	6	12SC27
	16	12SC26
	26	12SC35
Aug	5	12SC55
	15	13SC25
	25	14SC04
Sep	4	14SC52
	14	15SC48
	24	16SC50
Oct	4	17SC58
	14	19SC11
	24	20SC27
Nov	3	21SC46
	13	23SC06
	23	24SC26
Dec	3	25SC45
	13	27SC02
	23	28SC16

Stations	Date	
Retrograde	Mar	2
Direct	Jul	12

1999

Date		Long.
Jan	2	29SC25
	12	00SA29
	22	01SA25
Feb	1	02SA14
	11	02SA54
	21	03SA24
Mar	3	03SA44
	13	03SA53
	23	03SA51
Apr	2	03SA39
	12	03SA17
	22	02SA47
May	2	02SA10
	12	01SA29
	22	00SA45
Jun	1	00SA02
	11	29SC20
	21	28SC44
Jul	1	28SC14
	11	27SC52
	21	27SC39
	31	27SC36
Aug	10	27SC43
	20	27SC59
	30	28SC26
Sep	9	29SC01
	19	29SC45
	29	00SA37
Oct	9	01SA34
	19	02SA38
	29	03SA46
Nov	8	04SA57
	18	06SA11
	28	07SA26
Dec	8	08SA41
	18	09SA55
	28	11SA06

Stations	Date	
Retrograde	Mar	16
Direct	Jul	29

2000

Date		Long.
Jan	7	12SA14
	17	13SA17
	27	14SA15
Feb	6	15SA07
	16	15SA51
	26	16SA26
Mar	7	16SA52
	17	17SA08
	27	17SA14
Apr	6	17SA10
	16	16SA56
	26	16SA33
May	6	16SA03
	16	15SA27
	26	14SA47
Jun	5	14SA05
	15	13SA23
	25	12SA43
Jul	5	12SA08
	15	11SA40
	25	11SA18
Aug	4	11SA06
	14	11SA02
	24	11SA08
Sep	3	11SA23
	13	11SA48
	23	12SA21
Oct	3	13SA02
	13	13SA50
	23	14SA45
Nov	2	15SA44
	12	16SA48
	22	17SA55
Dec	2	19SA04
	12	20SA13
	22	21SA23

Stations	Date	
Retrograde	Mar	27
Direct	Aug	12

2001

Date		Long.
Jan	1	22SA31
	11	23SA37
	21	24SA39
	31	25SA37
Feb	10	26SA29
	20	27SA14
Mar	2	27SA52
	12	28SA21
	22	28SA42
Apr	1	28SA53
	11	28SA54
	21	28SA47
May	1	28SA30
	11	28SA06
	21	27SA35
	31	26SA59
Jun	10	26SA20
	20	25SA39
	30	24SA59
Jul	10	24SA22
	20	23SA50
	30	23SA23
Aug	9	23SA04
	19	22SA53
	29	22SA51
Sep	8	22SA58
	18	23SA13
	28	23SA38
Oct	8	24SA10
	18	24SA50
	28	25SA36
Nov	7	26SA28
	17	27SA24
	27	28SA25
Dec	7	29SA28
	17	00CA32
	27	01CA37

Stations	Date	
Retrograde	Apr	8
Direct	Aug	27

2002

Date		Long.
Jan	6	02CA41
	16	03CA44
	26	04CA44
Feb	5	05CA40
	15	06CA31
	25	07CA16
Mar	7	07CA54
	17	08CA25
	27	08CA48
Apr	6	09CA03
	16	09CA08
	26	09CA05
May	6	08CA53
	16	08CA34
	26	08CA07
Jun	5	07CA35
	15	06CA59
	25	06CA21
Jul	5	05CA42
	15	05CA04
	25	04CA30
Aug	4	04CA01
	14	03CA37
	24	03CA22
Sep	3	03CA14
	13	03CA14
	23	03CA23
Oct	3	03CA40
	13	04CA05
	23	04CA38
Nov	2	05CA17
	12	06CA03
	22	06CA53
Dec	2	07CA47
	12	08CA45
	22	09CA44

Stations	Date	
Retrograde	Apr	18
Direct	Sep	8

2003

Date		Long.
Jan	1	10CA45
	11	11CA45
	21	12CA44
	31	13CA41
Feb	10	14CA35
	20	15CA25
Mar	2	16CA09
	12	16CA47
	22	17CA19
Apr	1	17CA43
	11	17CA59
	21	18CA07
May	1	18CA07
	11	17CA59
	21	17CA43
	31	17CA20
Jun	10	16CA51
	20	16CA18
	30	15CA42
Jul	10	15CA05
	20	14CA28
	30	13CA53
Aug	9	13CA22
	19	12CA57
	29	12CA38
Sep	8	12CA26
	18	12CA21
	28	12CA25
Oct	8	12CA37
	18	12CA57
	28	13CA24
Nov	7	13CA58
	17	14CA38
	27	15CA23
Dec	7	16CA12
	17	17CA05
	27	18CA00

Stations	Date	
Retrograde	Apr	26
Direct	Sep	19

2004

Date		Long.
Jan	6	18CA56
	16	19CA53
	26	20CA49
Feb	5	21CA43
	15	22CA34
	25	23CA22
Mar	6	24CA05
	16	24CA43
	26	25CA14
Apr	5	25CA38
	15	25CA56
	25	26CA05
May	5	26CA07
	15	26CA01
	25	25CA48
Jun	4	25CA28
	14	25CA02
	24	24CA31
Jul	4	23CA57
	14	23CA22
	24	22CA46
Aug	3	22CA12
	13	21CA40
	23	21CA13
Sep	2	20CA52
	12	20CA38
	22	20CA30
Oct	2	20CA31
	12	20CA39
	22	20CA54
Nov	1	21CA17
	11	21CA46
	21	22CA21
Dec	1	23CA02
	11	23CA47
	21	24CA36
	31	25CA27

Stations	Date	
Retrograde	May	3
Direct	Sep	27

2005

Date		Long.
Jan	10	26CA20
	20	27CA13
	30	28CA06
Feb	9	28CA57
	19	29CA47
Mar	1	00AQ32
	11	01AQ14
	21	01AQ50
	31	02AQ21
Apr	10	02AQ46
	20	03AQ03
	30	03AQ14
May	10	03AQ17
	20	03AQ12
	30	03AQ01
Jun	9	02AQ43
	19	02AQ19
	29	01AQ51
Jul	9	01AQ19
	19	00AQ45
	29	00AQ10
Aug	8	29CA36
	18	29CA05
	28	28CA38
Sep	7	28CA16
	17	28CA00
	27	27CA50
Oct	7	27CA48
	17	27CA53
	27	28CA05
Nov	6	28CA24
	16	28CA50
	26	29CA22
Dec	6	29CA59
	16	00AQ41
	26	01AQ26

Stations	Date	
Retrograde	May	9
Direct	Oct	6

2006

Date		Long.
Jan	5	02AQ14
	15	03AQ04
	25	03AQ54
Feb	4	04AQ44
	14	05AQ33
	24	06AQ20
Mar	6	07AQ04
	16	07AQ44
	26	08AQ19
Apr	5	08AQ49
	15	09AQ13
	25	09AQ31
May	5	09AQ42
	15	09AQ45
	25	09AQ42
Jun	4	09AQ32
	14	09AQ16
	24	08AQ54
Jul	4	08AQ27
	14	07AQ57
	24	07AQ24
Aug	3	06AQ50
	13	06AQ18
	23	05AQ47
Sep	2	05AQ19
	12	04AQ57
	22	04AQ39
Oct	2	04AQ28
	12	04AQ24
	22	04AQ27
Nov	1	04AQ37
	11	04AQ54
	21	05AQ17
Dec	1	05AQ46
	11	06AQ21
	21	06AQ59
	31	07AQ42

Stations	Date	
Retrograde	May	16
Direct	Oct	13

2007

Date		Long.
Jan	10	08AQ27
	20	09AQ14
	30	10AQ02
Feb	9	10AQ50
	19	11AQ36
Mar	1	12AQ21
	11	13AQ03
	21	13AQ42
	31	14AQ16
Apr	10	14AQ45
	20	15AQ09
	30	15AQ26
May	10	15AQ37
	20	15AQ41
	30	15AQ38
Jun	9	15AQ29
	19	15AQ14
	29	14AQ53
Jul	9	14AQ27
	19	13AQ58
	29	13AQ27
Aug	8	12AQ55
	18	12AQ23
	28	11AQ52
Sep	7	11AQ25
	17	11AQ02
	27	10AQ44
Oct	7	10AQ33
	17	10AQ27
	27	10AQ29
Nov	6	10AQ37
	16	10AQ52
	26	11AQ13
Dec	6	11AQ40
	16	12AQ12
	26	12AQ49

Stations	Date	
Retrograde	May	21
Direct	Oct	20

2008		2009	
Date	**Long.**	**Date**	**Long.**
Jan 5	13AQ29	Jan 9	18AQ51
15	14AQ12	19	19AQ32
25	14AQ56	29	20AQ15
Feb 4	15AQ42	Feb 8	20AQ59
14	16AQ28	18	21AQ43
24	17AQ13	28	22AQ26
Mar 5	17AQ56	Mar 10	23AQ07
15	18AQ36	20	23AQ46
25	19AQ13	30	24AQ22
Apr 4	19AQ46	Apr 9	24AQ54
14	20AQ14	19	25AQ21
24	20AQ37	29	25AQ43
May 4	20AQ54	May 9	25AQ59
14	21AQ04	19	26AQ09
24	21AQ08	29	26AQ13
Jun 3	21AQ06	Jun 8	26AQ11
13	20AQ58	18	26AQ03
23	20AQ43	28	25AQ49
Jul 3	20AQ23	Jul 8	25AQ30
13	19AQ59	18	25AQ06
23	19AQ31	28	24AQ39
Aug 2	19AQ01	Aug 7	24AQ09
12	18AQ29	17	23AQ39
22	17AQ58	27	23AQ08
Sep 1	17AQ28	Sep 6	22AQ39
11	17AQ01	16	22AQ13
21	16AQ38	26	21AQ50
Oct 1	16AQ20	Oct 6	21AQ32
11	16AQ08	16	21AQ20
21	16AQ02	26	21AQ13
31	16AQ03	Nov 5	21AQ13
Nov 10	16AQ10	15	21AQ19
20	16AQ23	25	21AQ32
30	16AQ43	Dec 5	21AQ50
Dec 10	17AQ08	15	22AQ14
20	17AQ38	25	22AQ43
30	18AQ13		

Stations	**Date**		**Stations**	**Date**	
Retrograde	May	26	Retrograde	May	31
Direct	Oct	26	Direct	Nov	1

2010

Date		Long.
Jan	4	23AQ17
	14	23AQ53
	24	24AQ33
Feb	3	25AQ14
	13	25AQ56
	23	26AQ39
Mar	5	27AQ20
	15	28AQ00
	25	28AQ38
Apr	4	29AQ12
	14	29AQ42
	24	00PI09
May	4	00PI30
	14	00PI45
	24	00PI55
Jun	3	00PI59
	13	00PI57
	23	00PI48
Jul	3	00PI35
	13	00PI16
	23	29AQ53
Aug	2	29AQ27
	12	28AQ58
	22	28AQ28
Sep	1	27AQ58
	11	27AQ30
	21	27AQ04
Oct	1	26AQ41
	11	26AQ24
	21	26AQ11
	31	26AQ05
Nov	10	26AQ04
	20	26AQ10
	30	26AQ22
Dec	10	26AQ39
	20	27AQ03
	30	27AQ30

Stations	Date	
Retrograde	Jun	5
Direct	Nov	6

2011

Date		Long.
Jan	9	28AQ03
	19	28AQ38
	29	29AQ16
Feb	8	29AQ56
	18	00PI37
	28	01PI18
Mar	10	01PI58
	20	02PI37
	30	03PI13
Apr	9	03PI46
	19	04PI16
	29	04PI41
May	9	05PI01
	19	05PI16
	29	05PI25
Jun	8	05PI29
	18	05PI26
	28	05PI18
Jul	8	05PI04
	18	04PI46
	28	04PI23
Aug	7	03PI57
	17	03PI29
	27	03PI00
Sep	6	02PI31
	16	02PI03
	26	01PI37
Oct	6	01PI15
	16	00PI58
	26	00PI46
Nov	5	00PI39
	15	00PI38
	25	00PI44
Dec	5	00PI55
	15	01PI13
	25	01PI35

Stations	Date	
Retrograde	Jun	9
Direct	Nov	11

2012

Date		Long.
Jan	4	02PI02
	14	02PI33
	24	03PI08
Feb	3	03PI45
	13	04PI24
	23	05PI03
Mar	4	05PI43
	14	06PI22
	24	07PI00
Apr	3	07PI35
	13	08PI07
	23	08PI35
May	3	08PI59
	13	09PI19
	23	09PI33
Jun	2	09PI42
	12	09PI45
	22	09PI42
Jul	2	09PI34
	12	09PI20
	22	09PI02
Aug	1	08PI39
	11	08PI14
	21	07PI46
	31	07PI17
Sep	10	06PI49
	20	06PI21
	30	05PI56
Oct	10	05PI35
	20	05PI18
	30	05PI06
Nov	9	04PI59
	19	04PI59
	29	05PI04
Dec	9	05PI15
	19	05PI32
	29	05PI54

Stations	Date	
Retrograde	Jun	13
Direct	Nov	15

2013

Date		Long.
Jan	8	06PI21
	18	06PI51
	28	07PI25
Feb	7	08PI01
	17	08PI39
	27	09PI18
Mar	9	09PI57
	19	10PI35
	29	11PI11
Apr	8	11PI45
	18	12PI16
	28	12PI44
May	8	13PI07
	18	13PI26
	28	13PI39
Jun	7	13PI47
	17	13PI50
	27	13PI46
Jul	7	13PI38
	17	13PI24
	27	13PI06
Aug	6	12PI44
	16	12PI18
	26	11PI51
Sep	5	11PI23
	15	10PI54
	25	10PI27
Oct	5	10PI03
	15	09PI42
	25	09PI25
Nov	4	09PI14
	14	09PI08
	24	09PI07
Dec	4	09PI13
	14	09PI24
	24	09PI41

Stations	Date	
Retrograde	Jun	17
Direct	Nov	20

2014

Date		Long.
Jan	3	10PI03
	13	10PI29
	23	10PI59
Feb	2	11PI32
	12	12PI08
	22	12PI45
Mar	4	13PI22
	14	14PI00
	24	14PI37
Apr	3	15PI13
	13	15PI46
	23	16PI16
May	3	16PI43
	13	17PI05
	23	17PI23
Jun	2	17PI36
	12	17PI43
	22	17PI45
Jul	2	17PI41
	12	17PI33
	22	17PI19
Aug	1	17PI00
	11	16PI38
	21	16PI13
	31	15PI46
Sep	10	15PI18
	20	14PI50
	30	14PI23
Oct	10	13PI59
	20	13PI39
	30	13PI23
Nov	9	13PI12
	19	13PI06
	29	13PI06
Dec	9	13PI12
	19	13PI23
	29	13PI40

Stations	Date	
Retrograde	Jun	21
Direct	Nov	24

2015

Date		Long.
Jan	8	14PI02
	18	14PI28
	28	14PI57
Feb	7	15PI30
	17	16PI05
	27	16PI41
Mar	9	17PI19
	19	17PI56
	29	18PI32
Apr	8	19PI07
	18	19PI39
	28	20PI08
May	8	20PI34
	18	20PI55
	28	21PI12
Jun	7	21PI24
	17	21PI31
	27	21PI33
Jul	7	21PI29
	17	21PI19
	27	21PI05
Aug	6	20PI47
	16	20PI24
	26	19PI59
Sep	5	19PI32
	15	19PI05
	25	18PI37
Oct	5	18PI11
	15	17PI48
	25	17PI28
Nov	4	17PI12
	14	17PI01
	24	16PI56
Dec	4	16PI57
	14	17PI03
	24	17PI14

Stations	Date	
Retrograde	Jun	25
Direct	Nov	29

2016

Date		Long.
Jan	3	17PI31
	13	17PI53
	23	18PI19
Feb	2	18PI48
	12	19PI21
	22	19PI56
Mar	3	20PI31
	13	21PI08
	23	21PI45
Apr	2	22PI20
	12	22PI54
	22	23PI25
May	2	23PI54
	12	24PI19
	22	24PI40
Jun	1	24PI56
	11	25PI07
	21	25PI13
Jul	1	25PI14
	11	25PI10
	21	25PI00
	31	24PI45
Aug	10	24PI27
	20	24PI04
	30	23PI39
Sep	9	23PI12
	19	22PI45
	29	22PI18
Oct	9	21PI52
	19	21PI29
	29	21PI10
Nov	8	20PI55
	18	20PI45
	28	20PI40
Dec	8	20PI41
	18	20PI47
	28	20PI59

Stations	Date	
Retrograde	Jun	28
Direct	Dec	6

2017

Date		Long.
Jan	7	21PI17
	17	21PI38
	27	22PI04
Feb	6	22PI34
	16	23PI06
	26	23PI40
Mar	8	24PI16
	18	24PI52
	28	25PI28
Apr	7	26PI03
	17	26PI36
	27	27PI07
May	7	27PI35
	17	27PI59
	27	28PI19
Jun	6	28PI35
	16	28PI45
	26	28PI51
Jul	6	28PI51
	16	28PI46
	26	28PI36
Aug	5	28PI21
	15	28PI02
	25	27PI39
Sep	4	27PI14
	14	26PI47
	24	26PI20
Oct	4	25PI53
	14	25PI28
	24	25PI06
Nov	3	24PI47
	13	24PI32
	23	24PI23
Dec	3	24PI19
	13	24PI20
	23	24PI27

Stations	Date	
Retrograde	Jul	2
Direct	Dec	6

2018

Date		Long.
Jan	2	24PI39
	12	24PI57
	22	25PI19
Feb	1	25PI45
	11	26PI15
	21	26PI47
Mar	3	27PI21
	13	27PI56
	23	28PI32
Apr	2	29PI07
	12	29PI42
	22	00AR14
May	2	00AR45
	12	01AR12
	22	01AR35
Jun	1	01AR55
	11	02AR10
	21	02AR20
Jul	1	02AR24
	11	02AR24
	21	02AR18
	31	02AR08
Aug	10	01AR52
	20	01AR33
	30	01AR10
Sep	9	00AR45
	19	00AR19
	29	29PI51
Oct	9	29PI25
	19	29PI00
	29	28PI38
Nov	8	28PI20
	18	28PI06
	28	27PI57
Dec	8	27PI53
	18	27PI55
	28	28PI03

Stations	Date	
Retrograde	Jul	6
Direct	Dec	10

2019

Date		Long.
Jan	7	28PI16
	17	28PI34
	27	28PI56
Feb	6	29PI22
	16	29PI52
	26	00AR24
Mar	8	00AR58
	18	01AR33
	28	02AR09
Apr	7	02AR44
	17	03AR18
	27	03AR50
May	7	04AR20
	17	04AR46
	27	05AR09
Jun	6	05AR28
	16	05AR42
	26	05AR51
Jul	6	05AR56
	16	05AR55
	26	05AR48
Aug	5	05AR37
	15	05AR22
	25	05AR02
Sep	4	04AR39
	14	04AR14
	24	03AR47
Oct	4	03AR20
	14	02AR54
	24	02AR29
Nov	3	02AR08
	13	01AR50
	23	01AR37
Dec	3	01AR28
	13	01AR25
	23	01AR28

Stations	Date	
Retrograde	Jul	9
Direct	Dec	14

2020		2021	
Date	**Long.**	**Date**	**Long.**
Jan 2	01AR36	Jan 6	05AR08
12	01AR50	16	05AR22
22	02AR08	26	05AR41
Feb 1	02AR31	Feb 5	06AR04
11	02AR57	15	06AR31
21	03AR27	25	07AR01
Mar 2	03AR59	Mar 7	07AR34
12	04AR33	17	08AR08
22	05AR09	27	08AR43
Apr 1	05AR44	Apr 6	09AR18
11	06AR19	16	09AR52
21	06AR52	26	10AR26
May 1	07AR24	May 6	10AR57
11	07AR53	16	11AR26
21	08AR19	26	11AR52
31	08AR42	Jun 5	12AR13
Jun 10	09AR00	15	12AR31
20	09AR13	25	12AR44
30	09AR22	Jul 5	12AR52
Jul 10	09AR26	15	12AR55
20	09AR24	25	12AR53
30	09AR17	Aug 4	12AR46
Aug 9	09AR06	14	12AR34
19	08AR50	24	12AR17
29	08AR29	Sep 3	11AR57
Sep 8	08AR06	13	11AR33
18	07AR41	23	11AR07
28	07AR14	Oct 3	10AR40
Oct 8	06AR47	13	10AR13
18	06AR21	23	09AR48
28	05AR57	Nov 2	09AR24
Nov 7	05AR36	12	09AR03
17	05AR18	22	08AR46
27	05AR06	Dec 2	08AR34
Dec 7	04AR58	12	08AR27
17	04AR56	22	08AR26
27	04AR59		

Stations	Date		Stations	Date	
Retrograde	Jul	12	Retrograde	Jul	16
Direct	Dec	16	Direct	Dec	20

2022		2023	
Date	**Long.**	**Date**	**Long.**
Jan 1	08AR30	Jan 6	12AR01
11	08AR39	16	12AR11
21	08AR54	26	12AR26
31	09AR13	Feb 5	12AR46
Feb 10	09AR37	15	13AR10
20	10AR04	25	13AR38
Mar 2	10AR35	Mar 7	14AR09
12	11AR07	17	14AR42
22	11AR42	27	15AR16
Apr 1	12AR17	Apr 6	15AR52
11	12AR52	16	16AR27
21	13AR26	26	17AR01
May 1	14AR00	May 6	17AR34
11	14AR31	16	18AR05
21	14AR59	26	18AR34
31	15AR24	Jun 5	18AR58
Jun 10	15AR46	15	19AR20
20	16AR03	25	19AR36
30	16AR16	Jul 5	19AR48
Jul 10	16AR23	15	19AR55
20	16AR25	25	19AR57
30	16AR23	Aug 4	19AR54
Aug 9	16AR15	14	19AR45
19	16AR02	24	19AR32
29	15AR45	Sep 3	19AR15
Sep 8	15AR24	13	18AR53
18	15AR00	23	18AR29
28	14AR34	Oct 3	18AR03
Oct 8	14AR07	13	17AR36
18	13AR40	23	17AR09
28	13AR15	Nov 2	16AR43
Nov 7	12AR51	12	16AR20
17	12AR31	22	16AR00
27	12AR14	Dec 2	15AR44
Dec 7	12AR03	12	15AR33
17	11AR57	22	15AR27
27	11AR56		

Stations	**Date**	**Stations**	**Date**
Retrograde	Jul 20	Retrograde	Jul 24
Direct	Dec 24	Direct	Dec 28

2024		2025	
Date	**Long.**	**Date**	**Long.**
Jan 1	15AR27	Jan 5	19AR01
11	15AR33	15	19AR07
21	15AR44	25	19AR18
31	16AR00	Feb 4	19AR35
Feb 10	16AR20	14	19AR57
20	16AR45	24	20AR22
Mar 1	17AR14	Mar 6	20AR51
11	17AR45	16	21AR23
21	18AR18	26	21AR57
31	18AR53	Apr 5	22AR32
Apr 10	19AR28	15	23AR07
20	20AR04	25	23AR43
30	20AR38	May 5	24AR18
May 10	21AR11	15	24AR51
20	21AR42	25	25AR21
30	22AR10	Jun 4	25AR49
Jun 9	22AR35	14	26AR14
19	22AR55	24	26AR35
29	23AR12	Jul 4	26AR51
Jul 9	23AR23	14	27AR02
19	23AR30	24	27AR08
29	23AR31	Aug 3	27AR09
Aug 8	23AR28	13	27AR05
18	23AR19	23	26AR55
28	23AR05	Sep 2	26AR41
Sep 7	22AR47	12	26AR22
17	22AR25	22	26AR00
27	22AR00	Oct 2	25AR34
Oct 7	21AR33	12	25AR07
17	21AR06	22	24AR40
27	20AR39	Nov 1	24AR12
Nov 6	20AR13	11	23AR47
16	19AR50	21	23AR24
26	19AR31	Dec 1	23AR05
Dec 6	19AR15	11	22AR50
16	19AR05	21	22AR40
26	19AR00	31	22AR36

Stations	**Date**		**Stations**	**Date**	
Retrograde	Jul	27	Retrograde	Jul	31
Direct	Dec	30			

2026

Date		Long.
Jan	10	22AR37
	20	22AR44
	30	22AR56
Feb	9	23AR14
	19	23AR36
Mar	1	24AR02
	11	24AR32
	21	25AR04
	31	25AR38
Apr	10	26AR14
	20	26AR50
	30	27AR26
May	10	28AR01
	20	28AR34
	30	29AR05
Jun	9	29AR33
	19	29AR58
	29	00TA18
Jul	9	00TA34
	19	00TA45
	29	00TA51
Aug	8	00TA51
	18	00TA46
	28	00TA36
Sep	7	00TA21
	17	00TA02
	27	29AR39
Oct	7	29AR13
	17	28AR46
	27	28AR18
Nov	6	27AR50
	16	27AR25
	26	27AR02
Dec	6	26AR43
	16	26AR28
	26	26AR19

Stations	Date	
Retrograde	Jan	3
Direct	Aug	4

2027

Date		Long.
Jan	5	26AR15
	15	26AR17
	25	26AR25
Feb	4	26AR38
	14	26AR57
	24	27AR20
Mar	6	27AR47
	16	28AR17
	26	28AR50
Apr	5	29AR25
	15	00TA01
	25	00TA37
May	5	01TA14
	15	01TA49
	25	02TA23
Jun	4	02TA54
	14	03TA22
	24	03TA46
Jul	4	04TA07
	14	04TA23
	24	04TA33
Aug	3	04TA39
	13	04TA39
	23	04TA34
Sep	2	04TA23
	12	04TA08
	22	03TA48
Oct	2	03TA24
	12	02TA58
	22	02TA30
Nov	1	02TA02
	11	01TA34
	21	01TA08
Dec	1	00TA45
	11	00TA27
	21	00TA13
	31	00TA04

Stations	Date	
Retrograde	Jan	7
Direct	Aug	9

2028

Date		Long.
Jan	10	00TA01
	20	00TA03
	30	00TA12
Feb	9	00TA26
	19	00TA45
	29	01TA09
Mar	10	01TA36
	20	02TA08
	30	02TA41
Apr	9	03TA17
	19	03TA54
	29	04TA31
May	9	05TA08
	19	05TA43
	29	06TA17
Jun	8	06TA49
	18	07TA17
	28	07TA42
Jul	8	08TA03
	18	08TA18
	28	08TA29
Aug	7	08TA34
	17	08TA34
	27	08TA28
Sep	6	08TA17
	16	08TA01
	26	07TA41
Oct	6	07TA17
	16	06TA50
	26	06TA22
Nov	5	05TA53
	15	05TA25
	25	04TA59
Dec	5	04TA36
	15	04TA17
	25	04TA04

Stations	Date	
Retrograde	Jan	11
Direct	Aug	12

2029

Date		Long.
Jan	4	03TA55
	14	03TA53
	24	03TA56
Feb	3	04TA05
	13	04TA20
	23	04TA40
Mar	5	05TA05
	15	05TA33
	25	06TA05
Apr	4	06TA40
	14	07TA16
	24	07TA54
May	4	08TA32
	14	09TA09
	24	09TA46
Jun	3	10TA20
	13	10TA52
	23	11TA21
Jul	3	11TA46
	13	12TA07
	23	12TA23
Aug	2	12TA33
	12	12TA39
	22	12TA38
Sep	1	12TA32
	11	12TA21
	21	12TA04
Oct	1	11TA43
	11	11TA18
	21	10TA51
	31	10TA22
Nov	10	09TA53
	20	09TA24
	30	08TA58
Dec	10	08TA35
	20	08TA17
	30	08TA03

Stations	Date	
Retrograde	Jan	14
Direct	Aug	17

2030

Date		Long.
Jan	9	07TA55
	19	07TA53
	29	07TA57
Feb	8	08TA07
	18	08TA23
	28	08TA44
Mar	10	09TA09
	20	09TA39
	30	10TA12
Apr	9	10TA47
	19	11TA24
	29	12TA03
May	9	12TA42
	19	13TA20
	29	13TA57
Jun	8	14TA32
	18	15TA05
	28	15TA34
Jul	8	16TA00
	18	16TA21
	28	16TA37
Aug	7	16TA48
	17	16TA54
	27	16TA53
Sep	6	16TA47
	16	16TA35
	26	16TA18
Oct	6	15TA57
	16	15TA31
	26	15TA03
Nov	5	14TA34
	15	14TA04
	25	13TA35
Dec	5	13TA08
	15	12TA45
	25	12TA27

Stations	Date	
Retrograde	Jan	18
Direct	Aug	22

Notes

Introduction

1 In 1772 an astronomer called Bode noticed a mathematical relationship describing the planets' relative distance from the Sun. The position of Uranus was thus accurately predicted, and discovered in 1801; later Neptune was discovered fairly close to its expected place (8.75 astronomical units off). Neither Pluto nor Chiron fit into this pattern; furthermore both planets have highly elliptical orbits, and both cross the orbits of their inner neighbours.

2 From 1992 until 1997, six further bodies similar to Chiron were discovered, and the whole group has officially been classified as 'Centaurs'. See *To the Edge and Beyond* (CPA Press, London, 1996) by Melanie Reinhart for exploration of this important new development.

3 Dane Rudhyar, *The Pulse of Life*, pp. 1–2.

4 Nicholas Campion, 'Analysis, Counselling and Natal Astrology', *Astrological Journal*, January/February 1988.

5 James Hillman, *Facing the Gods*, p. 35.

6 Richard T. Tarnas, 'Uranus and Prometheus', *Spring*, 1984, p. 83.

Chapter 1

1 'Wilderness – A Way of Truth', in C. A. Meier *et al.*, *A Testament to the Wilderness*, p. 57.

2 Barbara G. Walker, *The Woman's Encyclopaedia of Myths and Secrets*, p. 24.

3 Robert Graves, *The White Goddess*, p. 384.

4 For a description of the ceremony, ibid., p. 384.

5 B. G. Walker, op. cit., p. 412. According to the *Encyclopaedia Britannica*, the historical Lady Godiva (Godgifu; c. 1040–80)

was an Anglo–Saxon gentlewoman, wife of Leofric, Earl of Mercia, with whom she founded and endowed a monastery in Coventry. The earliest extant source of this information is Roger of Wendova (d. 1236). In *Chronica* he reports that her husband, tired of her imploring him to reduce taxes, agreed to do so on condition that she ride naked through the town. This she duly did, with her long hair covering all but her legs; tolls on everything except horses were duly waived!

According to *The Woman's Encyclopaedia of Myths and Secrets*, Lady Godiva is the triple goddess. Mother Goda, or Gerd, is equivalent to Freya, fertility goddess and consort of Godan (Wotan), father of the Gods. *Diva* is the universal Indo-European word for 'goddess'. Every seven years a woman would ride naked through the streets of Coventry as her representative, this custom lasting until 1826, although periodically forbidden by the Puritans.

6 B. G. Walker, op. cit., p. 412.
7 *New Larousse Encyclopaedia of Mythology*, pp. 342–3.
8 See books by Carlos Castenada and Lynn Andrews, and *Lightning Bird* by Lyall Watson.
9 Ken Wilbur, *Up From Eden*, p. 42.
10 C. G. Jung, *Man and his Symbols*, p. 85.
11 Joseph Campbell, *The Masks of God: Primitive Mythology*, pp. 252–3.
12 See Joan Halifax, *Shamanic Voices*, for firsthand accounts of initiation processes.
13 Joan Halifax, *Shaman: The Wounded Healer*, p. 13.
14 ibid., pp. 66–9 for examples from North American indigenous cultures.
15 *The Tibetan Book of the Dead* contains a detailed description of the journey of the soul of the deceased. Tibetan Buddhism absorbed some elements of the indigenous Bon-po religion of Tibet, which was shamanic in character.
16 See the works of Stanislav Grof, as mentioned in the Bibliography.
17 Joan Halifax, *Shaman: The Wounded Healer*, p. 78.
18 ibid., p. 7.
19 ibid., p. 94.

Chapter 2

1 See Chapter 8, n. 1, for further details.
2 A. R. Hope Moncrieff, *Classic Myth and Legend*.
3 According to Grimm, the blossom of this tree will cause heroes to fall into an enchanted sleep, i.e. to 'lose their soul' or become unconscious. This foreshadows the theme of the reawakening of individuality which the planet Chiron represents in the natal chart. From classical times, the linden-blossom has also been used as a restorative. The inner bark was used for writing-tablets, and when torn into strips became a divinatory device. Chiron's name comes from the Greek word *cheir* meaning 'hand', and his daughter was a prophetess.
4 Robert Stein, *Incest and Human Love*, pp. 62–3.
5 M. Grant and J. Hazel, *Who's Who in Classical Mythology*.
6 Aeschylus, *Prometheus Bound*, trans. Philip Vellacott, pp. 26, 28.
7 Marie Louise Von Franz, *Puer Aeternus*, p. 114.
8 Richard T. Tarnas, op. cit., p. 83.
9 Notably Steven Arroyo, Liz Greene and Richard T. Tarnas; the last-mentioned suggests that the planet Uranus may even have been misnamed.
10 Joseph Campbell, op. cit., p. 281.

Chapter 3

1 K. Wilbur, *Up From Eden*, p. 27, quoting S. Arieti, *Interpretation of Schizophrenia*, Brunner, New York, 1955.
2 ibid., p. 233.
3 Mircea Eliade, *Shamanism: Archaic Techniques of Ecstasy*, p. 4.
4 K. Wilbur, *The Atman Project*, p. 55.
5 K. Wilbur, *Up From Eden*, p. 327n.
6 K. Wilbur, *The Atman Project*, p. 54, quoting R. Masters and J. Houston, *The Varieties of Psychedelic Experience*, Delta, New York, 1967.
7 K. Wilbur, *Up From Eden*, p. 323.
8 ibid., p. 328.

Chapter 4

1 Toni Wolff, 'Some Thoughts on the Individuation of Women', *Spring*, 1941, p. 90. For elaboration of these themes,

see also Nor Hall, *The Moon and the Virgin*, The Women's Press, 1980.

2 ibid., p. 93.

3 According to Plutarch; see *New Larousse Encyclopaedia of Mythology*, p. 149.

4 Barbara G. Walker, op. cit., pp. 732, 1048–9.

5 See Erminie Lantero, *The Continuing Discovery of Chiron*, pp. 30–31.

6 In *The Greek Myths*, vol. 1, p. 161, Robert Graves suggests that this seduction refers to the seizure of the pre-Hellenic horse-cults by the Aeolians, who were patriarchal Hellenes.

7 Traditionally, this episode is listed as Hercules' ninth labour, but Alice Bailey in *The Labours of Hercules* lists it as the sixth labour.

8 After I had completed this chapter, Tina Whitehead kindly showed me *The Illustrated Earth Garden Herbal* in which is illustrated a twelfth-century woodcut showing Chiron receiving healing herbs from Artemisia, a woman personifying the plant. The Artemisias family is described thus in the *Herbarium Apuleius* (AD 1050): 'it is said that Diana . . . delivered their powers . . . to Chiron the Centaur, who first from these Worts set forth a leechdom (a practice of herbal medicine), and he named these Worts from the name of Diana, Artemis, that is Artemisias.' The Artemisias family has long been used in magic and medicine, and this ancient reference to Chiron underlines the connection between the goddess Artemis and Chiron and his family.

9 See Carl Kerenyi, *Asklepios*, pp. 20, 25.

10 Florence Mary Bennett, *Religious Cults Associated with the Amazons*.

11 René Malamud, 'The Amazon Problem', *Spring*, 1971, pp. 1–21.

12 V. E. Robson, *The Fixed Stars and Constellations in Astrology*, Weiser, Maine, 1979.

13 René Malamud, op. cit., n. 32, pp. 20–21.

14 ibid., p. 12.

Chapter 5

1 Dane Rudhyar, *An Astrological Mandala*, pp. 86–7.
2 ibid., p. 284.
3 ibid., p. 284.
4 T. S. Eliot, 'Little Gidding', *Four Quartets*, p. 48.
5 C. G. Jung, *Four Archetypes*, p. 136.
6 Brian Masters, *Killing for Company*, Jonathan Cape, London, 1985, p. 257.
7 The reader is referred to Tad Mann's book *The Divine Plot*, which contains an intriguing list of historical periods and dates related to the degrees of the zodiac. I have found that if people are preoccupied with a certain historical period, or have fantasies or gifts which they attribute to a past life, these often relate to the degree of Chiron's natal placement.
8 Carl Kerenyi, op. cit., p. 99.
9 H. Hubert and M. Mann, *Sacrifice: Its Nature and Function*, p. 97.
10 Kahlil Gibran, *The Prophet*, p. 61.

Chapter 6

1 Zane Stein, *Essence and Application: A View from Chiron*, p. 44; also Al Morrison, quoted in Lantero, op. cit., p. 52.
2 See Lantero, op. cit., pp. 47–57 for discussion of the various opinions. Note that the three astronomical constellations associated with Chiron's story all lie near the zodiacal area Virgo through Sagittarius: Ophiucus (Asclepius immortalized), Sagittarius (the Centaur) and Centaurus (Chiron himself immortalized).
3 Richard Nolle, *Chiron: The New Planet in Your Horoscope*, pp. 76–7.
4 Barbara Hand Clow is also of the opinion that Chiron facilitates this shift. See *Chiron: Rainbow Bridge Between the Inner and Outer Planets*.
5 *Larousse Encyclopaedia of Astrology*, pp. 224–6.
6 Edward F. Edinger, *The Creation of Consciousness*, p. 9.
7 ibid., p. 11.
8 David Sox, *Relics and Shrines*, pp. 194–201.
9 ibid., p. 200.

10 *Larousse Encyclopaedia of Astrology*.

11 The esoteric ruler of Chiron's sign often seems to assume importance in the horoscope, especially during transits to it or to natal Chiron. At the time of writing I have not done sufficient research to comment further, but below for reference is a list of the esoteric rulers of each sign. See Alice Bailey, *Esoteric Astrology*, for further information. My gratitude to Margi Robinson for helpful discussions on this subject.

Aries	Mercury
Taurus	Vulcan
Gemini	Venus
Cancer	Neptune
Leo	Sun
Virgo	Moon
Libra	Uranus
Scorpio	Mars
Sagittarius	Earth
Capricorn	Saturn
Aquarius	Jupiter
Pisces	Pluto

12 See Charles Harvey, 'The Galactic Centre and Beyond: Signposts to Evolution?', *Journal of the Astrological Association*, vol. 25, no. 2, spring 1983, in which he discusses the work of Erlewine, Ebertin, Landscheidt and others.

13 Barbara Hand Clow, op. cit., pp. 39–40.

14 See the books of Ken Carey for an example of 'channelled' Uranian visions, and also C. G. Jung, 'Flying Saucers: A Modern Myth of Things Seen in the Sky', *Collected Works*, vol. 10, p. 307.

15 Laurens van der Post, 'Wilderness – A Way of Truth', in C. A. Meier, op. cit., p. 50.

16 W. Y. Evans-Wentz, ed., *The Tibetan Book of the Great Liberation*, pp. xxxii–xxxiii.

17 J. E. Lovelock, *Gaia: A New Look at Life on Earth*, Oxford University Press, New York, 1982.

18 Ken Carey, *The Starseed Transmissions*, p. 37.

Chapter 7

1 My gratitude to Eve Jackson for showing me her statistical study of Chiron in the charts of 115 healers and therapists, included in her contribution to a symposium on Chiron in the Astrological Association's Conference, September 1985. The house most frequently occupied by Chiron was the 10th, followed by the 1st and 12th, the 6th, and then the 8th. 'A high proportion of those with Chiron in the 8th and 12th were spiritual or psychic healers, or psychotherapists working with the unconscious.'

2 See Frank Lake, *Studies in Constricted Confusion: Explorations of a Pre- and Peri-natal Paradigm*, in which he discusses the phenomenon of the 'foetal therapist'. Available from Clinical Theology Association, Lingdale, Weston Avenue, Nottingham NG7 4BA.

3 Werner Heisenberg, *Physics and Beyond*, Allen and Unwin, 1971.

4 See works by Ken Wilbur and Stanislav Grof listed in the Bibliography. Note that Assagioli (Psychosynthesis) has Chiron in Gemini.

5 Goethe, *Faust*, trans. Theodore Martin, p. 59.

6 My gratitude to Margi Robinson for reading and commenting upon this section.

7 This term is from Howard Sasportas. For a full discussion of this topic see his book *The Twelve Houses*, pp. 56–8.

8 Dane Rudhyar, *The Astrological Houses*, p. 70.

9 See Ean Begg, *The Cult of the Black Virgin*.

10 See Liz Greene, *The Astrology of Fate*, pp. 211–20 for further material on the mythological aspects of this Virgoan theme.

11 Marion Woodman, *Addiction to Perfection*, p. 111.

12 C. G. Jung, *Aion, Collected Works*, vol. 9, p. 123.

13 Aeschylus, *The Oresteia*, trans. Robert Fagles, pp. 266–77.

14 Laurens van der Post, *The Heart of the Hunter*, p. 13.

15 C. G. Jung, *Aion, Collected Works*, vol. 9, pp. 72ff, 91, 111, 145.

16 Liz Greene, *The Astrology of Fate*, pp. 257–66.

17 C. G. Jung, *Psychology and Alchemy, Collected Works*, vol. 12, p. 318.

18 Jane Harrison, *Prolegomena to the Study of Greek Religion*, p. 481.

19 ibid., p. 489.

20 See David Lan, *Guns and Rain: Guerrillas and Spirit Mediums in Zimbabwe,* James Currey, London, 1985. See also Alec J. C. Pongeweni, *Songs That Won the War of Liberation,* The College Press, PO Box 3041, Harare, Zimbabwe, 1982.

Chapter 8

1 Ixion is sometimes said to have been the father of the Centaurs. He agreed to marry Dia, daughter of Eioneus, promising a rich dowry of bridal gifts. He invited them both to a banquet, but set a trap on the way, in which Eioneus was burnt to death. Zeus purified him of his crime and brought him to his house, where Ixion plotted to seduce Zeus' wife Hera. However, Zeus realized his mischief, and deceived him with a cloud made in the image of his wife. Ixion was caught in the act, and punished by having to repeat the words, 'Benefactors deserve honour', as he rolled eternally through the sky on his fiery wheel. From the union of Ixion and the cloud named Nephele the Centaurs were born.

2 Joan Halifax, *Shaman: The Wounded Healer*, p. 21.

3 Bradley te Paske, *Rape and Ritual*, pp. 59–62.

4 Keith Sagar, *From the Life of D. H. Lawrence*, p. 100.

5 Elwin Verrier, 'The Hobby Horse and the Ecstatic Dance', *Folklore*, pp. 209–13.

6 Joan Halifax, *Shaman: The Wounded Healer*, p. 94.

7 Manson quoted in Bradley te Paske, op. cit., pp. 59–62.

8 Mother Teresa, *A Gift for God*, pp. 22–3, 27, 32.

9 C. G. Jung, 'On the Psychology of the Trickster Figure', *Four Archetypes*, p. 136.

10 Joseph Campbell, op. cit., p. 274.

11 There is much uncertainty about the data for Maria Callas. However, in most of the variants, her Sun/Mercury conjunction is also conjunct the Ascendant.

12 Robert Johnson, *The Psychology of Romantic Love*, p. 133.

13 Those who wish to explore the myth and its implications in more depth are referred to two works in particular: *Amor*

and the Psyche bȳ Erich Neumann and *She* by Robert Johnson.

14 Eight horoscopes studied, from two generations of the Moffat and the Thomas family.

15 Gordon Le Sueur, *Cecil Rhodes, the Man and his Work*, John Murray, London, 1913.

16 See Eugene Monick, *Phallos: Sacred Image of the Masculine*, for a full discussion of this important topic.

17 D. H. Lawrence, *The Man who Died*, p. 13.

18 K. Sagar, op. cit., p. 105.

19 ibid., p. 241.

20 ibid., p. 60.

21 ibid., p. 243.

22 Kahlil Gibran, op. cit., p. 57.

23 Aeschylus, *Prometheus Bound*, trans. Philip Vellacott, pp. 30, 31.

24 Martin Luther King, *Strength to Love*, Foreword.

25 Dane Rudhyar, *An Astrological Mandala*, p. 74.

26 Thanks to astrologer Darby Costello for this evocative image.

27 N. E. Davis, *A History of Southern Africa*, pp. 20–21.

28 Genesis 9.25–7.

29 These observations were made by Richard Nolle in his book, *Chiron*. As Quinlan's death occurred after his book was published, I have updated the material by including astrological details of the time of her death.

30 Dane Rudhyar, *The Astrology of Personality*, p. 305.

31 M. R. Meyer, op. cit., p. 102.

32 See Alice Miller, *For Your Own Good*, Faber & Faber, 1983.

33 I studied sixty-seven charts of people of widely differing ages where profound and long-term commitment to a guru figure (not always the same one) was a central feature of their life. Chiron was conjunct either the North or South Node in sixteen of the sixty-seven charts, that is, 23.88%, which is a very high proportion.

Chapter 9

1 In a hymn possibly composed for the cult of Kairos, Ion of Chios (b. 490 BC) called Kairos 'the youngest son of Zeus',

meaning that opportunity is god-sent. Kairos appears to have been more substantial than many personifications, depicted in art as bald behind, but with a long forelock in front – hence the expression 'to take time by the forelock'.

2 Kahlil Gibran, op. cit., p. 1.

3 Frank Haronian, *The Repression of the Sublime*, Psychosynthesis Research Foundation, New York, 1972.

4 Dane Rudhyar, *The Astrology of Self-Actualization and the New Morality*, p. 27.

5 Dane Rudhyar, *New Mansions for New Men*, pp. 77–81.

6 Dane Rudhyar, *An Astrological Mandala*, p. 261.

7 David Sox, op. cit., p. 123 ff.

8 See Patrick Marnham, *Lourdes: A Modern Pilgrimage*, Heinemann, London, 1980.

Chapter 10

1 S. Grof, *Beyond the Brain*, p. 123.

Chapter 11

1 For a detailed discussion of Chiron in Kubler Ross's horoscope, see Lantero, op. cit., pp. 115–20.

2 M. R. Meyer, *A Handbook for the Humanistic Astrologer*, p. 102.

3 Charles A. Krause, *Guyana Massacre*, p. 79.

4 ibid., pp. 205–10.

5 Dane Rudhyar, *An Astrological Mandala*, p. 82.

6 Shortly after 5 pm. See Charles A. Krause, op. cit., p. 167.

7 ibid., pp. 153, 158.

8 My thanks to Christine Murdock for this perceptive observation.

9 Charles Darwin, *The Descent of Man*, John Murray, London, 1871, p. 660.

10 Rudhyar, *An Astrological Mandala*, p. 256.

11 Thompson, *The Political Mythology of Apartheid*, p. 74.

12 In 1607 Edward Topsell described Negroes as 'libidinous as Apes that attempt women, and having thick lippes the upper hanging over the neather, they are deemed fooles, like . . . asses and Apes'. (Quoted in Fagan, op. cit., p. 24.) Drawings of unfamiliar peoples encountered by explorers show clearly

the degree of fantasy with which they were imbued. They were always measured against European criteria and, found wanting, dismissed with contempt.

13 Killing Aborigines was considered a sport among some early Tasmanian settlers. Similarly, movies made in America turned killing Indians into a game played by children – 'Cowboys and Indians'. In Southern Africa, black and white people alike have committed virtual genocide of the Bushmen.

14 Thompson, op. cit., p. 127.

15 My thanks to Jean Elliott for a transcript of her lecture on the chart of South Africa, given at the Astrological Lodge, London, 1986; she pointed out the specific correlations ascribed to the planets in mundane astrology, and their aptness in the South African chart.

16 *United No More*, by Otto Friedrich, reported by Peter Hawthorne and Bruce W. Nelan, in *Time* magazine, 4 May 1987, p. 12.

17 Laurens van der Post, op. cit., pp. 55, 56.

18 C. A. Meier, op. cit., p. 13.

19 ibid., p. 2.

20 Laurens van der Post, op. cit., pp. 49–50.

21 C. A. Meier, op. cit., p. 6.

22 Personal communication from Dr Player, February 1988. See also Laurens van der Post, *A Walk with a White Bushman*, pp. 139–43 for reference to the work of the Wilderness Leadership School.

23 M. R. Meyer, op. cit., p. 100.

24 Robert Graves, *The Greek Myths*, vol. 1, Foreword. Note that the cover of the Penguin edition shows a carved relief from fifth-century-BC Greece, depicting two figures each holding up a mushroom.

25 See John Allegro, *The Sacred Mushroom and the Cross*, and Gordon Wasson, *Soma*.

26 *Centaurium umbellatum* is one of the Bach Flower Remedies, said to be for those who are unable to refuse the demands of others, and who thus become exploited, servile or enslaved. Although this is the 'classic' symptom picture, intuitive attunement also reveals a strong and genuine desire to be of

service, but a distorted idea of what that means; this is coupled with a strong, wild and angry energy reminiscent of the energy of the Centaurs, and usually indicating repressed self-assertion.

27 Wasson, Hofmann and Ruck, *The Road to Eleusis*, p. 38.

28 While completing this section, I heard on the radio that 'medical researchers' had announced that LSD might be present in significant quantities in muesli, and that muesli bars could be dangerously addictive. I wondered who had funded this research, and whether sales would either drop or soar – Chiron was within 1° of its first exact opposition to Neptune in Capricorn that week!

29 Dane Rudhyar, *An Astrological Mandala*, pp. 252–3.

30 Personal communication from Dr Hofmann, 1988.

31 Albert Hofmann, *LSD My Problem Child*, p. 209.

32 Dane Rudhyar, *An Astrological Mandala*, p. 55.

33 Aeschylus, *Prometheus Bound*, trans. Philip Vellacott, p. 20.

34 ibid., pp. 34–5.

35 Laurens van der Post, *Heart of the Hunter*, p. 124.

Appendix 1

1 Joelle K. D. Mahoney, 'A Question of Identity, *CAO Times*, vol. 3, no. 3, 1978.

2 *The Key*, no. 9, 23 April 1980.

3 *The Key*, no. 43, 14 October 1983.

4 Mahoney, op. cit.

5 *The Key*, no. 48, 16 March 1984.

Bibliography

Chiron and the Centaurs

Books

Clow, Barbara Hand, *Chiron: Rainbow Bridge Between the Inner and Outer Planets*, Llewellyn Publications, Minnesota, 1987.

Reinhart, Melanie, *To the Edge and Beyond*, CPA Press, London 1996.

Lantero, Erminie, *The Continuing Discovery of Chiron*, Weiser, Maine, 1983.

Nolle, Richard, *Chiron, The New Planet in Your Horoscope: The Key to Your Quest*, American Federation of Astrologers, Arizona, 1983.

Koch, Dieter and von Heeren, Robert, *Pholus: Wandler zwischen Saturn und Neptun*, Chiron Verlag, Mossingen, Germany, 1995.

Stein, Zane, *Essence and Application: A View from Chiron*, CAO Times, New York, 1986.

Internet Resources

http://ourworld.compuserve.com/homepages/
  RobertvonHeeren/astrolog.htm

http://www.omna.com/yes/zanestein/index.htm

http://cfa-www.harvard.edu/cfa/ps/lists/Centaurs.htm

Background Reading

Aeschylus, *The Oresteia*, trans. Robert Fagles, Penguin Books, Harmondsworth, 1979.

   Prometheus Bound, trans. Philip Vellacott, Penguin Books, Harmondsworth, 1961.

Bailey, Alice, *Esoteric Astrology*, (vol. 3 of *A Treatise on the Seven Rays*), Lucis Press, London, 1951.

Begg, Ean, *The Cult of the Black Virgin*, Arkana, London, 1985.

Bennett, Florence Mary, *Religious Cults Associated with the Amazons*, Columbia Studies in Classical Philology, New York, 1912.

Buhrmann, Vera, *Living in Two Worlds*, Human and Rousseau, Cape Town, 1984.

Burkert, Walter, *Greek Religion, Archaic and Classical*, trans. John Raffan, Basil Blackwell, Oxford, 1985.

Campbell, Joseph, *The Masks of God: Primitive Mythology*, Penguin Books, Harmondsworth, 1983.

Campion, Nicholas, *The Book of World Horoscopes*, Aquarian Press, Wellingborough, 1988.

Carey, Ken, *The Starseed Transmissions*, Starseed Publishing, Edinburgh, 1986.

Davis, N. E., *A History of Southern Africa*, Longman, Harlow, 1987.

Edinger, Edward E., *The Creation of Consciousness*, Inner City Books, Toronto, 1984.

Eliade, Mircea, *Shamanism: Archaic Techniques of Ecstasy*, Routledge & Kegan Paul, London 1972.

Eliot, T. S., *Four Quartets*, Faber & Faber, London, 1959.

Erlewine, Stephen, *The Circle Book of Charts*, American Federation of Astrologers, Tempe, Arizona, revised edition 1982.

Evans-Wentz, W. Y., ed., *The Tibetan Book of the Great Liberation*, Oxford University Press, New York, 1968.

Gibran, Kahlil, *The Prophet*, Heinemann, London, 1964.

Goethe, Johann Wolfgang von, *Faust*, trans. Theodore Martin, Dent, London, 1971.

Grant, M. and Hazel, J., *Who's Who in Classical Mythology*, Hodder & Stoughton, London, 1979.

Graves, Robert, *The Greek Myths*, 2 vols., Penguin Books, Harmondsworth, 1955.

    The White Goddess, Faber & Faber, London, 1984.

Green, Jeff, *Pluto: The Evolutionary Journey of the Soul*, Llewellyn Publications, Minnesota, 1986.

Greene, Liz, *Star Signs for Lovers*, Arrow Books, London, 1980.

    The Astrology of Fate, Allen & Unwin, London, 1984.

    The Outer Planets and Their Cycles, CRCS Publications, Nevada, 1983.

Grof, Stanislav, *Beyond the Brain*, State University New York Press, New York, 1985.

Halifax, Joan, *Shamanic Voices*, Penguin Books, Harmondsworth, 1979.
> *Shaman: The Wounded Healer*, Thames & Hudson, London, 1982.

Harrison, Jane, *Prolegomena to the Study of Greek Religion*, Merlin Press, London, 1962.

Heisenberg, Werner, *Physics and Beyond*, Allen & Unwin, London, 1971.

Hillman, James, *Facing the Gods*, Spring Publications, Dallas, 1980.

Hubert, Henri and Mann, Marcel, *Sacrifice: Its Nature and Function*, trans. W. D. Hall, University of Chicago Press, 1981.

Hume, R., trans., *Upanishads*, Oxford University Press, London, 1974.

Johnson, Robert, *The Psychology of Romantic Love*, Routledge & Kegan Paul, London, 1984.
> *She: Understanding Feminine Psychology*, Harper & Row, New York, 1977.

Jung, C. G., *Aion, Collected Works*, vol. 9, Routledge & Kegan Paul, London, 1959.
> *Four Archetypes*, Princeton University Press, New Jersey, 1970.
> *Man and his Symbols*, Dell Publishing, New York, 1968.
> *Psychology and Alchemy, Collected Works*, vol. 12, Routledge & Kegan Paul, London, 1971.

Jung, Emma and Von Franz, Marie Louise, *The Grail Legend*, Hodder & Stoughton, London, 1971.

Kerenyi, Carl, *Asklepios: Archetypal Image of the Physician's Existence*, Pantheon Books, New York, 1959.

Khan, Hazrat Inayat, *Gayan, Vadan, Nirtan*, Barrie & Jenkins, London, 1970.

King, Martin Luther, *Strength to Love*, Collins (Fount Paperbacks Edition), Glasgow, 1977.

Krause, Charles A., *Guyana Massacre*, London, Pan Books, 1979.

Landaw, Jonathan, ed. *Introduction to Tantra*, Wisdom Publications, London, 1987.

Lao Tzu, *Tao Te Ching*, Routledge & Kegan Paul, London, 1978.

Lawrence, David Herbert, *The Complete Poems of D. H. Lawrence*, ed. Vivian da solo Pinto, Heinemann, London, 1964.
  The Man Who Died, in *Short Novels*, vol. 2, Heinemann, London, 1959.

Lovelock, J. E., *Gaia: A New Look at Life on Earth*, Oxford University Press, New York, 1979.

Malamud, René, 'The Amazon Problem', trans. Murray Stein, *Spring*, Zurich, 1971.

Mann, Tad, *The Divine Plot*, Allen & Unwin, London, 1986.

Meier, C. A., *Ancient Incubation and Modern Psychotherapy*, Northwest University Press, Evanston, 1967.

Meier, C. A., et al., *A Testament to the Wilderness*, Daimon Verlag, Zurich and Lapis Press, Santa Monica, 1985.

Meyer, Michael R., *A Handbook for the Humanistic Astrologer*, Anchor Press/Doubleday, New York, 1974.

Miller, Alice, *For Your Own Good*, Faber & Faber, London, 1983.

Monick, Eugene, *Phallos, Sacred Image of the Masculine*, Inner City Books, Toronto, 1987.

Mother Teresa of Calcutta, *A Gift for God*, Collins, London, 1975.

Neumann, Erich, *Amor and the Psyche: The Psychic Development of the Feminine*, Princeton University Press, New Jersey, 1956.
  The Great Mother, Princeton University Press, New Jersey, 1972.

Rodden, Lois M., *The American Book of Charts*, Astro Computing Services, San Diego, California, 1980.

Rudhyar, Dane, *The Astrological Houses: The Spectrum of Individual Experience*, Doubleday New York, 1975.
  An Astrological Mandala, Vintage Books, 1974
  The Astrology of Personality, Servire, The Hague, 1963.
  The Lunation Cycle, Shambala, London, 1971.
  Pulse of Life: New Dynamics in Astrology, Shambala, Berkeley, California, 1970.
  New Mansions for New Men, Servire, Wassenaar, Holland, 1971.

Sagar, Keith, *From the Life of D. H. Lawrence*, Methuen, London, 1980.

Sanford, John A., *Healing and Wholeness*, Paulist Press, New York, 1977.

Sasportas, Howard, *The Twelve Houses*, Aquarian Press, Wellingborough, 1985.

Smith, Keith Vincent, *The Illustrated Garden Herbal*, London, Elm Tree Books/Hamish Hamilton, 1979.

Smith, Stevie, *Collected Poems of Stevie Smith*, Penguin Books, Harmondsworth, 1985.

Sox, David, *Relics and Shrines*, Allen & Unwin, London, 1985.

Stein, Robert, *Incest and Human Love: Betrayal of the Soul in Psychotherapy*, Spring Publications, Dallas, 1984.

Tarnas, Richard T., 'Uranus and Prometheus', *Spring*, 1984.

Te Paske, Bradley, *Rape and Ritual*, Inner City Books, Toronto, 1982.

Thompson, Leonard, *The Political Mythology of Apartheid*, Yale University Press, New Haven and London, 1985.

Tyler, Pamela H., *Mercury, The Astrological Anatomy of a Planet*, Aquarian Press, Wellingborough, 1985.

van der Post, Laurens, *The Heart of the Hunter*, Penguin Books, Harmondsworth, 1961.

Verrier, Elwin, 'The Hobby Horse and the Ecstatic Dance', *Folklore*, vol. 53, December 1942.

Von Franz, Marie Louise, *Projection and Recollection in Jungian Psychology*, Open Court Publishing, Illinois, 1978.

   Puer Aeternus, 2nd edn, Sigo Press, Santa Monica, 1981.

Walker, Barbara G., *The Woman's Encyclopaedia of Myths and Secrets*, Harper and Row, New York, 1983.

Weaver, Helen, Brau, Jean-Louis and Edmands, Allan, eds. *Larousse Encyclopaedia of Astrology*, trans. Librairie Larousse, New American Library, New York, 1982.

Wilbur, K., *The Atman Project*, Theosophical Publishing House, Illinois, 1980.

   Up From Eden, Routledge & Kegan Paul, London, 1981.

Wolff, Toni, 'Some Thoughts on the Individuation of Women', *Spring*, Zurich, 1941.

Woodman, Marion, *Addiction to Perfection*, Inner City Books, Toronto, 1982.

Copyright Permissions

Index of People

General Index